FOUNDATIONS OF
Kinesiology

FOUNDATIONS OF
Kinesiology

Carole A. Oglesby, PhD, AASP-CC
Professor Emeritus
Department of Kinesiology
Temple University
Philadelphia, PA

Kim Henige, EdD, CSCS, EP-C, EIM
Associate Professor
Department of Kinesiology
California State University, Northridge
Northridge, CA

Douglas W. McLaughlin, PhD
Associate Professor
Department of Kinesiology
California State University, Northridge
Northridge, CA

Belinda Stillwell, PhD
Associate Professor
Department of Kinesiology
California State University, Northridge
Northridge, CA

JONES & BARTLETT
LEARNING

World Headquarters
Jones & Bartlett Learning
5 Wall Street
Burlington, MA 01803
978-443-5000
info@jblearning.com
www.jblearning.com

Jones & Bartlett Learning books and products are available through most bookstores and online booksellers. To contact Jones & Bartlett Learning directly, call 800-832-0034, fax 978-443-8000, or visit our website, www.jblearning.com.

02665-8

Production Credits

VP, Executive Publisher: David D. Cella
Publisher: Cathy L. Esperti
Acquisitions Editor: Sean Fabery
Editorial Assistant: Hannah Dziezanowski
Production Editor: Kristen Rogers
Director of Marketing: Andrea DeFronzo
VP, Manufacturing and Inventory Control: Therese Connell
Composition: Cenveo® Publisher Services
Cover Design: Kristin E. Parker
Director of Rights & Media: Joanna Gallant
Rights & Media Specialist: Jamey O'Quinn
Media Development Editor: Troy Liston
Cover and Title Page Image: © Chris Ryan/Getty Images
Printing and Binding: LSC Communications
Cover Printing: LSC Communications

Library of Congress Cataloging-in-Publication Data
Names: Oglesby, Carole A., author. | Henige, Kim, author. | McLaughlin, Douglas W., author. | Stillwell, Belinda, author.
Title: Foundations of kinesiology / Carole A. Oglesby, PhD, AASP-CC, Professor Emeritus, Department of Kinesiology, Temple University, Philadelphia, PA, Kim Henige, EdD, CSCS, EP-C, EIM, Associate Professor, Department of Kinesiology, California State University, Northridge, Northridge, CA, Douglas W. McLaughlin, PhD, Associate Professor, Department of Kinesiology, California State University, Northridge, Northridge, CA, Belinda Stillwell, PhD, Associate Professor, Department of Kinesiology, California State University, Northridge, Northridge, CA.
Description: Burlington, MA : Jones & Bartlett Learning, [2018] | Includes index.
Identifiers: LCCN 2016028463 | ISBN 9781284034851 (pbk.)
Subjects: LCSH: Kinesiology—Textbooks. | Human mechanics—Textbooks.
Classification: LCC QP303 .O35 2018 | DDC 612/.04—dc23
LC record available at https://lccn.loc.gov/2016028463

6048

Printed in the United States of America
21 20 19 18 17   10 9 8 7 6 5 4 3 2

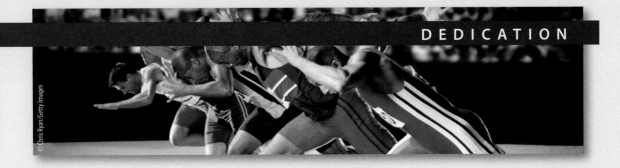

To the teachers who mentored me, and the students whom I have taught, who form a bridge honoring the past and building for a better future. The shining beauty of this bridge is what motivates me to carry and pass the torch.

To Emily Dell for excellent assistance in the technical preparation of the manuscript.

—Carole A. Oglesby

To the kinesiology students of California State University, Northridge, who inspire and motivate me every day.

—Kim Henige

To all the kinesiology students who take seriously the idea that our efforts to promote human flourishing through physical activity are best realized when they are undertaken with a play spirit.

—Douglas W. McLaughlin

To all kinesiology students who appreciate the importance of movement and its lasting benefit.

—Belinda Stillwell

PART I **KINESIOLOGY: ITS FUNDAMENTALS AND PARADOXES** 1

CHAPTER 1 **Fundamentals and Paradoxes** 3

CHAPTER 2 **Pathways to the Pillars** 17

CHAPTER 3 **A History of Kinesiology** 41

PART II **PILLARS OF THE DISCIPLINE: KINESIOLOGY SUBDISCIPLINES** 53

CHAPTER 4 **Biomechanics** 55

CHAPTER 5 **Exercise and Sport Psychology** 91

CHAPTER 6 **Exercise and Sport Physiology** 119

CHAPTER 7 **Motor Behavior** 141

CHAPTER 8 **Philosophy of Kinesiology** 155

CHAPTER 9 **Sport Pedagogy and Physical Activity** 179

© Chris Ryan/Getty Images

CHAPTER 10   Sociology of Sport, Exercise,
and Physical Activity   205

CHAPTER 11   Adapted Physical Activity   231

CHAPTER 12   Sport Management   261

PART III   INTEGRATION OF THE PILLARS   283

CHAPTER 13   Healthy Living   285

CHAPTER 14   Restoring Function   303

CHAPTER 15   Discovering Possibilities   329

CHAPTER 16   Diversity: Sport as Welcoming Space   343

CHAPTER 17   Promoting Excellence   371

CHAPTER 18   Inclusive Physical Education for Children
with Autism Spectrum Disorder   391

CHAPTER 19   Kinesiology and the Public's Health:
Collaboration Imperatives   417

EPILOGUE   Prelude to Your Career   429

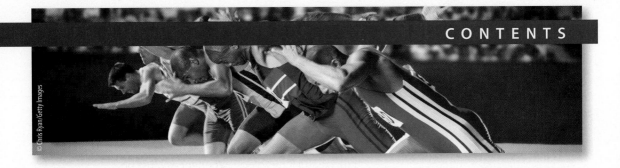

CONTENTS

Foreword xxi

Preface xxv

About the Authors xxix

About the Contributors xxxi

Reviewers xxxvii

PART I **KINESIOLOGY: ITS FUNDAMENTALS AND PARADOXES** 1

CHAPTER 1 **Fundamentals and Paradoxes** 3
Carole A. Oglesby

Introduction 4

Classic Definitions 8

Three Strata 10

    Core Scientific Domains 10

    Sociocultural-Based Forms of Movement 11

        Specialized Movement Forms 12

    Methods in Career Applications 14

Chapter Summary 14

Discussion Questions 14

References 15

CHAPTER 2 **Pathways to the Pillars** 17
Kim Henige, Douglas W. McLaughlin,
Carole A. Oglesby, and Belinda Stillwell

Introduction: Guiding Principles 18

A Competency Approach 20

Popularity of Kinesiology   20
Skills and Competencies   21
Learner-Centered Approach   23
Teacher-Centered vs. Learner-Centered Approaches   23
Five Basic Principles   24
Student is Center Stage   28
Commitment to a Holistic Approach   30
Successful Kinesiology Experiences Must be
as Diverse as the People Who Move   31
The Parts of Kinesiology Are Critical to the Whole   33
Implementing the Approaches   35
Chapter Summary   38
Discussion Questions   39
References   39

CHAPTER 3   **A History of Kinesiology**   **41**
Jaime Schultz

Introduction   42
The Embryonic Period: 1880s–1900s   42
The Profession of Physical Education: 1900–1960   44
The Academic Discipline of
Physical Education: 1960–1980   46
Kinesiology as a Unifying Title: 1990–Present   49
Chapter Summary   51
Discussion Questions   51
References   51

PART II   **PILLARS OF THE DISCIPLINE:
KINESIOLOGY SUBDISCIPLINES**   **53**

CHAPTER 4   **Biomechanics**   **55**
*Sean P. Flanagan, Shayna L. Kilpatrick,
and William C. Whiting*

What Is Biomechanics?   56
A Brief History of Biomechanics   58
The Anatomical Period   58

    The Theoretical Period   59
    The Experimental Period   59
    The Modern Period   60
Why Study Biomechanics?   61
Major Principles of Biomechanics   63
    Mechanical Principles   63
    Multisegment Principles   69
    Biological Principles   74
        Actions of the MTC   74
    Factors Affecting MTC Force   79
        MTC Length   79
        MTC Action   81
        Velocity   82
        The Stretch-Shortening Cycle   83
What Can You Do With a Degree in Biomechanics?   84
    Careers in Biomechanics   84
    Biomechanics for Everyone   84
        Observation   85
        Evaluation and Diagnosis   86
        Intervention   86
Areas of Research in Biomechanics   87
Chapter Summary   88
Discussion Questions   89
References   89

CHAPTER 5   **Exercise and Sport Psychology**   **91**
    Ashley A. Samson

What Is Sport Psychology?   92
History of Sport Psychology   92
What Do Sport Psychologists Do?   95
    Research   95
    Teaching   96
    Consulting   96
How Does One Become a Sport Psychologist?   96
    Clinical Sport Psychology   97
    Educational Sport Psychology   97

Orientations in Sport Psychology   98
   Psychophysiological Orientation   98
   Social-Psychological Orientation   98
   Cognitive-Behavioral   99
Major Topics in Sport Psychology   99
   Motivation   99
      Social Cognitive Theory   100
      Achievement Goal Theory   101
      Attribution Theory   101
   Psychological Skill Development   102
      Myths About Psychological Skill Development   103
      Delivery of PSD Programs   104
   Team/Group Dynamics   104
      Formation of Groups   105
      Factors Influencing Team Performance   106
Research Methods in Sport Psychology   108
Chapter Summary   114
Discussion Questions   115
References   115

CHAPTER 6   Exercise and Sport Physiology   119
Kim Henige

What Is Exercise and Sport Physiology?   120
The History of Exercise Physiology
in the United States   121
Why Study Exercise Physiology?   126
The Principles of Exercise Physiology   128
The Components of Physical Fitness   131
The Principles of Exercise Training   132
What Can You Do with a Degree in
Exercise Physiology?   134
Areas of Research in Exercise Physiology   137
Chapter Summary   139
Discussion Questions   139
References   140
Other Resources   140

CHAPTER 7   **Motor Behavior**   **141**
Nancy Getchell

What Is Motor Behavior?   142
   Basic Building Blocks of the Study of Motor Behavior   142
Contemporary History of Motor Behavior
as an Area of Inquiry   143
Major Topics in Motor Behavior and
Research Approaches   146
   Motor Control   147
   Motor Learning   148
   Motor Development   148
How Can You Use Motor Behavior in Your Career?   149
   Coaching   149
   Physical Education   150
   Physical or Occupational Therapy   150
Career Opportunities in Motor Behavior   151
Chapter Summary   152
Discussion Questions   152
References   152

CHAPTER 8   **Philosophy of Kinesiology**   **155**
Douglas W. McLaughlin

Introduction   156
What Is the Philosophy of Kinesiology?   156
A Brief History of the Philosophy of Kinesiology   160
Major Topics in the Philosophy of Kinesiology   161
Metaphysics   163
Epistemology   168
Values   169
Ethics   170
Aesthetics   172
What Can You Do with a Degree in the Philosophy
of Kinesiology?   174
Chapter Summary   176
Discussion Questions   177
References   177

CHAPTER 9   **Sport Pedagogy and Physical Activity**   **179**
Belinda Stillwell

What Is Sport Pedagogy?   180
The History of Physical Education   182
Why Study Sport Pedagogy?   188
Major Topics in Sport Pedagogy   188
  Opportunity to Learn   189
  Meaningful Content   190
  Appropriate Instruction   190
    Teacher Movement   190
    Meaningful Feedback   192
    Minimizing Instructional, Managerial, and Wait Time   192
  Student and Program Assessment   193
What Can You Do with a Degree in Sport Pedagogy?   194
Areas of Research in Sport Pedagogy   194
  Descriptive Research   195
  Experimental Research   196
  Action Research   198
  Research and Technology   200
  Analytic Research   200
The Future of Physical Education   201
  National Physical Activity Plan   201
  Comprehensive School Physical Activity Program   202
Chapter Summary   203
Discussion Questions   203
References   204

CHAPTER 10   **Sociology of Sport, Exercise, and Physical Activity**   **205**
Maureen Smith and Katherine M. Jamieson

What Is Sociology of Sport, Exercise, and Physical Activity?   206
A Brief History of the Sociology of Sport, Exercise, and Physical Activity   209
Major Topics in Sociology of Sport, Exercise, and Physical Activity   211

Preparing to Ask and Answer Sociological Questions
Related to Sport, Exercise, and Physical Activity   211

Why Apply Sociological Knowledge to Sport
and Physical Activity?   213

Theory and Practice in the Sociology of
Sport, Exercise, and Physical Activity   215

    Landscape Knowledge Techniques   219

    Experience Knowledge Techniques   220

    Analytic Knowledge Techniques   221

**Case Study: Applying Your Sociological
Imagination to Movement Settings**   223

    Emergent Sport: From CrossFit and
    Tough Mudders to the Biggest Loser   224

    Cultural Conditions   225

    Structural Conditions   226

    Historical Context   226

**What Can You Do with a Degree in Sociology
of Sport, Exercise, and Physical Activity?**   227

Chapter Summary   227

Discussion Questions   228

References   228

CHAPTER 11   **Adapted Physical Activity**   **231**

Taeyou Jung

What Is Physical Activity?   232

    What Is Adapted Physical Activity?   233

A Brief History of APA   235

Major Topics in APA   239

    What Is Adaptation?   239

    What Is Appropriate Language in APA?   239

    How Can APA Impact Aging and Disability?   240

    What Courses are Available in APA?   241

    What Do APA Service Programs Look Like?   242

What Can You Do with Training in APA?   245

    What Kind of Work Do You Actually Do in APA?   247

     APE Teacher   247

Adapted Aquatics Instructor — 248

APA Specialist at a Medical Center — 249

APA Coordinator in the Public Sector — 250

Adapted Fitness Business Owner — 250

APA Service Program Director at a Community College — 250

Adapted Fitness Trainer in a Recovery Exercise Program — 251

APA Researcher in a University — 251

Adapted Wellness Program Director at a Retirement Community — 251

What Credentials or Certifications Are Available in the Field of APA? — 252

Certified Adapted Physical Educator (CAPE) — 252

Certified Inclusive Fitness Trainer (CIFT) — 253

Aquatic Therapy and Rehabilitation Institute Certified (ATRIC) — 253

Areas of Research in APA — 254

Administrative and Epidemiological Approach — 254

Biomechanical Approach — 255

Motor Behavioral Approach — 255

Pedagogical Approach — 256

Physiological Approach — 256

Psychological Approach — 256

Chapter Summary — 257

Discussion Questions — 257

References — 257

CHAPTER 12   Sport Management — 261

Adam G. Pfleegor

What Is Sport Management? — 262

The History of Sport Management in the United States — 263

The Size of the Sport Industry in the United States — 266

Major Topics in Sport Management — 267

Intercollegiate, Interscholastic, and Amateur Athletics — 268

Sport Marketing and Revenue Generation 269
Sport Consumer Behavior 270
Sport Facility Management 272
Sport Management Ethics 274
Sport Law 275
**Career Opportunities with a Sport
Management Degree** 276
**Predominant Areas of Research in
Sport Management** 276
Chapter Summary 279
Discussion Questions 280
References 280

PART III | **INTEGRATION OF THE PILLARS** | 283

CHAPTER 13 | **Healthy Living** | **285**
Kim Henige

Case Study: Health and Wellness 286
Two Common Problems 288
A Solution? 289
Health Evaluation 290
Physician Clearance 292
Fitness Assessment 292
Goal Setting and Exercise Prescription 294
The Fitness Program 297
Post-Assessment, Reevaluation, and Revision 300
Chapter Summary 301
Discussion Questions 302
References 302

CHAPTER 14 | **Restoring Function** | **303**
Belinda Stillwell

Case Study: Care for Restoring Healthy Balance 304
Key Legislation 306
Extra IEP Content for Youth with Disabilities 309
Adapted Physical Education 311

Becoming an Adapted Physical Educator   312
Adapted Physical Activity   315
Career Possibilities   320
Allied Health Professions   321
Broader Issues in Therapeutic Exercise and
Allied Health   324
Chapter Summary   327
Discussion Questions   327
References   327

CHAPTER 15   **Discovering Possibilities**   **329**
Belinda Stillwell

Case Study: Personal and Cultural
Physical Activity   330
Understanding the Physical Activity Relationship   330
Life as a Stranger   331
Life as a Tourist   333
Life as a Regular   335
Life as an Insider   337
The Potential of the PAR   339
Chapter Summary   340
Discussion Questions   340
References   341

CHAPTER 16   **Diversity: Sport as Welcoming Space**   **343**
Carole A. Oglesby

Diversity, Safe Space, and Community   344
Difference to Discrimination   346
Individuals on the Margins: The Case
of Citizen's Fitness   350
Kroma   351
Viktor   352
Aodi   353
Aki   353
Julio   354

Strategies for Positive Inclusion   354
   Awareness and Appreciation   354
   Other Strategies for Fostering Unity in Diversity   357
Nature of Competition   359
Bullying   360
Gender Diversity   362
Chapter Summary   367
Discussion Questions   367
References   368

CHAPTER 17   **Promoting Excellence**   **371**
Douglas W. McLaughlin

Case Study: Personal and Shared Excellence   372
Foundations for Excellence   372
Sacrificing for Excellence   375
Models of Excellence   377
Barriers to Excellence   379
The Contribution of Kinesiology to Excellence   381
Setbacks and Challenges   382
Meaning and Relative Excellence   386
Excellence as an Unending Quest   388
Chapter Summary   389
Discussion Questions   390
References   390

CHAPTER 18   **Inclusive Physical Education for Children with Autism Spectrum Disorder**   **391**
Teri Todd and Melisa Mache

Case Study: Adapted Physical Education   392
Autism Spectrum Disorder in the Physical Education Setting   392
Overview of Autism Spectrum Disorder   395
Autism Spectrum Disorder and Physical Activity   397
Evidence-Based Strategies for Inclusive Physical Education for Children with ASD   401

Understanding Mark and Addressing His Needs   409
Red Light, Green Light Dribble Revisited   410
Conclusion   412
Chapter Summary   413
Discussion Questions   413
References   414

CHAPTER 19   Kinesiology and the Public's Health: Collaboration Imperatives   417
Steven Loy

Reaching Your Destination   418
Setting the Course   418
Strategic Planning for Success   419
Personal and Professional Goals   420
Assessing Your Progress   422
Facing Uncertainty: The Promising Future
of Kinesiology   423
  The Question We Must Ask   424
  The Methods We Use, the Answers We Offer,
  and the Opportunities We Seek and Develop   424
The Long Run   426
  Achieving Your Personal
  and Professional Goals   426
  Be an Advocate for Meaningful
  Physical Activity   426
A Journey Without End: Lifelong Learning   427
Chapter Summary   427
Discussion Questions   428
Reference   428

EPILOGUE   Prelude to Your Career   429
*Carole A. Oglesby, Kimberly Henige, Douglas W. McLaughlin,
and Belinda Stillwell*

Glossary   433
Index   453

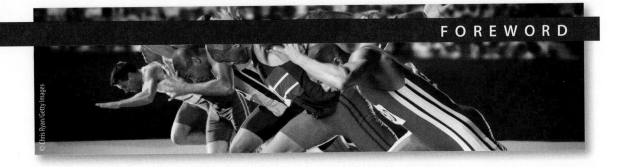

©Chris Ryan/Getty Images

Congratulations! I suspect that since you are reading this text, you are among the thousands of students that have been accepted into a kinesiology major program. Kinesiology is one of the fastest-growing majors across the country, and you are now among a growing number of students who will apply their skills in a variety of applications.

The purpose of this text is to orient new students to the field known today as *kinesiology*. The text will take you on a journey to explore the basic knowledge and essential skills needed by kinesiology professionals. The text consists of three parts, each with a series of chapters. I invite you to take the long view and examine the table of contents to develop a broad understanding of where this journey leads, as the authors and contributors have envisioned a specific approach with which you might begin to more fully realize the extent of the field.

Recognized scholars and professionals with broad expertise wrote the chapters here. Most important, however, is that they also teach an introduction to the major course at their home institution, which has familiarized them with the ever-changing and dynamic conditions produced by newly enrolled groups of students. They know the factors that will contribute to your success, as modeled in the adoption of a learning-centered approach for the text as described in Part I. By adopting this approach, you are expected to be active rather than passive in your learning. You will learn better, as evidenced by retention and transfer of knowledge, if you engage with the material. Part I also presents a competencies orientation that will assist you in beginning to realize the sets of skills necessary for earning a degree and moving toward professional practice. Furthermore, the faculty teaching your introductory classes can easily construct activities to help you identify competencies to assess your development. The authors demonstrate how the knowledge we have about how people learn and cutting-edge educational practice can be applied in kinesiology.

In Part II, the authors examine the foundations of kinesiology using a "pillars" metaphor to study the various subdisciplines of the field. Part II of the text also lays the groundwork for absorbing deeper-level coursework in biomechanics, exercise physiology, motor behavior, and sport psychology that you will encounter later in the core of your program of study.

Lastly, Part III of the text offers specific scenarios to support your understanding of the complexities of kinesiology as you move toward integration of subdisciplinary knowledge by applying a holistic approach. Apply these skills whenever learning new information, and always attempt to create meaning by connecting these new ideas with information you already have in your memory. This holistic and comprehensive approach will enable you to deeply and broadly understand kinesiology.

As a field that now leads to many different options for practice, kinesiology has realized enormous changes since its inception at the turn of the 20th century. Your journey launches here with an understanding of the roots of kinesiology in physical education and physical medicine. The programs that were designed over 100 years ago prepared teachers of physical education with the intention of improving the physical health and well-being of the populace. Today, kinesiology is a complex area of academic study. It has a body of knowledge with diverse forms of scholarship and numerous applications.

Broadly defined, kinesiology is the study of the art and science of movement, and because movement is the means by which as humans we interact with the world, many applications can be made from the knowledge gained in a kinesiology major. Today, kinesiology majors apply their knowledge in a wide range of practices, including as physical education teachers, physical therapists, occupational therapists, athletic trainers, human factors and ergonomics specialists, sport managers, adapted physical activity specialists, and medical doctors. Many more new applications of knowledge from kinesiology will be made as our society continues to discover new techniques for practice and new technologies to understand human motor performance. Some current-day examples of technological advances and applications in kinesiology include the use of an exoskeleton to afford upright posture while moving for people with paraplegia and quadriplegia, the use of a brain–muscle computer interface to control the movement of a robotic arm, and the use of brain stimulation techniques to produce new pathways for movement of affected limbs in those with brain injuries.

Reflected in this national transformation is how departments and professional organizations in higher education (e.g., American Academy of Kinesiology, American Kinesiology Association, National Association for Kinesiology in Higher Education) have incorporated the term *kinesiology*, and how our leaders have reenvisioned their purposes, what products they deliver, and the constituencies for whom they provide services. Although the term *kinesiology* is widely accepted to identify the broad area of study, some departmental structures use different names to emphasize specific components of kinesiology (such as *movement science*, *exercise science*, and *sport science*, to name only a few), or they outright reject the term *kinesiology* to describe the field. Progress and tensions can be observed in any transformative process.

Although our most prominent scholars have called for these transformations, external social and educational forces have also had an impact on kinesiology. In general, in an age of information implosion and an era where high degrees of specialization are valued, kinesiology has been impacted, as have all disciplines in academia. Faculty are now required to conduct and publish more data-based research, as evidenced by the proliferation of journals and journal manuscripts over the last 50 years. Learn more about the expertise of your faculty by conducting a search of the library databases and Google Scholar to see what they have published; you might even consider becoming actively involved in their research programs.

A consequence of the transformation is overspecialization and a lack of integration of information among the subdisciplines. We are at a crossroads though, because scholars in our field have envisioned the big picture. In January 2014, a historic congress, held in conjunction with at the National Association of Kinesiology in Higher Education annual conference in San Diego, brought together our most thoughtful and seasoned leaders to establish dialog on how and why we need to reunite our field. The proceedings can be found in an issue of *Quest* (2014, volume 66, number 3).

This is not the first time our field has needed uniting. As you unpack the history, you will learn that until the latter part of the 20th century our field was segregated by sex. In K–12 education, males and females were separated for physical activity in classes and in sports. Oftentimes, the curricula governing the segregated programs varied, too. In colleges and universities a variety of settings existed. Some programs had separate activity and theory classes, or various combinations of the above. In 1972, the passage of Title IX by the U.S. Congress enacted a more neutral playing field specifically for males and females in professional school admissions, such as law and medicine; however, the most formidable impact was on the real playing fields of athletics and physical education programs.

The merger of males and females is still being managed in many programs; as well, today we must accommodate many diverse principles and issues into our programs (e.g., race, religion, sexuality, gender assignment, disability, and age) and not make assumptions that one way is the right way. In this text the authors commit to successful inclusion of diversity in sport to offer you a holistic view, including global sport and its impact. Additionally, numerous scenarios are presented to direct your understanding of how diverse groups can be served and included in sport and kinesiology practice.

As with any journey, you must connect all of the pieces to make it successful. Follow the strategies contained in this text and use them so that you can become the next successful expert contributing to our field.

Emily H. Wughalter, EdD

Professor

Department of Kinesiology

San Jose State University

San Jose, CA

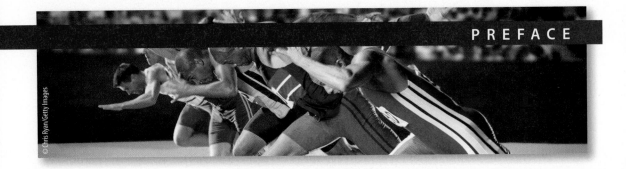

© Chris Ryan/Getty Images

Foundations of Kinesiology provides a guided journey into the discipline and profession of kinesiology. Its learner-centered approach is designed to give each reader a sense of relationship to its authors, whom you can consider to be mentors who care deeply about the progress of those choosing to enter the field. We have written this text for students in their first year as kinesiology majors or as transfer students who have entered kinesiology following earlier choices that were not the desired match.

The number of students choosing to study kinesiology is extraordinary. As just one example, consider that kinesiology is the seventh largest major in the entire California State University system, which numbers hundreds of thousands of students. This growth is nationwide, as the various postgraduate applications of kinesiology have stretched well beyond the traditional paths of teaching and coaching to include health and wellness and professions such as physical therapy, athletic training, physician assistants, fitness specialists, adapted specialists, and administrators. The kinesiology core is also expanding as research and scholarship embraces basic scientific theories and applies research in new areas.

A great challenge has emerged in the necessity to refine and maintain core scientific bases as well as to achieve relevance and cohesion in the emerging applications. This text is specifically designed to present an introduction to the holistic core features of the discipline of kinesiology along with real-life scenarios that dramatically illustrate how the entire discipline is useful in solving individual and social challenges. We offer evidence-based information utilizing both quantitative and qualitative approaches in the science-based formulations of chapters.

Why This Text?

The authors have years of experience teaching introductory courses, and it was in the teaching of these courses that we encountered frustration with other textbooks. While these other options were excellent, lengthy sections invariably went unread and unused in the structure of the course. There was either too much material for a typical introductory course, or the text went into detail about aspects of the discipline that were outside the parameters of particular departmental configurations. We were also dissatisfied with the impersonal, journal-style presentation of these texts that were to serve as a welcome and introduction to a lifetime of disciplinary study. We have sought to create a text that speaks to each student in a more personal, mentor-like fashion. The learner-centered approach completes this picture, as the readings and assignments make it necessary for the student to add her or his personal knowledge, views, and experiences to the content.

Organization of the Text

The content is organized as an exploration of a new cognitive structure—kinesiology. It is intended consciously to provide a foundation for the knowledge of the discipline to be acquired throughout the length of collegiate studies and a pathway to success through the full journey as a professional. This foundation has three sections and an epilogue: an introduction to the text and format, core subdisciplinary elements, applied real-life scenarios utilizing multiple subdisciplinary knowledge sources, and closing challenges concerning the way ahead.

Part I, "Kinesiology: Its Fundamentals and Paradoxes," comprises Chapter 1, "Fundamentals and Paradoxes," Chapter 2, "Pathway to the Pillars," and Chapter 3, "A History of Kinesiology." These three chapters serve as a preparation for the course and associated readings ahead. In Chapter 1, students are asked to consider the curiosity of never having encountered the label *kinesiology* in their elementary and secondary school coursework in physical education. Students are encouraged to get comfortable with the unique aspects of their discipline and profession. Chapter 2 introduces the bases of the text. It is in this chapter that we, as authors, give detail and meaning to the three commitments on which the text is based:

1. The holistic view of kinesiology, in which the discipline is seen not as a train with many separate and discrete cars that can be assembled and disassembled without effect, but as a unitary whole.

2. The learner-centered approach, wherein the student-reader is not perceived as an empty vessel into which the wisdom and knowledge of the professor is poured. Rather, ideas are presented for exploration and enhancement through the involvement of all.

3. A competency- and skill-based approach, wherein tools are presented in every chapter to enable the student-reader to be better able to serve themselves and society through lifelong endeavors.

Part II, "Pillars of the Discipline: Kinesiology Subdisciplines," offers nine chapters introducing the knowledge base of kinesiology. These chapters illustrate the remarkable reach of kinesiology, from contemplation of the meaning of the body (philosophy), to the biomechanical and chemical complexities of the body in motion (biomechanics and exercise physiology), to the behavioral and social realities of play and sport in our world (sociology and psychology of sport, motor behavior), to the complexities of teaching and managing sport and recreation in diverse institutional structures (pedagogy, sport management, adapted physical activity). This breadth and depth of knowledge ends the introduction to kinesiology in most texts.

Our text takes another step in illustrating the holistic nature of our comprehensive discipline in Part III, "Integration of the Pillars." In these chapters, real-life scenarios are narrated in detail, showing how the totality of kinesiology can be crucial in enabling a healthy and joyful course of life for diverse populations. These scenarios deal with life-long active habits, maintaining an active lifestyle while making transitions throughout the life span, overcoming injury and illness challenges in pursuing sport, being inclusive in our individual and community participation patterns, and building enduring excellence in performance. Again, for ease of comprehension, each of these diverse chapters follows a common path in which we find (1) a narrative description of the characters in the story, (2) a description of the situational context, (3) a description of the challenges, (4) the elements of possible solutions using knowledge from the subdisciplines, and (5) options for solutions and consequences.

The last three chapters offer a retrospective as the student completes the text. These chapters consider how the totality of this introduction to the field prepares the student-reader for the remainder of his or her collegiate experiences and provides ways of thinking about the career path ahead.

Features of the Text

This text has multiple aids and benefits built into its narrative.

Each chapter begins with Learning Objectives and Key Terms that help orient the reader to the chapter content. Key Terms are then defined in the margins of the text, as well as in the Glossary at the end of the text.

Within the body of each chapter, *Stop and Think* boxes provide questions that will help the student-reader fully grasp the significance of the content. Additional boxes scattered throughout the text also help to amplify content. Chapters within each part also feature a consistent heading structure designed to aid the acquisition of content

Each chapter ends with a Chapter Summary that recaps the chapter content, along with Discussion Questions.

Instructor Resources

Qualified instructors can receive the full suite of Instructor Resources, including the following:

- Test bank
- Slides in PowerPoint format
  - One set of standard slides for a traditional classroom experience
  - One set of discussion-based slides for a learner-centered classroom experience
- Instructor's Manual
- Sample syllabus

We, the authors, hope this text will have significant meaning to you as a cornerstone foundation to your professional library and the "story" of your career in kinesiology.

Carole A. Oglesby

Kim Henige

Douglas W. McLaughlin

Belinda Stillwell

© Chris Ryan/Getty Images

Carole A. Oglesby

Dr. Carole A. Oglesby has been in the professoriate for 45 years. She earned a PhD in Kinesiology from Purdue University in 1969 and a PhD in counseling at Temple University in 1999. She was a department chair at Temple from 1992–1995 and at California State University, Northridge, from 2003–2009.

She has been recognized through the Association for Intercollegiate Athletics for Women (AIAW) Award of Merit, the National Association for Girls and Women in Sport (NAGWS) Honor Fellowship, the Women's Sports Foundation Billie Jean King Award, the American Alliance for Health, Physical Education, Recreation and Dance (AAHPERD) R. Tait McKenzie Award, and the American Psychological Association, Division 47, Lifetime Achievement Award in Public Service.

Carole has published more than 55 chapters, articles, and essays, as well as four books/monographs. While at Temple, she advised 49 successful PhD students. She has performed consulting work for Olympic/Pan-American Game rowers and cyclists and for a race car driver, along with years of work with collegiate, high school, and youth teams and participants. She has been named a Distinguished Alumnus at both Purdue and Temple.

Kim Henige

Dr. Kim Henige received her BA (emphasis in Exercise Science) and MA (emphasis in Exercise Physiology) in Physical Education from CSU Northridge and her EdD in Education (emphasis in Learning and Instruction in Science Education) from the University of Southern California. Dr. Henige is a Certified Strength and Conditioning Specialist (National Strength and Conditioning Association) and a Certified Exercise Physiologist (American College of Sports Medicine).

At CSUN, Dr. Henige supervises the Peer Learning Facilitator Program for exercise physiology courses within the department. In addition, she supervises Commit to be Fit, a fitness program on campus for staff, faculty, students, and the local CSUN community.

Her research interests are in the area of science education, specifically improving the cognitive and affective domains of the learning experience for students in exercise physiology. She was inspired to write this book based on the needs of her students. She saw a need to present the big picture before students begin taking courses within the major. She also recognizes the need to help students apply their coursework to real life in order to make it meaningful to them.

Douglas W. McLaughlin

Dr. Douglas W. McLaughlin is an associate professor of kinesiology at California State University, Northridge. He earned his PhD in kinesiology from the Pennsylvania State University. His research focuses on ethical issues concerning the Olympic Games and the role of physical activity in promoting the good life. He holds the strong conviction that game playing is the central activity of a life most worth living. Playing Ultimate is his most cherished way to express his play spirit, though an arthritic knee has him considering new alternatives. This transition provides an opportunity to reflect on his own efforts to teach students ways to invite and support people to engage in physical activity in intrinsically meaningful ways.

Belinda Stillwell

Dr. Belinda Stillwell is an associate professor in the kinesiology department at California State University, Northridge. She received her PhD from Arizona State University in physical education/curriculum and instruction/secondary education. She works extensively with students who are pursuing their undergraduate degrees in kinesiology/physical education, as well as those going on to earn their Single-Subject Teaching Credential. Her research interests entail creating and delivering swimming instruction to those students who are afraid in water. In terms of the material in this text, it is her hope to catch and hold students' interest and motivation to learn about the broad nature of kinesiology as it applies to human movement across diverse populations.

Bonnie Berger, EdD, CC-AASP

Dr. Berger is a professor in the School of Human Movement, Sport, and Leisure Studies at Bowling Green State University in Bowling Green, Ohio, where she teaches undergraduate and graduate courses in exercise psychology and conducts research on the contributions of exercise to quality of life. Her research interests focus on the development of an exercise taxonomy designed to maximize the psychological benefits and complex interactions among mood alteration, exercise enjoyment, social physique anxiety, and life-satisfaction in diverse populations. Internationally recognized for her expertise on the contributions of exercise to quality of life, Dr. Berger has been an invited speaker and a visiting fellow at universities in numerous countries around the world, including Australia, China, the Czech Republic, England, Greece, Morocco, Singapore, and Thailand. Dr. Berger is a charter member, fellow, and Certified Consultant of the Association for Applied Sport Psychology (AASP). She also served as AASP's president and is a fellow and founding member of the American Psychological Association (APA) Division of Exercise and Sport Psychology (now Society for Sport, Exercise and Performance). She also is a fellow in the prestigious National Academy of Kinesiology (NAK), and is a charter member of the North American Society for the Psychology of Sport and Physical Activity (NASPSPA), from which she received the Outstanding Dissertation Award.

Robert A. Bucciere, MSW, LCSW

Robert A. Bucciere is currently a mental health and healthcare consultant in North Carolina. Prior to being a consultant, he was a hospital manager for the Department of Clinical Social Work and Chaplaincy Program at the University of Utah: Health Care. Prior to his position as a manager, he was the lead licensed clinical social worker at the University Health Care: Neurobehavior HOME Program. He graduated from the University of Maryland at Baltimore and the University of North Carolina at Greensboro.

Sean P. Flanagan, PhD, ATC, CSCS

Dr. Flanagan is a professor at California State University, Northridge. He received his BS in exercise science (with an emphasis in athletic training) from the Pennsylvania State University, an MS in exercise and sport science (with an emphasis in exercise physiology) from the University of Dayton, and a PhD in biokinesiology (with an emphasis in biomechanics) from the University of Southern California. He is a certified Athletic Trainer (National Athletic Trainers Association), Strength and Conditioning Specialist (National Strength and Conditioning Association), and Exercise Physiologist (American College of Sports Medicine). Additionally, he is a member of the American Society of Biomechanics. His research interests are in the biomechanics of kinetic chains, compensatory motions as a cause and a result of musculoskeletal injury, and the use of resistance exercise to restore, maintain, or improve human function.

Nancy Getchell, PhD

Dr. Getchell is a professor at the University of Delaware, where she focuses her research on the development and learning of motor control in children with disabilities not usually associated with motor dysfunction, such as autism spectrum disorder and learning disabilities. Recently, she has begun to use functional near-infrared spectroscopy to better understand brain–behavior connections.

Katherine M. Jamieson, PhD

Dr. Jamieson is Professor and Chair in the Department of Kinesiology and Health Science at California State University, Sacramento. Her teaching and research interests are focused on issues related to sport, power, and social stratification, including feminist, postcolonial, and queer analyses of transnational sporting spaces that operate at spectacular and non-spectacular levels. Dr. Jamieson's research has been published in the *Sociology of Sport Journal*, the *Journal of Sport and Social Issues, AVANTE*, the *Women in Sport and Physical Activity Journal*, the *Journal of Lesbian Studies*, the *Journal of Physical Education, Recreation and Dance*, and *Read-ing Sport: Critical Essays on Power and Representation* (Northeastern, 2000).

Taeyou Jung, PhD, ATC, CAPE
Dr. Jung is a professor in the Department of Kinesiology at California State University, Northridge and serves as a director at the Center of Achievement through Adapted Physical Activity, which provides internationally recognized adapted exercise and aquatic therapy programs. His research focuses on studying movements of people with neuromuscular disabilities and investigating clinical outcomes after therapeutic exercise. He teaches classes in adapted physical activity and therapeutic exercise.

Shayna Kilpatrick, BS, BASI Certified
Shayna Kilpatrick received her bachelor's degree from California State University, Northridge, in kinesiology with an emphasis in exercise science. Her love for biomechanics and human movement, in general, has pushed her to continuously expand her knowledge in the kinesiology field. Shayna's passion for helping others comes through in her instructing of fitness and Pilates classes. In addition, she loves to compose textbooks and manuals, allowing her to share her knowledge with others.

Steven Loy, PhD
Dr. Loy has years of experience as an exercise physiologist. In the first decade of his career he focused on teaching and completing publications based on traditional laboratory research. With the recognition of exercise as a significant part of the solution to many of the diseases that are prevalent in today's society, he shifted his attention to the public health arena, which has been his focus for the past 15 years. His intentions are to have professionals in public health recognize the contributions kinesiology can make to improve population health and the importance of creating jobs for kinesiology professionals. Throughout his career he has emphasized the importance of experiences gained and professionalism demonstrated by the students he teaches.

Melissa Mache, PhD
Dr. Mache is currently an assistant professor in the Department of Kinesiology at California State University, Chico, where she teaches courses in biomechanics, biomechanical analysis, and research design. Melissa is an applied biomechanist whose research interests focus on enhancing the safety and skill of human movement for movers of all ages and abilities. Melissa holds

a doctorate in exercise and sport sciences from Oregon State University and a master's degree in kinesiology from California State University, Chico.

Adam G. Pfleegor, PhD

Dr. Pfleegor currently serves as an assistant professor of sport administration at Belmont University in Nashville, Tennessee. His research emphasis involves the utilization of ethical theory and historical methods to examine a variety of issues in sport, such as leadership, management ethics, and heritage management. Dr. Pfleegor is a member of the executive board for the International Association for the Philosophy of Sport. He was named a 2014 Gerald "Gerry" D'Agostino Distinguished Scholar by his alma mater, The College at Brockport, State University of New York.

Justine J. Reel, PhD, LPC, CC-AASP

Dr. Reel is a professor and associate dean of research and innovation at the University of North Carolina, Wilmington (UNCW). Prior to UNCW, she was an associate professor and director of graduate studies in the Department of Health Promotion and Education at the University of Utah. She received her bachelor's degree from North Carolina State University and her master's and doctoral degrees from the University of North Carolina, Greensboro. Dr. Reel has published several books, including *Filling Up: The Psychology of Eating* (Greenwood, 2016); *Working Out: The Psychology of Sport and Exercise* (Greenwood, 2015); *The Hidden Faces of Eating Disorders and Body Image* (AAHPERD, 2009); and *Eating Disorders: An Encyclopedia of Causes, Treatment, and Prevention* (Greenwood, 2013).

Ashley A. Samson, PhD, CC-AASP

Dr. Samson is an associate professor in the Department of Kinesiology at California State University, Northridge, where she teaches courses on sport psychology and sport sociology and conducts research on athletes. Dr. Samson works with individual student-athletes, teams, and coaches on a variety of topics, including competition anxiety, confidence building, team cohesion, and communication. She received her doctorate from Louisiana State University and completed her dissertation on self-perceptions of distance runners, which is a line of research that she continues today. She has published in internationally and nationally recognized scientific journals and has been interviewed for both television and radio programs about her work.

Jaime Schultz, PhD

Jaime Schultz is an associate professor of kinesiology and women's, gender, and sexuality studies at the Pennsylvania State University. She has published or edited five books: *Women in Sport* (Oxford University Press, forthcoming); *Women and Sports in the United States: A Documentary Reader* (with Jean O'Reilly and Susan K. Cahn; Northeastern University Press, forthcoming); *Moments of Impact: Injury, Racialized Memory, and Reconciliation in College Football* (University of Nebraska Press, 2016); *American National Pastimes—A History* (co-edited with Mark Dyreson; Taylor & Francis, 2015); and *Qualifying Times: Points of Change in U.S. Women's Sport History* (University of Illinois Press, 2014); as well as numerous journal articles and essays in edited collections.

Maureen Smith, PhD

Dr. Smith teaches sport sociology and sport history at California State University, Sacramento. She is an active member of the North American Society for the Sociology of Sport, as well as the North American Society for Sport History. Her research interests are varied, and include material culture in sport, such as sport statues, African American sporting experiences in the 20th century, as well as topics related to women in sport, including the Olympics and Paralympics.

Teri Todd, PhD

Dr. Todd is an associate professor in the Department of Kinesiology at California State University, Northridge, as well as the director of clinical operations at the Center of Achievement where she develops and oversees adapted physical activity programs for children. She completed her master's and PhD at McGill University, Montreal, Quebec, in the areas of adapted physical activity and educational psychology. Her passion is working with individuals with developmental disorders. Her research has focused on encouraging physical activity for people with autism spectrum disorder.

William Whiting, PhD, FACSM, CSCS

Dr. Whiting earned a bachelor's degree in mathematical sciences from Stanford University and his master's and PhD degrees in kinesiology from UCLA. He has been a professor in the Department of Kinesiology at California State University, Northridge, since 1994, and also serves as an adjunct professor in the Department of Integrative Biology and Physiology at UCLA. He has numerous journal publications and has coauthored two textbooks. His research interests include the biomechanics of the human musculoskeletal system, with particular interest in performance enhancement and injury reduction.

Emily Wughalter, EdD
Dr. Wughalter is a professor at San Jose State University. Her major area of specialization is motor behavior. She teaches a variety of classes in the undergraduate and graduate programs on motor learning, research methods, measurement and evaluation, and writing. Dr. Wughalter has been involved in professional writing and service in the kinesiology field for over 35 years.

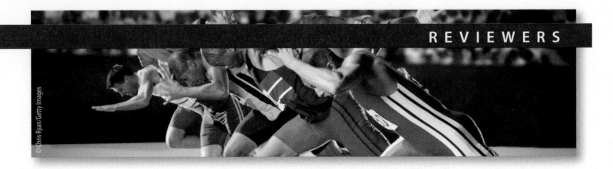

Diana Avans, PhD
Professor
Vanguard University
Costa Mesa, CA

Randy J. Dietz, PhD
Program Head
Our Lady of the Lake University
San Antonio, TX

K. Randell Foxworth, PhD
Associate Professor
Mississippi University for Women
Columbus, MS

Elizabeth Kelley, EdD
Professor
Grossmont College
El Cajon, CA

James F. Kern, PhD
Associate Professor
Lincoln University
Jefferson City, MO

Doris Lu-Anderson, PhD
Associate Faculty
Mira Costa College
Oceanside, CA

Bryan A. McCullick, PhD
Professor
The University of Georgia
Athens, GA

Jesse Lee Rhoades, PhD
Associate Professor
University of North Dakota
Grand Forks, ND

Jennifer Spry-Knutson, MA
Fitness/Sports Management Program Chair
Des Moines Area Community College
Boone, IA

Ash Walker, MA, ACSM-RCEP, FAACVPR
Manager, Cardiopulmonary Rehabilitation Services
Southeastern Health
Lumberton, NC

Dr. Will Walker, PhD
Associate Professor
East Texas Baptist University
Marshall, TX

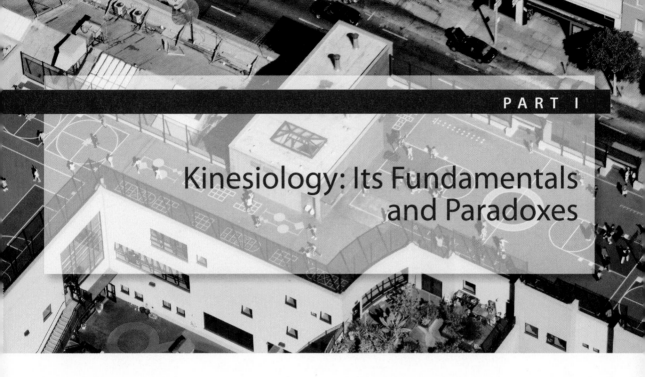

PART I

Kinesiology: Its Fundamentals and Paradoxes

CHAPTER 1

Fundamentals and Paradoxes

CAROLE A. OGLESBY

LEARNING OBJECTIVES

1. Identify and describe four paradoxes found in the discipline of kinesiology.
2. Define *kinesiology*.
3. Identify the various forms of movement.
4. Describe the subdisciplines of kinesiology.
5. Identify and define the three strata into which kinesiology is organized.
6. Explain the differences between physical education of the past and kinesiology as it is taught in universities today.

KEY TERMS

fundamental movement skills

human movement

kinesiology

kinesiology administrative location

medical gymnastics

"rolling-out-the-ball" methods

subdisciplines

Introduction

What brings you here? We hope that this is a question that intrigues you. How have you arrived at this point where you are reading this page right now, attending this university, and choosing this major? Perhaps you have a quick and easy answer that you use to fend off the many people who have asked these questions of you since you made the decisions that have brought you here. Perhaps there are some deeper aspects to these questions that you would prefer not to face right now, because the answers are not that clear. We are writing this text, in large part, because we have taught the "foundations" courses over many years and have witnessed hundreds and hundreds of students struggling with such questions. Worse yet have been those instances of students who have shrugged off these questions as "unknowable" and just plowed ahead into a great unknown with nothing on their side but blind trust. We are committed to each of you having much more than blind trust as you go forward with us.

Life's big choices, such as what course of study will be the fundamental grounding of one's career and life work, tend to be complicated with networks of explanations running in all directions. Additionally, these explanatory networks may be based on emotion, subjective, and not completely obedient

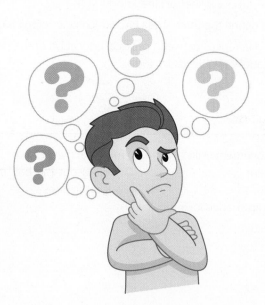

to the laws of logic. It is highly probable that one reason you are reading this text is that it is required for a course you are taking. It is also highly likely that the course you are taking is an introduction to your choice of major—**kinesiology**.

Many paradoxes and curiosities are to be found in kinesiology and the choice of this area of study as a major. We think it is important to name some of these paradoxes right from the start. It is a good first step in knowing and appreciating the path you have chosen. Of course, we think you have made the choice of a lifetime in becoming a kinesiology major (but more about that as we go along).

Paradox 1: If you are new to a college campus, it is quite possible that you have chosen to major in a field in which you have never taken a class. In secondary schools, students take courses in physical education but not kinesiology. Chemistry is still chemistry in high school, and biology is still biology. Why is kinesiology different? Some of your fellow kinesiology majors are extraordinarily fit and athletic; some may be scholarship athletes; and others may seem somewhat ungainly and not able to move comfortably for any number of reasons. The athletes say they chose the major because of their "love of sport" and that they want the opportunity to bring it to everyone. The less-abled say they love sport as well and are committed to bringing sport opportunities to all those who, like themselves, are in danger of missing it completely.

Paradox 2: How can people come to a common mission in kinesiology from vantage points that are as different from one another as chemistry, biology, psychology, and philosophy? Are there ways to discern commonality in the face of great diversity? In kinesiology, *diversity* can have many different meanings.

Paradox 3: How can a discipline that began as being apparently limited to the physical realm ever be understood as actually one of the most holistic ones in the academic community?

We will deal more directly with the history of physical education and kinesiology in later sections, but it is

kinesiology
The study of the art and science of human movement.

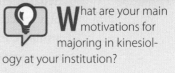
STOP AND THINK

What are your main motivations for majoring in kinesiology at your institution?

STOP AND THINK

Team A was heavily favored to defeat Team B in an important tournament, but Team B won.

- How would a kinesiology major who focuses on the physiology and biomechanics of performance explain this outcome?

- How would a kinesiology major who focuses on psychology explain this outcome?

- How would a philosophy-oriented kinesiology major explain this outcome?

- What is gained by looking at all of these factors in explaining the outcome?

important to mention a bit about our history here as an aspect of our exploration of the complexity of the field. If we could go back to a time as recent as the 1960s, it was easy to find people in our field on college campuses. We were called "PE" or "physical education," and we were usually physically housed in a "gym." We might have shared the space with the athletic department, and, in fact, athletics may have gotten the prime offices and play spaces. Our unit was either housed in the athletics department; part of a small college that included professionals in health, recreation, and dance; or we were included in a college of education. We were considered to be immersed in squats (exercise) and sports. Lastly, we existed as two separate departments—one for men and one for women—and the programs of study for each were different from one another.

Kind of amazing isn't it? As a consequence of many diverse forces (which will be explored later), male and female professionals merged into one field and (often) took on the identity of kinesiology. Leaders in the field decided it was better that our academic colleagues, as well as the lay public, become confused for a time about who we were and where we belonged administratively, rather than remain as woefully misunderstood and misperceived as we were in earlier times. Forty years later, a kind of 'name game' persists with regard to the labeling of our discipline on university campuses. It has not been easy to achieve widespread understanding and consensus concerning our new identity. As one small example, take a look at the **kinesiology administrative location** (or the equivalent) on numerous campuses in just one state university system in California (**TABLE 1-1**). There are five variants! Yet, kinesiology is one of the most popular majors in the California State University (CSU) system. This is a real tribute to student persistence and ingenuity concerning how to find the housing of their major!

One last paradox for kinesiology is that a student's devotion to his or her chosen work can become a limitation to the full appreciation of the discipline itself. How can this be? Kinesiology is complex in its taxonomy, and among its important components are the various movement forms that exist in our culture and that in fact are almost objects of worship. For example, American football, global football (soccer), basketball, marathon, track, and tennis are just a few of the movement forms that engage us. Great numbers of professionals in kinesiology enter the field because of

kinesiology administrative location
The place where kinesiology is housed within the organizational structure of a university.

STOP AND THINK

Did you personally have any difficulty locating information on the kinesiology department when you were exploring what school or major you would choose? Describe any difficulties you encountered.

TABLE 1-1 Institutional Housing of Kinesiology

University	College	Department
Cal Poly Pomona	Science	Kinesiology and Health
Cal State Fullerton	Health/Human Development	Kinesiology
Cal State LA	Health/Human Services	Kinesiology
Cal State Northridge	Health/Human Development	Kinesiology
Cal State Stanislaus	Education	Kinesiology (Physical Education and Recreation)
Humboldt State	Professional Studies	Kinesiology and Recreation
San Diego State	School of Exercise and Nutritional Sciences	Kinesiology
San Jose State	Applied Science and Art	Kinesiology
Sonoma State	Science and Technology	Kinesiology

their devotion to one or more of these forms and the place it holds, or once held, in their lives. People coach a particular sport or a particular age group for decades or an entire career. Likewise, athletic trainers are frequently completely devoted to the rehabilitation of injured athletes. This commitment

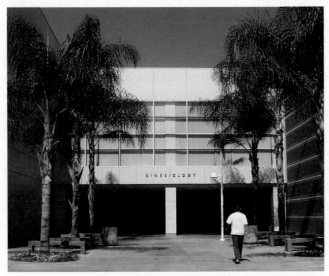

Courtesy of California State University, Northridge, College of Health and Human Development.

and desire motivates them to spend countless hours throughout their career (often volunteering) in keeping athletes whole and in the game. We would never maintain that this is a bad thing; however, a love affair with specific, tiny pieces of kinesiology can mask an observer's understanding of the whole and how the tiny pieces fit together into a unified discipline.

You are reading this text in the context of a foundations course. Enrollment could be 30, 60, or over 100. Imagine if, on the first day of class, each student is asked to introduce him- or herself and describe why he or she is taking the class. We predict that almost all will say they have chosen the major because of something (usually professionally) each wants to *do* with it—teach, promote, research, heal, perform. Who will say, "I am here because I love and want to study kinesiology"? We hope this book will be a stepping-stone to more students understanding the nature of kinesiology and how it is the "whole of it" that allows us to do all the things we want to do with the important pieces and parts.

Classic Definitions

human movement
The change of position of the individual in time-space resulting from force developed from expending energy in interaction with the environment.

Kinesiology is the study of the art and science of human movement, where **human movement** "is the change in position of the individual in time-space resulting from force developed from the expenditure of energy interacting with the environment" (Brown & Cassidy, 1963, p. 33). The cornerstones of kinesiology as an academic discipline and field of study, with an agreed-upon structure of knowledge, have been built upon these definitions.

Here we are, however, with that same old "bad penny" showing up: what is our consensus view of the structure of knowledge in kinesiology? In the decades since the 1960s, a great deal of progress has been made in unifying the disciplinary study for men and women in our field and in exemplifying that the study of human movement is not limited to the physical realm. Of primary importance has been the transformation in our understanding of what elements form the core of kinesiology, but even our most fundamental core is not something about which we all agree.

medical gymnastics
The first organized school activities involving human movement in the United States. The most popular types were those based on German, Danish, and Swedish programs.

In the early 1900s, school exercise programs were introduced in the United States that were often referred to as **medical gymnastics**. The primary purpose of these programs was to enable students to tolerate the loss of activity associated with the hours spent in required public education. In the 1920s and 1930s, the program focus shifted from prescribed exercise to so-called natural sports and games (Spears, 1973), where the fundamental core of physical education was sports and dance activities. Let us refer to these activities as *forms of movement*. Programs for boys and girls emphasized greatly differing forms of movement. However, even in times where the focus of attention was on sports and games, professionals in the field and curriculum visionaries were consistently clear that what was of crucial import in preparation of qualified teachers was the grounding of sport/games instruction in adherence to scientific and medical principles that would guarantee that the consequences of participation would be healthy and developmentally appropriate growth (Brown & Cassidy, 1963). Throughout the first 60 years of the 20th century, the attention to quality physical education based on cutting-edge research and science was in stark contrast to "rolling-out-the-ball" methods, where simply playing the game was sufficient.

Once leaders such as Henry (1964) and Brown and Cassidy (1963) began to speak out, a paradigm shift was begun that had striking results. The sport/dance forms of

"rolling-out-the-ball" methods
Physical activity programs focused only on play rather than on planned human movement using scientific methods.

STOP AND THINK

Did you ever have a physical education class in which the teacher just distributed equipment and told everyone to go play? What was the result? Is this practice widespread today, or is it "past history"?

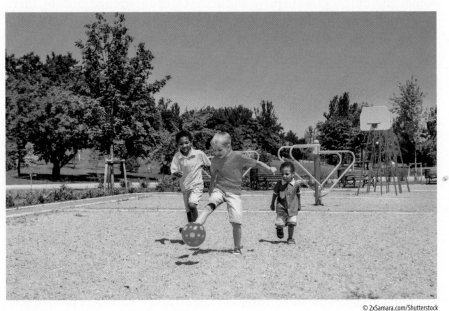
© 2xSamara.com/Shutterstock

movement were moved from the programmatic core and were replaced by concepts directly drawn from the scientific domains underlying, explaining, and predicting human movement behavior. University programs featured sequences of courses in exercise and sport science, with movement forms appearing as applications requiring professional training in the latter stages of baccalaureate work. Masters and doctoral programs grew for those who were interested in the scientific underpinnings of kinesiology. However, primary and secondary school programs continued to focus on popular sports, games, and dance.

Three Strata

The study of the art and science of human movement can be organized into three multifaceted strata: (1) core scientific domains, (2) sociocultural-based forms of movement, and (3) methods in professional (career) applications. Our purpose here is to give a brief overview of the whole of kinesiology and a sense of its breadth and complexity.

CORE SCIENTIFIC DOMAINS

subdiscipline
Field within a discipline. Kinesiology has a number of subdisciplines, including biomechanics, exercise physiology, neurophysiology of performance, and others.

Although from program to program, in the United States and globally, there may be modest variations in scope and terminology, what follows are the agreed-upon foci of inquiry in kinesiology. You may notice that many of the core elements are rooted in or have overlap with traditional and ancient disciplines. Our core domains are often referred to as subdisciplines, because they share commonalities with the so-called parent disciplines (**TABLE 1-2**). In each instance, time and exercise/sport science research **has** revealed significant and unique elements of the kinesiology subdisciplines that distinguish them from disciplines. This can be seen most dramatically in the subdiscipline of biomechanics. Biomechanics is the study of the principles that govern the human body in motion. It requires a combination of knowledge concerning the physics of objects and the anatomy of human motion. Biomechanics, dealing as it does with our familiar movement forms, also concerns itself with the human moving in relation to inanimate objects (e.g., ball, bat, javelin) and animate cocreators of movement (e.g., dogs/sleds, horses in equestrian). Neither anatomy, nor physics, nor any other scientific domain covers the subject area of biomechanics. This same pattern (i.e.,

TABLE 1-2   Subdisciplines in Kinesiology

Biomechanics
Exercise physiology
History of sport and dance
Neurophysiology of performance
Philosophy of sport
Psychology of performance (developmental, learning, self-regulation, and performance)
Sociology of sport
Sport medicine

overlap with other disciplines but with extensive uniqueness) holds true for the variety of sport/exercise subdisciplines that overlap in limited ways with more traditional disciplines in the arts and sciences.

SOCIOCULTURAL-BASED FORMS OF MOVEMENT

Country by country, around the world, thousands of game, sport, and dance forms exist as part of ethnic or national cultures. Canadians love their curling. In the United States, sport sociologists have analyzed the shift of our "national pastime" of baseball over time from its original rural, agrarian orientation, as well as our current fascination with football and its corporate structure and basketball as an urban, fast-paced, diverse sport (Woods, 2007).

No human movement specialist could possibly possess expert skills and understanding of all of our myriad forms of sociocultural-based movement. In the past, physical education preparation was devoted to producing a teacher/coach with all the capabilities necessary for the most commonly practiced movement forms. Today, the credit hours necessary for the science core of the major makes this kind of skills focus impractical. These diverse movement forms serve an important purpose in potentially offering opportunities for people of all sizes, shapes, conditions, strengths and vulnerabilities, personal temperaments, and interests to find activities for health and vitality throughout the lifetime. One of the challenges of kinesiology today is to find avenues for schools, local governments, and public health agencies to provide as many options as possible to engage as many citizens as

TABLE 1-3   Examples of Common Sociocultural-Based Forms of Movement

Aquatics (all types)
Combatives (boxing, fencing, martial arts, shooting)
Equestrian activities
Individual sports (racket, handball)
Running (marathon, triathlon)
Team (basketball, baseball, football, softball, soccer)
Vertigo sports (diving, gymnastics)
Winter sports (skiing, skating)

possible in an active lifestyle. Additionally, the professional workforce for staffing these options must be produced. **TABLE 1-3** lists some of the most common sociocultural-based forms of movement in the United States and most other developed countries. Kinesiology departments usually feature processes by which students in the major can develop and demonstrate knowledge and proficiencies in some number of these forms.

SPECIALIZED MOVEMENT FORMS

Two specialized types of movement forms are crucial in schools, public recreational spaces, hospitals, and private facilities. The first of these specialized types is often referred to as **fundamental movement skills**, or *basic movement skills*. These are the childhood building blocks on which sophisticated sport skills are based. Such skills include catching, hopping, jumping, kicking, skipping, running, throwing, twirling, and walking. Elementary school physical education focuses on these fundamentals, and low-organized games and rhythmic activities put these skills to use. Some believe that these basic skills are "natural" and do not need to be formally taught and practiced. In many states today, physical education has all but disappeared from elementary schools. However, motor development research has shown that the acquisition of basic movement skills is far from natural or automatic for all children.

A second important specialized type of movement falls under the category of exercise. Research has shown that specially designed movement

fundamental movement skills Building blocks of human movement upon which sport skills are based, including catching, hopping, jumping, kicking, skipping, running, throwing, twirling, and walking.

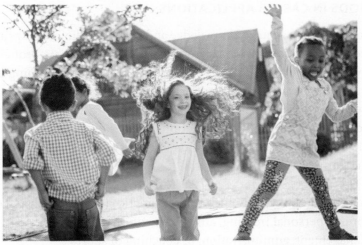

© Tony Tallec / Alamy Stock Photo

patterns are ideally suited for building capacities such as strength, cardio-vascular endurance, muscular endurance, flexibility, agility, and the like. Today, well-designed exercise programs are an important part of kinesiology in restoring capacity in those who are wounded or disabled, increasing their capacity for high-level skill performance and maintaining fitness levels throughout the lifespan.

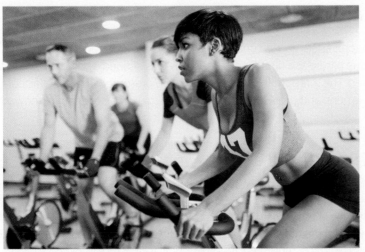

© iStock.com/ Cristian Casanelles at Tempura

METHODS IN CAREER APPLICATIONS

Once a student has acquired knowledge and understanding of the principles derived from the subdisciplinary domains and appropriate proficiencies in movement forms common in our culture, professional training begins. Generally, in kinesiology a student will complete some upper-division baccalaureate work and possibly some graduate work to acquire certifications and licenses that enable the application of kinesiology in a profession or career. Five general areas of professional training are rooted in kinesiology knowledge and skills:

1. Capacity building and/or restorative practice (e.g., strength and conditioning, personal training, athletic training)
2. Management, administration, or coaching of sport
3. Performance enhancement (e.g., sport psychology consulting)
4. Instruction in physical education
5. Research (career in academics)

This text presents three pathways to accomplish our purpose, which is to enable you to understand, describe, and appreciate the discipline of kinesiology. These three pathways include a competency orientation, a learning-centered focus, and a holistic perspective. Your journey is opening up before you.

CHAPTER SUMMARY

This chapter asked you to consider four paradoxes in kinesiology that contribute to its unique nature as a discipline. Kinesiology was defined, and its key subdisciplines identified. The three strata of kinesiology were presented: the scientific core, forms of movement, and professional practice. The chapter also identified how contemporary kinesiology differs from its historical precursors.

DISCUSSION QUESTIONS

1. What is kinesiology? Discuss what the concept of kinesiology entails.
2. Describe the paradoxes found in kinesiology. Have you had personal experience with any of these paradoxes?
3. Are you more drawn to the core scientific domains of kinesiology, sociocultural-based forms of movement, or professional (career) applications? What area drew you to the major? What area are you most excited about learning more about?

REFERENCES

Brown, C., & Cassidy, R. (1963). *Theory in physical education*. Philadelphia: Lea & Febiger.

Henry, F. (1964). Physical education: An academic discipline. *Proceedings of the 67th annual conference of NCPEAM*, 6–9. (Reprinted in *Journal of Health, Physical Education and Recreation*, 1964, *35*, 32–33, 69.)

Spears, B. (1973). The emergence of sport as physical education. In *Coping with controversy*. Washington, D.C.: American Alliance of Health, Physical Education, Recreation and Dance.

Woods, R. (2007). *Social issues in sport*. Champaign, IL: Human Kinetics.

CHAPTER 2

Pathways to the Pillars

KIM HENIGE, DOUGLAS W. McLAUGHLIN,
CAROLE A. OGLESBY, AND BELINDA STILLWELL

LEARNING OBJECTIVES

1. Describe the popularity of kinesiology as a college major.
2. Identify two of the most highly valued qualities that employers look for in new college graduates.
3. Describe three important skills that you will be expected to master during the course of the major in kinesiology.
4. Explain the differences between teacher-centered and learner-centered approaches to learning.
5. List the five principles of the learner-centered approach and describe how these principles may be used in class to enhance learning.
6. Describe the differences between the dualistic and holistic views of human beings.
7. Describe how actions, such as running, holistically involve all of the subdisciplines of kinesiology.
8. Describe how both "good" and "bad" (pleasant/unpleasant) movement experiences can deepen your commitment to bring kinesiology and movement activity to everyone.

KEY TERMS

American Kinesiology Association (AKA)

communication

competency approach

competency skills

desired skills

dualistic interpretation of a person

empowered learner

experiences of physical activity

focus

guiding principles

holistic approach

holistic interpretation of a person

interpersonal skills

learner centered

learner-centered strategies

learning skills

mentor

physical activity

prepared

professionalism

self-assessment

teamwork

unprofessional qualities

Introduction: Guiding Principles

guiding principles
Core ideas and concepts that direct and influence a plan of action.

When we set out to write an introductory textbook to the field of kinesiology, we discussed what our **guiding principles** would be. Some of the principles we identified apply to us as authors and teachers. Some of the principles we identified apply to you as readers and learners. Our decision to incorporate these principles was based on our combined experiences as teachers and learners. Our hope is that we have written, through our collective wisdom, a text that is as interesting and engaging as it is informative. Our goal is to start you off on the right path as you begin your journey into the field of kinesiology. Therefore, we believe it is important to share our principles with you so that you can understand why the text is written the way it is and how you can get the most out of it.

mentor
An individual who will guide and support you on various aspects of your life journey.

Four principles guided our writing of this text. First, we want you to think of us as **mentors** who respect and support you and your pursuit of kinesiology. Although we bring several combined decades of experience and knowledge to this text, we are not merely presenting information about kinesiology. In this spirit, we encourage you to become apprentice learners by engaging with the activities we have incorporated throughout the text. Second, we have written a text that is accessible but rigorous. We have attempted to write in a manner that is not too technical but that prepares you for advanced levels of study. Although this is an introduction to kinesiology, it is important that you be properly prepared for the challenging road ahead. Third, we want to make manifest that we have a deep regard for the field of kinesiology. We love **physical activity**, the different ways we can examine it, and the ways it can provide meaning in both personal and professional contexts. Just as our mentors shared this passion with us, we now pass it on to you. We hope that you will share this passion with others as you become more involved in the field of kinesiology in practical settings. Last but not least, we have written this text in a shared voice that incorporates the above principles and speaks to you directly in both a personal and professional way. We have selected many different authors to contribute to this book so that you get the best introduction possible. In one sense, each author has a unique voice because of his or her unique history within the field of kinesiology. However, all the authors recognize the importance of mentoring, maintaining rigorous standards, and loving the field of kinesiology. We hope that you can hear this as a consistent voice, like the beautiful song of a choir. The individuals may have different parts and different voices, but they join together in a way that the whole is more than the parts.

In addition to our own guiding principles, we have also identified guiding principles for you. These principles are intended to prepare you to be successful both inside and beyond the classroom. If you can incorporate these guiding principles into your education, then you will be well prepared upon graduation. These guiding principles are (1) developing **competency skills**, (2) becoming **learner centered**, and (3) maintaining a **holistic approach** to the

physical activity
Any bodily movement that requires the use of energy by the individual.

competency skills
The set of skills required to efficiently and successfully participate in a professional setting.

learner centered
Information exchange and knowledge enhancement produced through the shared effort of the professor, student, and classmates.

holistic approach
View that different course experiences and practical applications are parts of a whole, with each part interacting with and influencing the others.

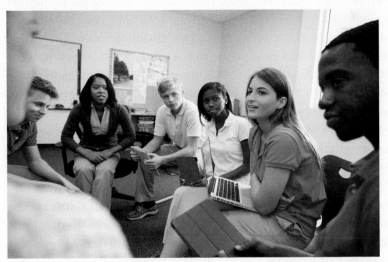

© Monkey Business Images/Shutterstock

field of kinesiology. Because we want you to adopt these principles, we will explain each one in detail, starting with the competency approach.

A Competency Approach

POPULARITY OF KINESIOLOGY

People choose to seek a college degree for a variety of reasons, but one important objective is generally to prepare to be marketable for, and successful in, their desired career. According to the **American Kinesiology Association (AKA)**, 820 U.S. institutions of higher education offer a bachelor's degree in kinesiology (AKA, 2013). Twenty-one (2.5%) of those 820 institutions are in the California State University (CSU) system, the largest and most diverse university system in the United States (The California State University, 2016). Student enrollment in CSU kinesiology programs alone was more than 17,000 in 2014, and more than 2,400 students received bachelor's degrees in kinesiology in the 2011–2012 academic year (The California State University, 2013). Kinesiology has also been identified as one of the fastest-growing majors in academia today (AKA, n.d.). These numbers translate into hundreds, if not thousands, of new kinesiology graduates each year, adding rapidly to the hundreds of thousands of other individuals who already hold kinesiology degrees. With so many people meeting the minimal qualification of a degree in kinesiology, what will make you stand out among the numerous other job candidates you will compete with for jobs once you graduate?

Recent surveys of U.S. employers reveal valuable information in this regard. One survey of 225 employers from a pool of 100,000 companies found that two of the most **desired skills** are in the areas of **communication** (98%) and **teamwork** (92%) (Millennial Branding, 2012). Communication, in this context, was defined to include the ability to write, compose emails, give presentations, and have conversations with people across the generations. Interestingly, the same survey revealed that these skills are also among the hardest to find among job candidates. The York College of Pennsylvania's (YCP) Center for Professional Excellence conducts an annual survey of professionalism in the workplace (YCP, 2013). In 2013, it surveyed more than 400 human resources professionals nationwide, with questions focusing on their experiences with recent college graduates. Almost half of those surveyed reported that less than 50% of new employees exhibited

American Kinesiology Association (AKA) Professional organization whose mission is to promote and enhance "kinesiology as a unified field of study and advances its many applications."

desired skills The ability to do something through practice or training that is highly valued in professional settings.

communication The ability to write, compose emails, give presentations, and have conversations with people across the generations.

teamwork The ability to work with other people to accomplish a shared task.

professionalism during the first year on the job. This statistic has risen 10% since 2009. College is traditionally thought to be a place to learn content knowledge, but perhaps just as important it should be a place to learn how to become a successful professional.

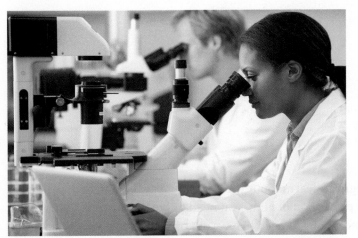

© Monkey Business Images/Shutterstock, Inc.

STOP AND THINK

The competency approach in this text takes seriously the notion that each student is concerned with his or her chances for a successful career with this major. At this point you should be asking yourself a number of different questions regarding a person's marketability in the field:

- What are employers looking for when hiring, retaining, and promoting?

- What makes one person more hirable than another?

- What makes one person more successful than another?

SKILLS AND COMPETENCIES

Many of the skills and characteristics valued by employers can be learned and practiced during the college years as part of coursework. You might be wondering what characteristics contribute to **professionalism**. **TABLE 2-1** lists the professional and **unprofessional qualities** mentioned most consistently by YCP survey respondents.

One of the objectives of this text is to consistently use a competency approach to present the material and guide you through the course. A **competency approach** involves an emphasis on skill development. Throughout your years as a kinesiology major, you will learn the core competencies of kinesiology within multiple subdisciplines, such as biomechanics, exercise physiology, exercise prescription, human and functional anatomy, motor learning and development, sport/kinesiology history, sport/kinesiology philosophy, and sport psychology. Kinesiology competencies include kinesiology-specific content knowledge and skills. This text will additionally

professionalism
The demonstration of conduct, behavior, and qualities that are expected in a professional setting.

unprofessional qualities
A failure to demonstrate conduct and behavior that is expected in a professional setting.

competency approach
An emphasis on skill development that will help you become an exceptional professional.

TABLE 2-1   Perceived Professional/Unprofessional Qualities

Qualities of a Professional	Unprofessional Qualities
Work until a task is completed competently	Inappropriate appearance
Interpersonal skills including civility	Poor work ethic
Appropriate appearance	Unfocused
Punctuality and regular attendance	Apathetic
Communication skills	Sense of entitlement
Honesty	Disrespectful and rude
Focused/attentive	Lack of time management

Reproduced from Center for Professional Excellence at York College of Pennsylvania. (2013). 2013 National Professionalism Survey Workplace Report. Retrieved from http://www.ycp.edu/media/york-website/cpe/York-College-Professionalism-in-the -Workplace-Study-2013.pdf (accessed March 28, 2016).

help you to begin to learn about the competencies involved in becoming an exceptional professional. First, you need to know what it is to be such a professional, and then you need to have opportunities to learn and practice those skills. Specifically, this text focuses on enabling you to learn and practice your communication skills (listening, verbal, and written), interpersonal and teamwork skills, work ethic and quality, and time management. Other skills from Table 2-1 will also be woven into the chapters.

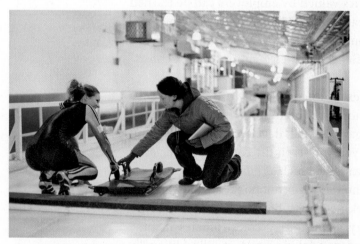

© Hero Images Inc. / Alamy Stock Photo

It is your responsibility to take advantage of the opportunity to begin the process of becoming an exceptional professional. Skills are not mastered overnight. You are now early in your college career, with years ahead to practice and refine your professional skills. If you take this seriously you will graduate with a degree in kinesiology and possess the qualities of a good professional, making you a more desirable candidate in the job market.

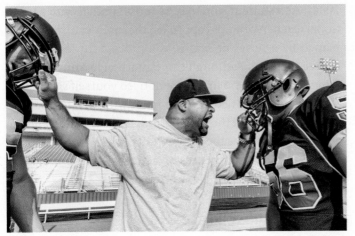

© TerryJ/Getty Images

Learner-Centered Approach

TEACHER-CENTERED VS. LEARNER-CENTERED APPROACHES

This text takes a learner-centered approach; that is, the emphasis is on learning: "Learning should be seen as a qualitative change in a person's way of seeing, experiencing, understanding, conceptualizing something in the real world—rather than as a quantitative change in the amount of knowledge someone possesses" (Weimer, 2002). Rather than simply *covering* the course content, you will *use* it to expand your knowledge base; while doing so, you will simultaneously improve your **learning skills** and heighten your learner awareness. Examples of common learning skills include time management, study skills, and computational skills. More sophisticated learning skills involve "the ability to apply theoretical information to complex practical problems and integrate information from different areas creatively in order to explain particular phenomena better" (Weimer, 2002, p. 54). Learner awareness focuses on your ability to reflect on how you learn—what your tendencies and preferences are. Also important is your ability to assess your own strengths and weaknesses. All of this is geared toward you developing your confidence as a student.

This particular format is often contrasted with that of teacher-centered delivery. In the teacher-centered approach, the focus is primarily on what the teacher *does* compared to what the students are *learning* (Blumberg,

learning skills
Skills such as time management, study skills, and computational skills that facilitate engagement with course content to expand one's knowledge base.

STOP AND THINK

Reflect on your past physical activity experiences (e.g., physical education classes, sport teams, dance groups, recreational activities, etc.). What factors contributed to high levels of engagement and promoted participation? What factors contributed to low levels of engagement and discouraged participation?

2004). As a student, you may be most familiar with a traditional teacher-centered approach that uses lectures accompanied by a series of exams as a process for learning the course material. Although this pattern of learning has certain advantages, you may have noticed yourself sitting passively in your seat taking some notes while the teacher was *on stage* for most of the class period. In the learner-centered approach, you have the opportunity to play a much larger role in the learning process by actively participating both inside and outside the classroom (**TABLE 2-2**).

FIVE BASIC PRINCIPLES

In order to achieve this deeper level of learning, you will utilize the five principles of the learner-centered approach

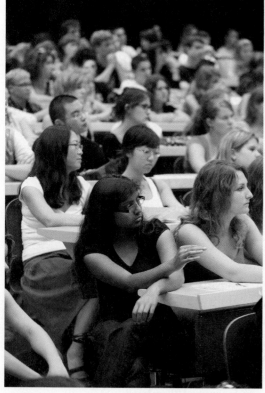

© Agencja Fotograficzna Caro / Alamy Stock Photo

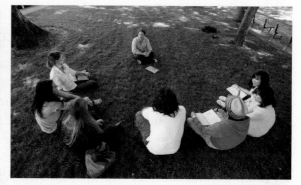

© Robert Crum / Alamy Stock Photo

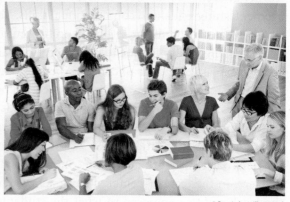

© Rawpixel.com/Shutterstock

TABLE 2-2   Comparison of Teacher- vs. Learner-Centered Paradigms on College Campuses

Teacher-Centered Paradigm	Learner-Centered Paradigm
Knowledge is transmitted from professor to students.	Students construct knowledge through gathering and synthesizing information and integrating it with the general skills of inquiry, communication, critical thinking, problem solving, and so on.
Students passively receive information.	Students are actively involved.
Emphasis is on acquisition of knowledge outside the context in which it will be used.	Emphasis is on using and communicating knowledge effectively to address enduring and emerging issues and problems in real-life contexts.
Professor's role is to be primary information giver and primary evaluator.	Professor's role is to coach and facilitate. Professor and students evaluate learning together.
Teaching and assessing are separate.	Teaching and assessing are intertwined.
Assessment is used to monitor learning.	Assessment is used to promote and diagnose learning.
Emphasis is on right answers.	Emphasis is on generating better questions and learning from errors.
Desired learning is assessed indirectly through the use of objectively scored tests.	Desired learning is assessed directly through papers, projects, performances, portfolios, and the like.
Focus is on a single discipline.	Approach is compatible with interdisciplinary investigation.
Culture is competitive and individualistic.	Culture is cooperative, collaborative, and supportive.
Only students are viewed as learners.	Professor and students learn together.

Reproduced from J. E. Huba & M. E. Freed. (2000). *Learner-centered assessment on college campuses.* Boston: Allyn & Bacon.

as they relate to kinesiology: (1) the balance of power, (2) the function of the content, (3) the role of the teacher, (4) the responsibility for learning, and (5) the purpose and processes of evaluation (Weimer, 2002). Although the balance of power, the function of the content, and the role of the teacher are primarily determined by your instructor, there are still steps you can take to develop a more learner-centered approach for yourself. This is because the responsibility for learning and the purpose and processes of evaluation rests on changes you, the student, can and will undertake. During this course, you will personally interact with your peers and the course content in ways that will result in better retention of the information, increased motivation, higher achievement, greater school satisfaction, and ultimately becoming a better-prepared professional (Blumberg, 2004). This results in a cooperative learning environment versus a competitive one. The following paragraphs cite examples of how these principles might translate to everyday life in the classroom.

The balance of power principle leans heavily on who is making decisions about learning. In a teacher-centered classroom, the teacher makes most, if not all, of the decisions about learning. This can be readily seen in most course syllabuses. Topics controlled by the teacher usually include what textbook will be used for the course, what assignments will be completed, or what constitutes participation. A teacher committed to a learner-centered classroom may seek your input regarding topics such as these. For instance, the teacher may solicit your help in determining what textbook will be used for the course. To do this, the teacher might select five textbooks that would accomplish the course expectations and then create student textbook review committees and as a group project ask students to make and justify a textbook recommendation (Weimer, 2002). The teacher could also provide you with an opportunity to choose from a menu of course assignments designed to reach the total point value for the course. This means that each student would have the chance to select what items he or she wanted to be evaluated on. Additionally, the teacher could involve you in classroom policy making, such as determining how points are earned for classroom participation. In groups, your teacher would ask you to address specific questions that relate to credit for participation, such as "What behaviors should count positively toward participation credit? Should some participation behaviors count more? And if so, which ones?" (Weimer, 2002). After answers are generated, class discussions follow to resolve any disagreements as well as provide needed refinements. The process concludes with a class vote. The participation policy then becomes a part of the course syllabus.

Even when a teacher does not engage in these types of strategies, you can still do a number of things to be an **empowered learner**. Knowing the difference between adequate and inadequate preparation for assignments and exams, you can take responsibility for your own preparation. Once given a course outline, you can develop your own schedule that allows you time to meet deadlines. Rather than waiting until the last minute to complete assignments or projects, you can plan ahead. Something as simple as becoming familiar with the course syllabus and schedule can empower you to take responsibility for and develop strategies for meeting your goals for the class.

empowered learner
A learner who can take responsibility for preparing for course requirements and distinguish between being adequately prepared and being underprepared.

With regard to the function of the content, you should be prepared to interact with the course material differently than you may have experienced in past classes. Even if little attention is given to teaching learning skills (e.g., note-taking, summarizing) and learner awareness (e.g., self-assessment, personal learning style) while building your knowledge, a learner-centered approach links these two concepts intimately with the course content. A learner-centered approach means you will experience the content firsthand through active-learning strategies that are designed to engage and motivate you throughout the class. For instance, when learning about career possibilities in kinesiology, you might elect to observe and interview a working professional. During this activity, you will practice vital learning skills such as note-taking, generating meaningful questions, and summarizing what you have found. In terms of learner awareness, you would complete a self-assessment that discusses your strengths and weaknesses as they relate to performing successfully in that job. Active-learning strategies do not need to be developed by the teacher. You should always be thinking about ways you can better engage the material. If you find an active-learning strategy particularly helpful in one class, perhaps you can incorporate that strategy into your other classes.

Some teachers assume that students know what learning strategies work for them. This may not be a good assumption to make, because we can always refine and improve our learning strategies. In contrast, some teachers provide so many different learning strategies that it can feel overwhelming. When trying to understand new learning strategies interferes with our ability to understand course content, it is as much as a problem as not having enough resources or appropriate strategies to enhance learning.

STOP AND THINK

Identify someone who works in a professional setting related to kinesiology. What qualities does the person believe contribute to professional and personal success? What qualities does he or she believe create problems that can inhibit success?

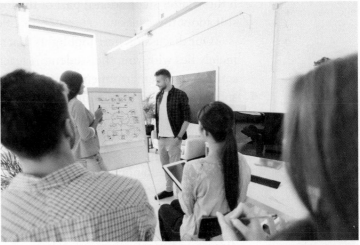

It is important that you become critically engaged in and self-aware of how your own strategies and habits promote successful learning of the content.

STUDENT IS CENTER STAGE

In a traditional college course, the role of the instructor is that of an actor—on stage and the center of focus for students. In other words, in traditional instruction, teachers dominate the activities that occur in the classroom, such as selecting and preparing the materials; leading and controlling discussions; and providing notes, diagrams, and graphs (Weimer, 2002). When you are committed to a learner-centered approach, you can situate the teacher's role as a guide who facilitates learning. With this approach, you are putting yourself alongside the teacher as a partner in the learning process. When a teacher sets up guidelines to conduct a debate in class, it is you, rather than the teacher, who is at the center of the activity. During the debate, the teacher is positioned *off center stage* by recording the arguments each side constructs on the board. Once the arguments are cited, the teacher may have each side meet and discuss the strongest argument on their side as well as how to address the best arguments from the opposing side. Finally, volunteers from each side role-play these arguments. Time can be taken at the conclusion of class to enhance your learner awareness by completing a peer-assessment on each of your group members (Weimer, 2002). Even if these latter steps are not part of the formal classroom activities, you can still adopt these **learner-centered strategies**.

learner-centered strategies
Activities and behaviors that enable you to take responsibility for and maximize your learning.

   Our discussion here highlights that the responsibility for learning ultimately lies with you, the student. A teacher can facilitate your learning by setting up an environment that is welcoming and productive—an atmosphere that helps to maximize learning. This may include fewer rules and requirements than you may be accustomed to, but the idea is to help you move toward becoming a responsible class member who understands that there are logical consequences involved when making decisions about your learning. You do not need your teacher to ask you to write about your experiences in classes where you believed you learned a lot and classes you may have not. You can identify these conditions on your own and discuss them with other students outside of class. It would be an interesting experience to discuss and summarize in the classroom these conditions and use them to establish a set of guidelines that promote learning (Weimer, 2002). Regardless of whether these guidelines become part of the syllabus and course website or become your own personal guidelines, they can serve as daily reminders about how learning can be promoted rather than simply a list of disciplinary procedures.

Letter grades are part of learner-centered classrooms just as much as they are in teacher-centered classrooms. Although the purpose and processes of evaluation may be different, if you are committed to a learner-centered approach, then you are concerned about the larger picture. Rather than focusing on the grade itself, you should focus on how evaluation and learning are closely linked so that your grade more accurately reflects what you have learned throughout the semester. Oftentimes, students take a course and receive a high grade but find out that this knowledge is forgotten soon after the final exam. You can adopt a learner-centered approach through the use of a variety of strategies to generate opportunities to deepen your knowledge by applying it later in the course and throughout your academic career.

> **STOP AND THINK**
>
> The purpose of a course is to learn/master content. The letter grade is only symbolic of the learning that has occurred. What would happen if students did *not* receive a grade in a teacher-centered environment? Would the outcome be different in a learner-centered environment?

Imagine your teacher designs a **self-assessment** activity after the first exam to help you reflect on your study skills. You are asked to respond to the following set of prompts:

1. What content did you know best? Why?
2. What content did you struggle with? Why?
3. Discuss three strategies you used to prepare for this exam. Which ones worked? Why do you think they worked?
4. Which ones did not work? Why?
5. Outline a plan to improve your preparation for the next exam.

self-assessment
An activity that allows you to reflect on how well you are learning and identify what learning-centered strategies work best for you.

Completing this exercise should not only improve your next exam score, but also point out any content you may need to relearn as well as enlighten you on the best ways that you learn.

If you have not experienced the learner-centered approach before, then you may be hesitant or resist when asked to participate in this way. You are not alone. Resistance is a natural occurrence when dealing with these sorts

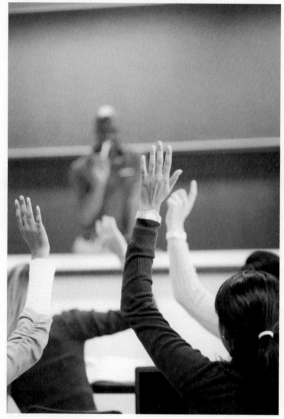

© Hongqi Zhang / Alamy Stock Photo

of changes. Keep in mind that being a successful learner requires many of the same features as excelling in sport: consistent training, development of advanced skills, acquisition of good habits, and evaluation of performance. You can seek guidance from your teachers and classmates on the process, but be patient, because the journey will be slow and gradual.

In a classroom environment that focuses on the learner-centered approach, your teacher will put several things in place to ease your transition from a traditional to a learner-centered classroom so that you become a fully independent and self-directed student. First, your teacher will communicate with you frequently and clearly about what is going on in class. Second, this communication will positively encourage and reinforce what you will be asked to do in class. Third, your teacher will often solicit feedback from you, especially at the end of an assignment or exam or during a semester-long project (Weimer, 2002). Your teacher wants to know how things are going, what is working well, what is not, and how these activities are affecting your learning. Be ready; learning is hard work. It will require you to take on more responsibility than you may be comfortable with, but the rewards are far-reaching.

Commitment to a Holistic Approach

Although interdisciplinary in nature, kinesiology is best understood from a holistic approach. The term holistic approach is used to refer to many different things, so it is important to understand the specific context used here. Simply put, a holistic approach considers the whole to be greater than the sum of its parts. For kinesiology, the "whole" refers to all forms of human movement/physical activity; not only sport, dance, exercise, or rehabilitative forms. A holistic approach influences how we understand experiences of physical activity, the nature of persons, and the field of kinesiology. Our commitment to a holistic approach will enable us to improve how we get people moving.

The first step is to recognize how **experiences of physical activity** are holistic in themselves. Many of us chose kinesiology because of the meaningful experiences we had with physical activity. Our own passion for physical activity is something that we want to share with others. Because physical activity has made a difference in our lives, we want to help others learn how it can make a difference in their lives. But it is important to recognize that it is the coherent, complex, and unique experiences we have with our physical activity that make it so meaningful. We have to recognize the dynamic social and cultural forces that are at play when people decide to be physically active. We have to be careful not to diminish or discredit other people's experiences because we could mistakenly discourage them from an activity they already enjoy or deter them from taking up a new movement form.

experiences of physical activity The variety of ways that people participate in physical activity that are coherent, complex, diverse, and meaningful.

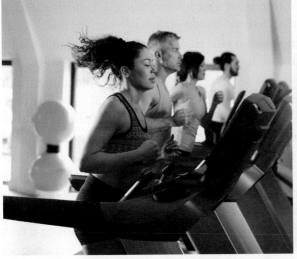

© Monkey Business Images/Shutterstock

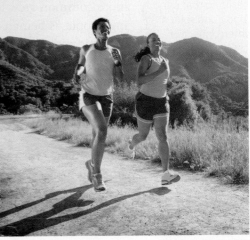

© Blend Images / Alamy Stock Photo

SUCCESSFUL KINESIOLOGY EXPERIENCES MUST BE AS DIVERSE AS THE PEOPLE WHO MOVE

Having a holistic approach means that we recognize the need for a variety of physical activity experiences based on the variety of personal experiences. We need to recognize and appreciate people's diverse interests and capabilities. Some people like competition, whereas others do not. Some people are energetic, whereas others are not. Some people love to dance, while others do not. Some people have many skills, whereas others have few. Some need social support and encouragement, whereas others need time and space to figure it out on their own. Some are enthusiastic; others are intimidated. Some require special accommodations. Some require access. When rehabilitating from an injury, some require motivation just to do the minimum, whereas others may need to be restrained so that they do not do too much. This list is by no means exhaustive. The list illustrates that the physical activity experiences of those we will be working with, and for, are often very different from our own. We do not need to ignore, or deny, that our experiences of physical activity are personally meaningful, but we need to be thoughtful about how we can help others develop new experiences so that they can find richer and more meaningful experiences as well.

holistic interpretation of a person
The view that we must take seriously and account for all aspects of a person's experience, realizing that mind, body, and spirit are interconnected.

dualistic interpretation of a person
The view that body and mind are separate and distinct parts of human beings and that we can isolate one aspect from the other within a person.

If we are able to consider experiences of physical activity holistically, then we are well on our way to having a **holistic interpretation of a person**; mind, body, and spirit interrelated and interconnected. Unfortunately, a more common view is the **dualistic interpretation of a person**; that is, seeing people as being composed of two parts: a body and a mind. From a dualistic perspective, the kinesiologist is thought to work on the body. This perspective can lead to several negative consequences, the most important being that our field is undervalued because it does not deal with the mind. This pressure is usually exerted from people outside our field, but within our field, we need to worry about a reductive, materialist interpretation that views people as nothing more than their material substance. Investigating the matter (or material body) of persons to see how they respond to different types of training can lead to important findings, but it is insufficient. In order to determine the best training program, taking a reductive account of the training responses of bodies is insufficient. Although it tells us important information, we need to remember that people's experiences matter, too. The best training program is based on the individual's needs and values. A holistic interpretation of a person requires us to take seriously all aspects of a person's experience. Although there might be things we can rule out (e.g., because they are unsafe) or rule in (e.g., the need to achieve a minimum fitness level) across the board, the specifics of how to engage people in physical activity requires that we know who they are and who they want to become.

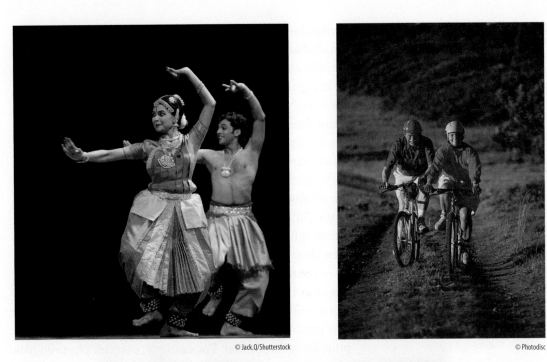

© Jack.Q/Shutterstock   © Photodisc

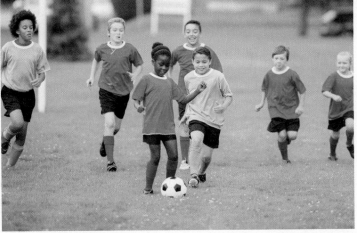

© iStock.com/ Christopher Futcher

THE PARTS OF KINESIOLOGY ARE CRITICAL TO THE WHOLE

This leads us to the importance of taking a holistic approach to the field of kinesiology. As you progress through your major, you will likely take specific classes in subdisciplines such as exercise physiology, motor learning,

- Review your campus and/ or community newspaper over the course of a few weeks. How often are references made to different forms of physical activity?

- What topics received the most attention?

- What forms of physical activity did not receive adequate coverage?

- In your view, how does this media coverage influence how people think about physical activity?

- Does media coverage generally make the work of kinesiology professionals easier or more difficult?

biomechanics, and sport psychology. It is important to remember that the insight and knowledge that these subdisciplines bring to our understanding of physical activity are interconnected. If we are serious about promoting meaningful physical activity experiences and we understand those experiences holistically, then we cannot help but recognize that subdisciplines are mutually informing. As an example, consider a basic physical activity experience such as running. There are lessons to be learned from all the subdisciplines. People do not need to know about any of the subdisciplines to experience running or experience meaningful running, but if they are curious or interested, then they could turn to any or all of the subdisciplines to learn more and deepen their experience. As professionals, it is important for us to have some sense of how the subdisciplines are interrelated. As we deepen our own knowledge, it is important to recognize ways in which one subdiscipline informs another. For example, exercise physiologists often say that fitness should be fun. Unfortunately, how they operationalize fun often does not hold for everyone. Exercise, such as running on a treadmill, may never be fun for some people. Thus, many trainers are at a loss to figure out how to make it fun. Physical educators can help people develop skills in activities that meet demands for fitness but that are also fun. Sport philosophers can help define concepts that allow us to better understand how physical activity is personally meaningful. But exercise physiologists can also inform sport philosophy. When developing ethical arguments relating to the fairness of a Paralympic athlete using a prosthetic device to compete in the Olympics, it is necessary to understand the physiological and biomechanical aspects of the issue. Are the physiological attributes of the Paralympic athlete equivalent to the other runners? Do the mechanisms of the prosthetic device enable the Paralympic runner to achieve similar results by doing more or less work? Exercise physiologists and biomechanists must answer these questions, and their answers should inform the sport philosophers' analysis. On your own, as you read this text, you should identify ways in which the subdisciplines are mutually informing and interconnected.

A commitment to a holistic approach in kinesiology begins with recognizing the importance of people's experience of physical activity. In large part, our good (and sometimes bad) experiences are what made us want to be involved in a profession that focuses on forms of movement. We recognize how our physical activity experiences can make our lives more meaningful and want to help others

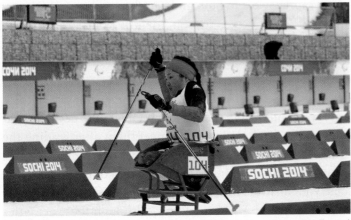

© Martynova Anna/Shutterstock

experience that same enthusiasm for physical activity. Based on the holistic approach to physical activity, we now recognize how we should assume a holistic approach to persons and the field of kinesiology. In doing so, we best prepare ourselves to utilize the insight and knowledge of kinesiology to help others achieve their goals and experience meaningful forms of physical activity.

STOP AND THINK

Coach A thinks the main function of a coach is to get the players physically ready to play at the highest level possible. Coach B thinks the main function of a coach is to get the players holistically ready (as individuals and as a team) to play at the highest level possible.

- Identify all the differences between Coach A and Coach B in regards to their coaching philosophy. How would their different approaches and beliefs shape their coaching decisions?
- Identify the differences between coaching practices between Coach A and Coach B.
- How might they structure their day-by-day interactions with athletes differently?
- What are the strengths and weaknesses of their different approaches?

Implementing the Approaches

It is one thing to know what the three different approaches are. It is quite another thing to adopt these approaches as guiding principles and implement them in academic preparation. So as you get started on your journey in this introduction to the field, make sure to practice these approaches on a regular basis. Once you incorporate these approaches into your daily study habits, your initial hard work will pay off by making future hard work easier and more manageable. So how can you implement these strategies?

You can develop your competency skills in a number of different ways through your use of this text. You can set aside time to actively **focus** on both the content and the activities in each chapter. You can do assigned readings and activities before class so that you are **prepared** to actively engage in classroom discussions. You can develop your communication and **interpersonal skills** by discussing your answers to Stop and Think activities and Discussion Questions with other students. You can identify your strengths and weaknesses in regards to competency and professionalism (see Table 2-1) and take time to improve upon your weaknesses now in order to be better prepared for advanced classes.

You can develop your learner-centered skills by engaging in features that are part of every chapter. Note the Learning Objectives at the beginning of each chapter and check that you can meet them after reading the chapter. Take time to understand the bold key terms in your own words. Use the Discussion Questions to think more about the course content and take time to discuss your answers with other students. Most important, take time to complete the Stop and Think activities. Although these activities vary, they all have several things in common. First, they prevent you from being a passive reader by asking you to actively engage the chapter content. Second, they challenge you to think about the content in ways that deepen your comprehension and promote your ability to apply that content in different settings. Most important, they promote learning strategies that are learner centered, because ultimately you are responsible for engaging with and completing the Stop and Think activities. If you find some Stop and Think activities particularly helpful, you can modify them for the content of other chapters or implement them in other classes. For example, a chapter does not need to have a Stop and Think activity that asks you to locate a research article focused on its content. You can take the initiative to find a research article related to the main content of each and every chapter. This activity can serve to deepen your understanding of the field of kinesiology. Another learner-centered approach you could adopt is to look for additional academic and educational resources that inform the course content. For example, the website "The Science of Sport" (*sportsscientists.com*) is a good example of a resource that applies

focus
Directing sustained attention toward an area of interest.

prepared
Making an organized effort to skillfully or knowledgably engage in an activity.

interpersonal skills
The ability to effectively relate to and communicate with other people in a given context.

"sports science concepts and insights to the sports news you see every day, and to the training and performance challenges you face." Finding and reviewing resources like these not only improves your research skills, but also informs you about different ways that the course content can be put to practical use. You are not only learning new information, but also new applications of that information.

You can develop a holistic approach by thinking seriously about how the multiple subdisciplines inform each other. Every chapter on the subdisciplines identifies several ways that a particular subdiscipline relates to other subdisciplines. Every Case Study not only discusses an issue central to the field of kinesiology, but also demonstrates how a holistic approach is the best strategy for addressing that issue. Many of the Stop and Think

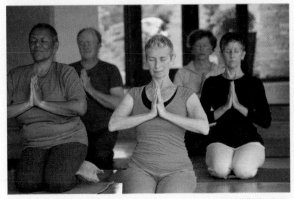

© Olivia Drew/National Geographic/age fotostock

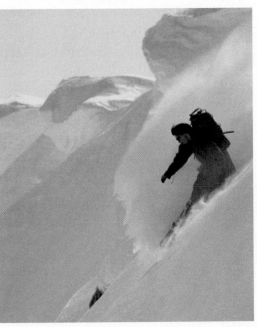

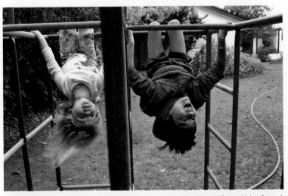

© Ariel Skelley/Getty Images

© Photodisc

activities and Discussion Questions challenge you to holistically integrate your knowledge. Although you will likely specialize or focus on a few subdisciplines by your senior year, it is important to remember and value how the subdisciplines are mutually informing. Potential solutions to difficult issues facing the field of kinesiology may actually require an integrated, holistic approach rather than a limited, specialist approach. Ultimately, if we have a deep respect and love for physical activity, then we should have a corresponding respect and admiration for the contributions that each subdiscipline provides to a comprehensive understanding of kinesiology.

CHAPTER SUMMARY

We used four guiding principles in writing this text. First, we sought to be mentors in your development as kinesiology students. Second, we sought to provide rigorous standards so that you are prepared for your future academic work. Third, we sought to share our love for physical activity and the field of kinesiology. Finally, we sought to use a shared voice that is personal yet professional in conveying the above principles and the necessary content for an introduction to the field of kinesiology.

We also had three guiding principles for you as readers. First, that you develop professional competency skills. Second, that you practice learner-centered strategies. Third, that you adopt a holistic understanding of the field of kinesiology.

The popularity of kinesiology as a major was described, and the growing numbers in the field provide the justification for a competency approach. Developing competency skills and qualities are essential for career success and finding fulfillment in your personal and professional dealings with kinesiology.

The essential qualities of a learning-centered approach were presented. The special responsibilities and powers of students in promoting a learning-centered environment were also described.

What it means to approach kinesiology in a holistic manner and how this differs from dualistic approaches was discussed. The importance of each element of kinesiology was emphasized, as well as how the integration of these elements enables kinesiology professionals to serve students and clients in the most effective manner possible.

Finally, strategies for implementing each of these approaches were explained. Actively engaging with the activities in the text has benefits not only for this course, but also for establishing the skills, strategies, habits, and perspectives that will lead to success in your academic pursuits.

DISCUSSION QUESTIONS

1. What professional traits and competency skills are necessary for success given your career ambitions? What traits and skills do you already possess? What traits and skills do you need to develop? Identify the benefits of possessing certain traits and skills. Identify the liabilities of not possessing certain traits and skills.

2. What learner-centered strategies do you already utilize? What steps can you take to improve your learner-centered approach? Compare and contrast a student who adopts a learner-centered approach with a student who does not.

3. Does a holistic approach to kinesiology make sense to you? Is it difficult to comprehend? Explain how it can make a difference in a professional setting when addressing a particular problem in the field of kinesiology.

4. What steps will you take to incorporating these approaches? Can you see them becoming guiding principles beyond this course? Are you concerned about your ability to implement these approaches?

REFERENCES

American Kinesiology Association. (2013, June). Kinesiology Institution Database. Retrieved from http://www.americankinesiology.org/kinesiology-institution-database

American Kinesiology Association. (n.d.). Position statement #1: Kinesiology on the move: One of the fastest growing (but often misunderstood) majors in academia. Retrieved from http://www.americankinesiology.org/white-papers/white-papers/kinesiology-on-the-move–one-of-the-fastest-growing-but-often-misunderstood-majors-in-academia

Blumberg, P. (2004). Beginning journey toward a culture of learning-centered teaching. *Journal of Student Centered Learning*, 2(1), 68–80.

The California State University. (2016). Facts about the CSU. Retrieved from http://www.calstate.edu/csufacts/2016Facts/

The California State University. (2013). Infocenter: Quick facts. Retrieved from http://www.calstate.edu/datastore/quick_facts.shtml?source=homepage

Huba, J. E., & Freed, M. E. (2000). *Learner-centered assessment on college campuses*. Boston: Allyn & Bacon.

Millennial Branding. (2012, May). Millennial Branding and Experience Inc. study reveals an employment gap between employers and students. Retrieved from http://millennialbranding.com/2012/millennial-branding-student-employment-gap-study/

York College of Pennsylvania. (2013, January). 2013 National Professionalism Survey: Workplace report. Retrieved from http://www.ycp.edu/media/york-website/cpe/York-College-Professionalism-in-the-Workplace-Study-2013.pdf

Weimer, M. (2002). *Learner-centered teaching: Five key changes to practice*. San Francisco: Jossey-Bass.

CHAPTER 3

A History of Kinesiology

JAIME SCHULTZ

LEARNING OBJECTIVES

1. Understand the importance of context in understanding historical change.
2. Describe the difference between physical education as a profession and physical education as a discipline.
3. Explain why departments of physical education became departments of kinesiology.
4. Recognize the importance of integrating kinesiology's subdisciplines.

KEY TERMS

academic discipline
disciplinary specialization
embryonic period

kinesiology
profession of physical education

Introduction

What we call ourselves matters. The discipline we know today as kinesiology has gone through several different names, and with each change came debate, contention, and a particular emphasis that gives the field its current meaning. We are now well into the second century of kinesiology's many evolutions, and a brief historical analysis is important to understanding where we came from, who we were, who we are, and where we might be going.

To appreciate the history of kinesiology requires recognizing its key precursor—physical education. In this case, physical education does not refer to the classes you took in elementary or high school, or even the skill or lifestyle classes you may take in college. Instead, it represents academic departments of physical education in higher education, many of which are now called departments of kinesiology. These are units dedicated to creating and sharing knowledge about physical activity and human movement, and as you will find in this chapter, these departments now include a variety of subdisciplines—specialized domains of study within the broader subject.

The Embryonic Period: 1880s–1900s

embryonic period
The first stage of the development of kinesiology (1880–1900) in the United States.

Sport studies scholar Joan Paul (1996) classifies the era between 1880 and 1900 as the **embryonic period** for physical education. In other words, the field was in the very beginning stages of development. During this time, advocates recognized the value of activities such as gymnastics (which then referred to a series of precise and regimented exercises), calisthenics, physical culture, and physical training to encourage health and physical fitness. However, physical education did not have a central mission, and multiple, competing philosophies and exercise systems created a lack of organization and coherence.

What encouraged the need for formalized physical education? Historical understanding requires situating the phenomenon in question within its historical context. It is important to ask what the larger social, cultural, political, and economic issues were at the time, how those issues affected physical education and, in turn, how physical education influenced those historical circumstances. For example, the modernization and industrialization of society in the 19th century reduced the amount of physical activity required in the average American's day. Activists therefore worried about the lack of "vigor" in people's lives, and promoted exercise as the antidote to a "soft" life. At the same time, lingering concerns about military preparedness resulted in the establishment of physical training programs. And with the large increase in immigration during this time, reformers turned to sport and physical activity to address their anxieties about health, assimilation, and Americanization. Thus, physical education developed within the context of great historical change and was designed to meet numerous social needs.

In the 1880s and 1890s, most programs aimed at training physical educators were located in private normal (or teachers') colleges. Instructors of these programs were often physicians, illustrating the close ties between the field and medicine and the biological sciences. Accordingly, the curriculum included aspects of anatomy and physiology, physics, and anthropometry (the scientific study of the measurements and proportions of the human body), as well as educational theory.

Physicians made up the majority of the first members of the Association for the Advancement of Physical Education, established in 1885 as a way to begin to institutionalize and legitimize the area of study. The following year, the organization (which had changed its name to the American Association for the Advancement of Physical Education, or AAAPE; see **TABLE 3-1** for a series of name changes that offer historical insight) published the *American Physical Education Review* (now the *Research Quarterly for Exercise and Sport*), a journal that disseminated and encouraged professional knowledge. At the 1890 AAAPE conference, physician Luther Halsey Gulick declared physical education a "new profession" that involved "a profound knowledge

TABLE 3-1 The Evolution of SHAPE America

1885	Association for the Advancement of Physical Education
1886	American Association for the Advancement of Physical Education
1903	American Physical Education Association
1937	American Association for Health and Physical Education
1938	American Association for Health and Physical Education and Recreation
1974	American Alliance for Health, Physical Education and Recreation
1979	American Alliance for Health, Physical Education, Recreation and Dance
2013	Society of Health and Physical Educators (SHAPE) America

of man [*sic*] through physiology, anatomy, psychology, history and philosophy" (p. 65). Although many think that the subdisciplinary movement of kinesiology is something that originated in the mid-20th century, it is clear that it has deeper roots (Park, 1989).

The Profession of Physical Education: 1900–1960

In the early 1900s, physical education also included elements of nutrition and hygiene, which originally signified elements of exercise, but later aligned more with what we think of today as health education. Before long, however, physical educators began to emphasize the value of play, games, and sport, leaving behind the gymnastic tradition. This happened in both men's and women's programs, which were almost always separate from one another.

Men's intercollegiate sport grew evermore popular during this time, and physical education programs extended their training to the preparation of coaches. After a brief period of intercollegiate sport for women, the majority of women physical educators advocated intramural and interclass athletics and, more often, dance, instruction in posture, hygiene, and "play days." These activities were supposed to promote cooperation, instead of the type of competition that would damage participants' bodies and minds. The "play attitude" promoted the "ideal of universal opportunity for participation in athletic activities" (Sefton, 1941, pp. 7–8). In this way, physical educators kept tight control over the development of women's sport, a situation that lasted throughout much of the 20th century.

Initially, many programs, for both men and women, operated under the name "physical culture," but in the late 1920s and early 1930s, the term **physical education** became the dominant title for the field. Most faculty "did not carry active programs of research in any area of specialization," but instead focused on teaching and advising their students (Massengale & Swanson, 1997, p. 7). Education "was dedicated to acquiring motor skills and methods of teaching these skills, planning curriculum, and the organization and administration of programs in athletics, health, and recreation as well as physical education" (Corbin, 1993, p. 84).

Times of war offer occasions to assess the physical fitness of the nation and often highlight the importance of physical education. This happened during World War I, when military officials rejected an alarming number of young men drafted into service due to "lack of fitness." As a result, many

profession of physical education
The second stage of the development of kinesiology that occurred in the 1920s and 1930s, when *physical education* became the dominant title for the field.

states enacted mandatory physical education instruction in public schools, which, in turn, created a need for trained and qualified teachers.

It happened again during World War II, when physical assessments deemed many potential draftees unfit to serve. Events in the postwar era also pointed to the need to bolster national health. The 1953 Kraus-Weber tests demonstrated that American youth were less fit than their European counterparts. President Dwight D. Eisenhower suffered a heart attack, which directed greater attention to the benefits of exercise for both health and rehabilitation. For these and other reasons, in 1956 President Eisenhower initiated the President's Council on Youth Fitness (now the President's Council on Physical Fitness, Sports, and Nutrition—once again, what we call ourselves matters). This high-profile, government-sanctioned program boosted the profession of physical education.

The end of World War II marked the beginning of Cold War hostilities between the United States and the Soviet Union. In the absence of "hot war" (or actual fighting), political and ideological tensions spilled over into symbolic arenas in which the two sides could compete for dominance. Sport was one such arena. In fact, the Cold War helped convince women physical educators and others to revise their views on women's sport and begin to promote elite-level training and competition. During this same time, administrators of high-profile men's athletic programs began to move into separate units and away from their historical homes within physical education. As coaches left physical education, it became possible for administrators to hire faculty dedicated to teaching and research.

Like sport, scientific innovation provided another place where Cold War opponents could compete. In 1957, the Soviets successfully launched Sputnik 1, the first artificial satellite, sparking a great deal of concern about the status of science education in the United States. This affected physical education and incited calls to "scientize" the field.

Physical educators added their voices to these calls. Some of this impulse came on the heels of James Conant's 1963 book, *The Education of American Teachers*. Conant, the former president of Harvard University, was critical,

STOP AND THINK

- What do you know about the 1980 "Miracle on Ice"? As dramatized in the 2004 film *Miracle*, the U.S. men's Olympic hockey team defeated the heavily favored team from the Soviet Union, which had won six of the seven previous games. What was the historical importance of this event?

- This movie was produced by Walt Disney Pictures. Why did this story grab Disney's attention? It was a game to get to the medal round, not the final showdown for the gold medal.

- Can you think of other examples where the politics of different groups or countries play out on sport's symbolic stage?

writing, "I am far from impressed by what I have heard and read about graduate work in the field of physical educations … To my mind, a university should cancel graduate programs in this area" (p. 201). As you might imagine, this alarmed physical educators, who already felt as though their work did not receive academic respect (see Twietmeyer, 2012).

The year after Conant published *The Education of American Teachers,* Franklin Henry, a professor at the University of California at Berkeley, pushed the idea that physical education should be an **academic discipline**, or a branch of knowledge designed to produce and disseminate expert knowledge, as opposed to a program that trained future physical educators and coaches for a *profession*. Henry (1964) claimed "that the proper academic study for physical education would only come by grounding the discipline in theory." He continued:

academic discipline
A branch of knowledge designed to produce and disseminate expert knowledge.

An academic discipline is an organized body of knowledge collectively embraced in a formal course of learning. The acquisition of such knowledge is assumed to be an adequate and worthy objective as such, without any demonstration or requirement of practical application. The content is theoretical and scholarly as distinguished from technical and professional. (p. 32)

Henry defined the "scholarly field" of physical education as one that includes "anatomy, physics and physiology, cultural anthropology, history and sociology, as well as psychology" (p. 33). No matter the students' career goals, he argued, they should be educated in these areas that would provide a broad-based understanding of human physical activity.

STOP AND THINK

- What are the "core," or required, courses in the department of kinesiology at your school?

- Why do you think you have to take these courses?

- What do they contribute to your understanding of human movement and physical activity?

The Academic Discipline of Physical Education: 1960–1980

In the early 1960s, prodded by the words of Conant and Henry, members of the American Academy of Physical Education sought to determine what should constitute the discipline's "body of knowledge." The subsequent Big Ten Body-of-Knowledge Symposium identified six areas of specialization:

(1) administrative theory in athletics and physical education, (2) biomechanics, (3) exercise physiology, (4) history and philosophy of physical education, (5) motor learning/sport psychology, and (6) sociology and sport education. These subdomains, along with several others, are currently recognized within kinesiology.

Consequently, the 1960s and the 1970s fostered specialization within physical education (**TABLE 3-2**). Members of the various subgroups formed their own organizations, journals, texts, and specialized courses within the major. With this trend came greater respect for the field and the production of new knowledge, but "disciplinization" also had some negative consequences. First, the move devalued the importance of physical education as it pertained to the preparation of teachers and coaches—suggesting that practitioners of physical education were somehow worth less than those who researched it.

Second, **disciplinary specialization** brought fragmentation, such that the subdomains too often acted independently, rather than in concert. Instead of integrating their knowledge for a more holistic understanding of human movement, scholars became isolated from one another. This lack of integration and unification troubled physical educators, who worried that students would fail to appreciate and, more important, assimilate the depth and

disciplinary specialization
The fragmenting of the components of a discipline into multiple subdomains.

TABLE 3-2   The Evolution of Subdisciplinary Organizations

1953	American College of Sport Medicine
1967	International Society of Biomechanics in Sports
1968	North American Society for the Psychology of Sport and Physical Activity
1972	North American Society for Sport History
1972	Philosophic Society for the Study of Sport
1973	International Society of Biomechanics
1974	The Association for the Study of Play
1978	North American Society for the Sociology of Sport
1983	Sport Literature Association
1985	North American Society for Sport Management
1985	Association for the Advancement of Applied Sport Psychology

breadth of information in their respective programs. They also worried that researchers in the subdisciplines could just as easily belong in departments of physiology, physics, biology, history, sociology, philosophy, and psychology as they could in physical education, which might, in turn, render departments of physical education obsolete in the eyes of campus administrators.

The number of programs dedicated to teacher training, often called *pedagogy*, started to decline. Some departments even eliminated the programs altogether. In time, "physical education" no longer seemed an appropriate title for the discipline. One by one, different units began to change their names, becoming departments of exercise science, sport science, sport studies, human movement, human kinetics, and kinesiology, to name a few.

In the 1980s, colleges and universities used as many as 100 different names for the area of study once known as physical education (Corbin, 1993, p. 85). By 1990, wrote Karl Newell, it was not "an overstatement to suggest that physical education in higher education is in a state of chaos" (1990a, p. 228). One way to remedy this, Newell (1989) argued, was to bring everyone together under the umbrella of *kinesiology*. He offered the following rationale for this name:

- It was representative of the entire field.
- It sounded academic.
- It was succinct.
- It was neutral with respect to the major subdomain debates on each dimension.
- It was already established as the departmental title in a number of leading academic institutions.

Not everyone has agreed with the wholesale change to kinesiology, and several departments have resisted the trend.

As we consider the subdisciplinary movement, it is important to understand that kinesiology not only *has* a history—it also *includes* history. Sport history is an important subdiscipline that emerged in the late 1960s and

STOP AND THINK

- What comes to mind when you think of the term *physical education*?

- What are the stereotypes associated with someone who studies physical education? Are they different for men and women?

- Where do you think those stereotypes came from?

early 1970s. Sport historians consider a range of fascinating topics, including organized athletics, physical education, physical culture, active leisure, dance, recreation, and other physical practices. Historians look at these topics as they relate to technology, media, education, religion, the military, race, ethnicity, class, sex, gender, sexuality, disability, popular culture, politics, the environment, public policy, geography, and ideas about the body. In the United States and Canada, the North American Society for Sport History has been the most important organization for work in this area, although sport historians are often involved with other organizations in kinesiology, sport studies, history, American studies, women's and gender studies, and popular culture.

Kinesiology as a Unifying Title: 1990–Present

The word **kinesiology** can be broken down into the Greek words *kinesis*, which means "movement," and *ology*, or "the study of." Newell was certainly not the first to suggest the word. Within physical education, it has been used since at least 1886 (Paul, 1996, p. 534). However, the 1990s brought a concerted quest for a common professional identity and, according to Newell (1990b), "*kinesiology* provides the best option in promoting a broad-based disciplinary, professional, and performance approach to the study of physical activity" (p. 273). Debates about the title and focus of kinesiology continue to rage. Some critics contend that the word is too esoteric for the general population. Others find the term's focus too narrow, aligned more with structural–functional research, particularly biomechanics, and divorced from practical application. Still others contend that guiding concepts, such as "movement" and "physical activity," are too broad and will lead (indeed, have led) to topics of study that deviate far afield from the field's roots in physical education. We continue to question what areas should constitute our collective body of knowledge.

STOP AND THINK

Take a look at the top sports stories of today. These stories have a history. Maybe it is a story about doping in sport.

- When did athletes first start using performance-enhancing drugs?

- What types of drugs did they use?

- How have methods to test for those drugs changed over time?

Maybe you find a story about a top woman athlete. Did you know that organized sport for women did not really gain popularity and acceptance until the 1970s? A historical perspective helps us understand contemporary issues.

- Why did it take so long for organized sport for women to gain acceptance?

- What were the reasons for keeping women out of sport?

---

kinesiology
The study of the art and science of human movement.

TABLE 3-3   The Evolution of the National Academy of Kinesiology

1904	Academy of Physical Education
1926	American Academy of Physical Education
1993	American Academy of Kinesiology and Physical Education
2010	National Academy of Kinesiology

However, kinesiology is frequently, though not entirely, the overriding title for the many things we do, study, and promote. If you take a look at **TABLE 3-3**, for example, you can see that what was once the American Academy of Physical Education gradually added "kinesiology" to its title and eventually dropped the phrase "physical education" altogether to become the National Academy of Kinesiology (NAK). The organization's dual purpose is

> to encourage and promote the study and educational applications of the art and science of human movement and physical activity and to honor by election to its membership persons who have directly or indirectly contributed significantly to the study of and/or application of the art and science of human movement and physical activity (NAK, 2016).

Embedded in this description is an appreciation of the field as both a profession and a discipline.

It bears mention that the need for unity also extends to work done within departments of kinesiology—not just among them. Kinesiology is composed of many subdisciplines; it is therefore *multidisciplinary.* But multi- and even cross-disciplinarity falls short, argues Gill (2007): "*Inter-*disciplinary implies actual connections among subareas, and an interdisciplinary kinesiology that integrates subdisciplinary knowledge is essential" (p. 275). As you move forward in your studies, your challenge is to start to see the many ways that kinesiology's subdisciplines inform one another—to see cross-disciplinary and interdisciplinary connections. Your ultimate goal is to take an integrative perspective to consider the many ways that knowledge from each area informs, enhances, and complements your understanding of human movement.

CHAPTER SUMMARY

From its humble beginnings in the 19th century, the field we know today as kinesiology has gone through many changes. From unorganized efforts to provide health and fitness opportunities for children, to the profession and eventual discipline of physical education, to the move toward kinesiology, physical activity and human movement have remained our core concerns. Kinesiology includes subdisciplines from the natural sciences, social sciences, and humanities, all of which help us understand how, when, and why people move.

DISCUSSION QUESTIONS

1. Kinesiology has not always been called kinesiology. What was the field called in the late 1800s and early 1900s?
2. During physical education's "embryonic period" (1880s–1900s), what were some of the larger social, cultural, political, and economic issues that encouraged the need for formalized physical education?
3. How did physical educators feel about intercollegiate sports for women in the first half of the 20th century?
4. How did the various wars in the 20th century influence physical education?
5. Do you think physical education is a discipline or a profession? Is there a difference between a discipline and a profession?
6. What are the positive and negative aspects of specialization and disciplinization?
7. Do you think *kinesiology* is the best name for your department?
8. What is the difference between multidisciplinary and subdisciplinary?

REFERENCES

Conant, J. B. (1963). *The education of American teachers*. New York: McGraw-Hill.

Corbin, C. B. (1993). The field of physical education: Common goals, not common roles. *Journal of Physical Education, Recreation and Dance*, 6(1), 79, 84–87.

Gill, D. L. (2007). Integration: The key to sustaining kinesiology in higher education. *Quest*, 59(3), 270–286.

Gulick, L. H. (1890). Physical education: A new profession. In *Proceedings of 5th Annual Meeting of the American Association for the Advancement of Physical Education* (pp. 59–66). Ithaca, NY: Andrus & Church.

Henry, F. (1964). Physical education: An academic discipline. *Journal of Health, Physical Education, and Recreation*, 35(7), 32–33.

Massengale, J. D., & Swanson, R. A. (1997). *The history of exercise and sport science*. Champaign, IL: Human Kinetics.

National Academy of Kinesiology (NAK). (2016). *AKA*. Retrieved 23 September 2016, from http://www.americankinesiology.org/affiliated-associations/affiliated-associations/american-academy-of-kinesiology-and-physical-education-aakpe

Newell, K. M. (1989). Kinesiology. *Journal of Physical Education, Recreation and Dance*, 60(8), 69–70.

Newell, K. M. (1990a). Physical education in higher education: Chaos out of order. *Quest*, 42, 227–242.

Newell, K. M. (1990b). Kinesiology: The label for the study of physical activity in higher education. *Quest*, 42, 269–278.

Park, R. J. (1989). The second 100 years: Or, can physical education become the renaissance field of the 21st century? *Quest*, 41, 1–27.

Paul, J. (1996). Centuries of change: Movement's many faces. *Quest*, 48(4), 531–545.

Sefton, A. A. (1941). *The Women's Division, National Amateur Athletic Federation*. Palo Alto, CA: Stanford University Press.

Twietmeyer, G. (2012). What is kinesiology? Historical and philosophical insights. *Quest*, 64(4), 4–23.

PART II

Pillars of the Discipline:
Kinesiology Subdisciplines

CHAPTER 4

Biomechanics

SEAN P. FLANAGAN, SHAYNA L. KILPATRICK,
AND WILLIAM C. WHITING

LEARNING OBJECTIVES

1. Define the following terms: *biomechanics*, *kinematics*, *kinetics*, *mechanics*, *force*, *torque*, *work*, and *energy*.

2. Explain why you should study biomechanics.

3. Explain how understanding biomechanics can assist in improving performance and decreasing injury risk.

4. Describe the three sets of principles that are used in biomechanics.

5. Distinguish between a propulsive force and a braking force.

6. Explain how you can increase or decrease torque.

7. Explain the work–energy principle.

8. Differentiate between a flexion/extension pattern and a swing/whip pattern, and specify when you would use each.

9. Describe scenarios where you would use a proximal-to-distal sequence and scenarios where you would use a distal-to-proximal sequence.

10. Discuss the three different actions and four different functions of the muscle–tendon complex.

This chapter was adapted from the text *Biomechanics: A Case-Based Approach*, also published by Jones & Bartlett Learning.

11. Describe the factors involved in producing muscle force.

12. Explain the steps in implementing a program to improve performance or reduce injury risk.

KEY TERMS

biomechanics
body
braking force
classical mechanics
clinical biomechanics
concentric action
dynamics
eccentric action
energy
extension pattern
flexion pattern
force
forensic biomechanics
impairment
in silico
in vitro
in vivo

isometric action
kinematics
kinetic energy
kinetics
mechanopathology
muscle–tendon complex
occupational biomechanics
pathomechanics
potential energy
propulsive force
sport and exercise biomechanics
statics
stretch-shortening cycle (SSC)
swing pattern
torque
whip pattern
work

What Is Biomechanics?

In the 1999 Warner Brothers movie *The Matrix*, Neo (played by Keanu Reeves) learns from Morpheus (played by Laurence Fishburne) that he has been living in a sort of virtual reality of computer-generated code. While in the Matrix, Morpheus is capable of doing incredible things, and he tells Neo that he can, too, as long as he understands the rules under which the Matrix operates (**FIGURE 4-1**): "What you must learn is that these rules are no different than the rules of a computer system. Some of them can be bent, others broken."

Although we do not live in a virtual reality programmed by machines (at least we do not think we do), we do live in a world that is governed by rules. And while we may not be able to bend or break these rules, we are

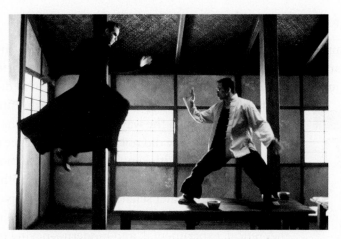

FIGURE 4-1   Neo is capable of doing incredible things once he understands the rules of the Matrix.

© Moviestore Collection LTD/Alamy

capable of doing some pretty amazing things with our bodies if we understand them. **Biomechanics** is a branch of science that looks to discover these rules by applying the methods of mechanics to the study of the structure and function of biological systems (Hatze, 1974).

As you may have guessed from the definition, biomechanics is a pretty broad field that includes analyses of all living things: humans, animals, and plants. In this chapter, we will limit our discussion to the human body and the application of biomechanics to four main areas:

- **Sport and exercise biomechanics**: Examination of the cause-and-effect mechanisms of sport movements and exercises.
- **Occupational biomechanics**: Examination of the interactions of workers with their tools, machines, and materials.
- **Forensic biomechanics**: Examination of accidents and failures.
- **Clinical biomechanics**: Examination of the causes of musculoskeletal disorders and evaluation of various treatment methods.

In all cases, the principles are the same, and they are extensions of physics and engineering. The desire to uncover these principles, and understand how we move, is nearly as old as man.

biomechanics
The application of the methods of mechanics to the study of the structure and function of biological systems.

sport and exercise biomechanics
Examination of the cause-and-effect mechanisms of sport movements and exercises.

occupational biomechanics
Examination of the interactions of workers with their tools, machines, and materials.

forensic biomechanics
Examination of accidents and failures.

clinical biomechanics
Examination of the causes of musculoskeletal disorders and evaluation of various treatment methods.

A Brief History of Biomechanics

The complete history of biomechanics is a long one, starting in ancient Greece and extending to the present day, but our tour will be brief. Here, we will just introduce you to some of the major "players" who developed the field of biomechanics; that is, those who uncovered the rules that govern the way we move. Biomechanics as a specialized discipline did not come into existence until the middle part of the 20th century, but its foundations lie in anatomy, mathematics, physics, photography (both still and motion), and computer science. We will trace this development through four periods (Thurston, 1999)—anatomical, theoretical, experimental, and modern—paying tribute to certain individuals in each one.

STOP AND THINK

- Describe the study of biomechanics in your own words.

- Do you understand what is studied within the four areas of biomechanics? How are the areas similar? Different?

THE ANATOMICAL PERIOD

Much of the history of biomechanics is the history of science and mathematics. And it all started with the ancient Greeks. One Greek, in particular, stands out: Aristotle (384–322 B.C.). In 334 B.C., Aristotle authored *De Motu Animalium* (*On the Movement of Animals*), which is considered to be the first book on biomechanics ever written (Thurston, 1999). Although he was somewhat mistaken in his views of anatomy (later corrected by the anatomists mentioned below) and mechanics (later corrected by Galileo during the theoretical period), he made some astute observations about the way animals and people move. Some of these observations include that people have to push against the ground to move, will run faster if they swing their arms, jump further if they have weights in their hands, and have their heads moving up and down in a sinusoidal fashion (as opposed to a straight line) when they walk (Baker, 2007; Thurston, 1999).

Our early understanding of anatomy was due to those who took it upon themselves to dissect corpses in an effort to understand what was going on under the skin. Galen (129–200), Leonardo da Vinci (1452–1519), and Andreas Vesalius (1514–1564) are considered the pioneers in this area. da Vinci was also legendary for his ability to link structure and function; that is, anatomy to mechanics.

THE THEORETICAL PERIOD

The theoretical period is synonymous with the Scientific Revolution. Galileo Galilei (1564–1642) is considered the founder of the scientific method, upon which almost all science is currently based. His studies of mechanics are particularly noteworthy, because he used empirical evidence to discredit many of things Aristotle believed to be true based on observation, intuition, and reason alone. He also set the stage for Sir Isaac Newton (1642–1726), who uncovered the mechanical principles described later in this chapter and published them in his famous book, *Philosophiae Naturalis Principia Mathematica* (*Mathematical Principles of Natural Philosophy*). Known as *The Principia* for short, it was published in 1687. However, another man, Giovanni Alfonso Borelli (1608–1679), whose life overlapped those of both Galileo and Newton, is considered the father of biomechanics. A student of Galileo's, Borelli extended Galileo's methods to the study of biology (Pope, 2005). In his book, also titled *De Motu Animalium* (it must have been a popular title), Borelli equated animals with machines and used the concept of levers to analyze movement (Thurston, 1999). Published after his death, the book was written in two parts: The first part (published in 1680) dealt with external motions; the second part (published in 1861) examined internal motions (Pope, 2005). Due to the significance of Borelli's work, the American Society of Biomechanics's top award is named after him.

> **STOP AND THINK**
>
> Which of these "players" had the greatest impact on biomechanics by the end of the theoretical period? Explain.

THE EXPERIMENTAL PERIOD

The experimental period occurred during the 19th century and was characterized by the study of the human gait, particularly walking. The Weber brothers—Eduard (1806–1871), Ernst Heinrich (1795–1878), and Wilhelm (1804–1891)—are credited with making many observations about gait (published in 1894 by Wilhelm and Eduard as *The Mechanics of the Human Walking Apparatus*), including annotating the phases of stance and swing (Thurston, 1999). However, they were limited in their ability to measure many gait characteristics. Eadweard Muybridge (1830–1904) was one of the first to change that. Muybridge was able to set up cameras in such a way so that he was able to take serial photographs, thus beginning the technique of cinematography (Braun & Whitcombe, 1999; Thurston, 1999). Legend has it that he did this to settle a wager as to whether all four hooves of a horse are airborne at the same time while trotting (they are). His techniques were further refined by Etienne-Jules Marey (1830–1904), who had subjects dress in black garb with white markers, similar to techniques used in modern motion analysis with digital computers. Marey also developed the chronophotograph, where several images are captured on the same photo plate rather than on different plates with different cameras (Baker, 2007; Braun & Whitcombe, 1999). Wilhelm Braune (1831–1892) and Otto Fischer (1861–1917) extended Marey's techniques to include three-dimensional analyses and the forces that produced the movements that were being recorded during gait.

Although typically remembered for his work in motor control and neuroscience, Nikolai Bernstein (1896–1966) also made several contributions to the field of biomechanics. He used techniques similar to those of Braune and Fischer in his study of coordination, upon which many multisegment principles are based.

Although technically a physiologist, A. V. Hill (1886–1977) was a pioneer in muscle mechanics. Hill uncovered many of the biological principles discussed in the later sections of this chapter, and his "muscle model" is still used today by biomechanists modeling movement.

STOP AND THINK

Although improvements have been made since the experimental period, what techniques were invented during the period that are still in use today?

THE MODERN PERIOD

Beginning in the mid-20th century and with the advent of the modern computer, the field of biomechanics experienced tremendous growth. We will follow the lead of a past-president of the American Society of Biomechanics (Martin, 1999), and refrain from naming individuals who have made outstanding contributions to the discipline in the present day; there are just too many, and any list would be incomplete and fraught with the risk of offending those who would be inadvertently omitted. Rather, we would like to highlight the major organizations and publications that emerged in this period:

In 1968, the first issue of the *Journal of Biomechanics* was published.
In 1973, the International Society of Biomechanics was formed.
In 1977, the American Society of Biomechanics was formed.
In 1983, the International Society of Biomechanics in Sports adopted its first constitution.

In 1985, the first issue of the *International Journal of Sports Biomechanics* was published.

In 1986, the first issue of *Clinical Biomechanics* was published.

In 1991, the first issue of the *Journal of Electromyography and Kinesiology* was published.

In 1992, the *International Journal of Sports Biomechanics* changed its name to the *Journal of Applied Biomechanics*.

In 1993, the first issue of *Gait & Posture* was published.

In 2002, the first issue of *Sports Biomechanics* was published.

These are certainly not the only organizations and journals promoting and publishing biomechanics research. Organizations such as the American College of Sports Medicine (which publishes *Medicine & Science in Sports and Exercise* and *Exercise and Sport Sciences Reviews*), the American Orthopaedic Society for Sports Medicine (which publishes the *American Journal of Sports Medicine*), the American Physical Therapy Association (which publishes *Physical Therapy* and the *Journal of Orthopaedic and Sports Physical Therapy*), the Institute for Ergonomics and Human Factors (which publishes *Ergonomics*), the National Athletic Trainers' Association (which publishes the *Journal of Athletic Training*), and the National Strength and Conditioning Association (which publishes the *Journal of Strength and Conditioning Research*), are but a few of the organizations whose members specialize in biomechanics. This should give you an indication of the number of areas where knowledge of biomechanics—knowing the rules that govern the way we move—is being used to help people move better!

Why Study Biomechanics?

As you can see, the history of biomechanics is a quest to uncover the rules by which we move. Two questions should immediately come to mind:

1. Why should I study the rules of biomechanics?
2. Who needs to know these rules?

The answer to the first question is to help people move better. To be fair, many biomechanists study more than just people, and some do not necessarily study movement. However, the study of biomechanics to help someone move better is the focus of this chapter. And by move better, we mean to improve performance or reduce the risk of injury.

Performing better can have several different connotations, depending on the task. For example, you may wish to have someone jump higher or throw farther. These are obvious examples of improved performance. But you may also wish to help someone perform their job better, decrease the amount of energy necessary to walk across a room or up a flight of stairs, or simply be able accomplish a task such as buttoning a shirt or combing hair. Do not think that performance is limited to high-achieving athletic competitions. Performance occurs during any human activity, including those that are a part of everyday life.

A lot of human activities are inherently risky, and you will never be able to eliminate all injuries that can occur as a result of participating in a particular activity. But there are a lot of ways that you can decrease the *potential* for injury. For example, certain ways of moving can place loads on the body that it was not designed to handle (**mechanopathology**). Alternately, an injury or disease can change the way a person moves as he or she attempts to "work around" the condition (**pathomechanics**), placing inappropriate loads on different structures (and/or degrading performance). Additionally, environmental (e.g., a slippery floor) and other external factors (e.g., being hit by an opponent) can be potentially injurious.

In general, these two objectives—improving performance and decreasing injury risk—are achieved by either modifying a person's technique (the way he or she moves) or the equipment that is used as part of the activity (**FIGURE 4-2**). It stands to reason that if the way a person moves limits his or her performance or exposes the person to potentially injurious forces, then changing the way the person moves can improve his or her performance or decrease the risk of injury. Similarly, if environmental or external factors impede performance or increase the potential for injury, then equipment may help. As with performance, you should not use too narrow a definition for equipment. Biomechanists have certainly been involved in the design and modification of athletic equipment, such as helmets and ski poles, but they also study shoes and the characteristics of floors or machines in industrial settings. So consider performance and equipment in the broadest sense of the terms.

If the answer to the first question is that knowledge of biomechanics is used to help people move better, then the answer to second question should

---

mechanopathology
Mechanics that cause injury.

---

pathomechanics
Mechanics that are a result of an injury.

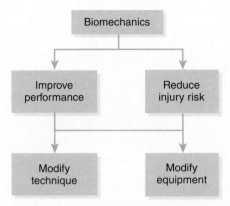

FIGURE 4-2 Biomechanics is used to improve performance or prevent injury by modifying either technique or performance.

S. P. Flanagan. (2014). *Biomechanics: A case-based approach.* Burlington, MA: Jones & Bartlett Learning.

be obvious: Anyone who is involved with the movement of people needs to understand the rules governing those movements. If you are (or are going to be) involved with teaching skills (e.g., a physical educator, personal trainer, dance instructor, or coach), preventing or rehabilitating from injury (e.g., an athletic trainer, physical therapist, chiropractor, or physician), designing equipment to be used by people (e.g., an ergonomist or engineer), or modifying the structure of the body (e.g., an orthopedic surgeon), then you need to study and understand biomechanics.

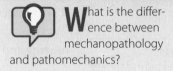

STOP AND THINK

What is the difference between mechanopathology and pathomechanics?

Major Principles of Biomechanics

Now that you understand why you should know the rules of human movement, you can begin to study them. The rules can be roughly grouped into three sets of principles: mechanical, multisegment, and biological (**FIGURE 4-3**; Lees, 2002).

MECHANICAL PRINCIPLES

Mechanical principles are derived from physics or, more specifically, classical mechanics. **Classical mechanics** is interested in the motion of bodies under the action of a system of forces, and basically deals with motion on

classical mechanics
The study of the motion of bodies under the action of a system of forces.

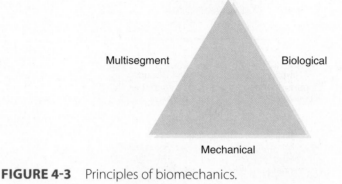

FIGURE 4-3   Principles of biomechanics.

S. P. Flanagan. (2014). *Biomechanics: A case-based approach*. Burlington, MA: Jones & Bartlett Learning.

a physical (size and speed) scale, involving everyday things that you can potentially see. It is called "classical" because it was developed from the work of Sir Isaac Newton and those who followed him, but it excludes such "modern" topics as quantum mechanics (which deals with physics on an extremely small size scale) and the work of Einstein and relativity (which deals with physics on an extremely fast speed scale). As a side note, in classical mechanics, a **body** is any collection of matter that you are examining. It is not necessarily synonymous with the human body.

Classical mechanics is usually divided into two areas: things that are moving and things that are not (**FIGURE 4-4**). **Dynamics** is the study of things

body
Any collection of matter that is being examined.

dynamics
The study of things that are moving.

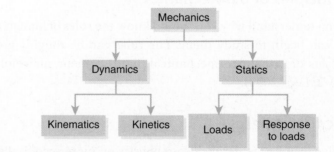

FIGURE 4-4   The areas of classical mechanics.

S. P. Flanagan. (2014). *Biomechanics: A case-based approach*. Burlington, MA: Jones & Bartlett Learning.

that are moving, and can be further broken down into kinematics and kinetics. **Kinematics** is the study of motion without consideration of the causes of that motion. In other words, kinematics measures the motion that you are examining. **Kinetics** examines the causes of that motion. **Statics** deals with loads on things that are not moving. Closely related to statics is *materials science*. Whereas statics deals with the loads applied to a body, materials science examines the material properties of that body and its response to a load. In biomechanics, materials science is often referred to as *tissue mechanics*.

The rules of classical mechanics revolve around the concept of force. A **force** is simply a push or pull by one body on another. A force will not always be in the direction of movement. It is useful to think of a **propulsive force** as one that is in the direction of movement and causes the body to speed up (or accelerate). In contrast, a **braking force** is in the direction opposite of the movement and causes the body to slow down (or decelerate). Think of a propulsive force as stepping on the gas and a braking force as stepping on the brakes when driving a car. Although there are several important rules that revolve around force, here we will only emphasize force's role in the production of torque and energy.

Torque is the turning effect of a force. It is sometimes called a *moment of force* (or *moment*, for short). Basic ideas about torque are exemplified by using a wrench to either tighten or loosen a nut on a bolt. To turn (rotate) the nut, you must apply a torque. The torque comes from applying a force (your hand) to a lever (the wrench) some distance from an axis of rotation (the bolt). But not just any force will do. Consider four forces, each equal in magnitude, applied to the wrench in different directions, as shown in **FIGURE 4-5**. From your everyday experience, you should be able to immediately recognize that the forces applied in Figure A and B will not turn the nut. The forces in Figure C and D will turn the nut, but in opposite directions.

What is the main difference between the forces in C and D compared to those in A and B? The forces in the latter two were applied parallel to the wrench, whereas the forces in the former were applied perpendicular to the wrench. The only forces (or components of forces) that create a torque are the ones that are perpendicular to the rigid body. If a force is applied at any angle other than perpendicular, the amount of torque it produces decreases: the further away from the perpendicular, the less amount of force. Forces parallel to the body end up producing zero torque. Additionally, the further away from the axis of rotation the force is applied (i.e., the longer the lever

kinematics
The study of motion without consideration of the cause of the motion.

kinetics
The study of the causes of motion (i.e., forces).

statics
The study of loads applied to a stationary body.

force
A push or pull by one body on another body.

propulsive force
A force that causes a body to speed up.

braking force
A force that causes a body to slow down.

torque
The turning effect of a force.

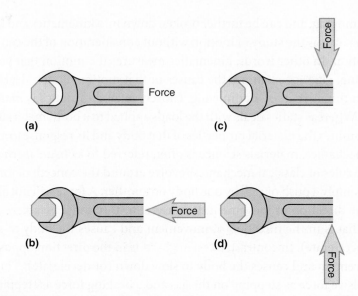

FIGURE 4-5   Each of the forces have the same magnitude, but different directions. The force in A and B will not produce torque. The force in C and D will produce torques in opposite directions.

S. P. Flanagan. (2014). *Biomechanics: A case-based approach.* Burlington, MA: Jones & Bartlett Learning.

arm), the larger the torque it will produce. Again, you should note this from your everyday experience. If the nut is stuck, you would grab a wrench with a longer handle (**FIGURE 4-6**). Door handles are placed at the outer edge of the door, not next to the hinges, so that the force applied to the handle maximizes the torque turning the door.

Although from a performance standpoint you would want to maximize the torque on an external object (such as the aforementioned nut or door), minimizing the torque an external object creates about your joints is an important consideration in injury prevention. Consider holding a package either close to your body or at arm's length (**FIGURE 4-7**). Even though the package weighs the same in both positions, holding the package at arm's length would create greater torque about the lumbar spine. Keeping external loads close to the trunk will decrease the stresses placed on the low back and help prevent injury.

Forces (and torques) are also involved with the exchange of energy. **Energy** is a state of matter that makes things change or has the potential to make things change (Watson, 2011). Note that energy is a *state* that

energy
The state of matter that makes things change or has the capacity to make things change.

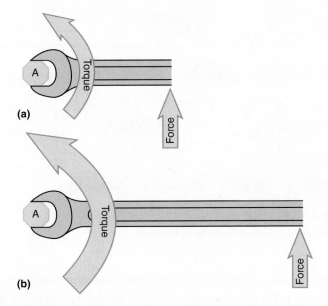

FIGURE 4-6   Torque is enhanced by increasing the length of the lever arm.

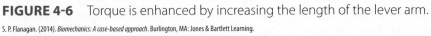

S. P. Flanagan. (2014). *Biomechanics: A case-based approach*. Burlington, MA: Jones & Bartlett Learning.

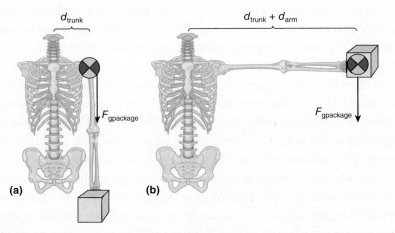

FIGURE 4-7   The external torque (A) when the package is held close to the body, and (B) when it is held at arm's length.

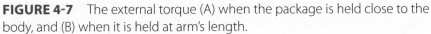

S. P. Flanagan. (2014). *Biomechanics: A case-based approach*. Burlington, MA: Jones & Bartlett Learning.

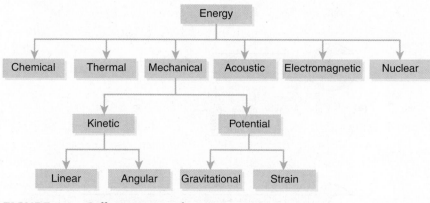

FIGURE 4-8 Different types of energy.

S. P. Flanagan. (2014). *Biomechanics: A case-based approach*. Burlington, MA: Jones & Bartlett Learning.

---

kinetic energy
The energy of motion.

potential energy
The energy of position.

work
The process by which energy is either added to or subtracted from a body.

---

characterizes a body or system. For a body or system to change, there needs to be energy. If there is no energy, the body or the system will not change. There are many different types of energy (for different types of changes): nuclear, chemical, electromagnetic, acoustic, and mechanical (**FIGURE 4-8**). The one that you are most interested in for biomechanics is mechanical energy (in physiology, you are probably more interested in chemical energy), because mechanical energy is needed to change the mechanics of a body or system, and that change could be in position, velocity, or shape. The two types of mechanical energy that we are interested in here are kinetic energy and potential energy. **Kinetic energy** is the energy that a body has because it is moving. If a body is moving, it is changing (position), and if it is changing, the body has to have energy. Gravitational **potential energy** is the potential an object has to change due to its position relative to the Earth. Think about a rock lying on the ground. Currently, it has no potential to change its position: It is just lying there. If you pick up the rock and hold it at shoulder height, it now has potential energy; if you let go of the rock, it will fall to the ground. The potential is there. All you have to do is release it.

The process of changing the amount of energy in the system is called mechanical work. **Work** is defined as a change in energy. In other words, work is changing (either increasing or decreasing) the amount of energy in the system. So whereas energy defines the *state* of a system, work is the *process* of moving energy into or out of that system. Work is equal to the product of force and displacement. Work is positive when the force and the displacement are in the same direction (a propulsive force). When work is positive, the energy of the system increases. Work is negative when the work and displacement are in opposite directions (a braking force). When work is negative, the energy of the system decreases. The energy of the system is transferred to objects outside of the system or lost to the environment as heat.

The work–energy concepts tell you that force has to be applied over a distance to be effective in changing energy, and a bigger change occurs if the either the magnitude of the force and/or the distance over which the force is applied increases. You are probably familiar with this idea already. Winding up before throwing increases the distance over which energy is generated, and consequently the ball is thrown farther. In much the same way, performing a countermovement (rapidly squatting down) prior to jumping increases the distance over which you can generate energy, leading to a higher jump. Assuming that you are already producing your maximum force (torque), the only way to increase energy is to increase the distance over which that force (torque) is applied.

How can you use this principle to decrease injury risk? You can decrease the amount of force for the same change in energy if you increase the distance over which that force is applied. If you have ever played the egg toss or water-balloon toss at a family picnic, you know that the egg (or balloon) will break if you stop it abruptly with your hand. To be successful, you have to "give" with it after impact, increasing the distance over which the braking force is applied. You would see the same thing in landing from a jump (**FIGURE 4-9**). Stiffer landings have a smaller distance over which the braking force is applied, and consequently subject your body to greater forces. Softer landings apply a smaller force over a longer distance.

MULTISEGMENT PRINCIPLES

If you have ever taken a high school physics class, you probably learned some basic principles of classical mechanics (such as Newton's laws of motion), or what we just referred to as the first set of rules. The second set of rules is a bit more complicated, but they are an extension of the first.

STOP AND THINK

- Name two mechanical principles, and apply them to familiar movements.

- Explain the difference between kinematics and kinetics.

- What are the two types of forces? List and describe each one in detail.

- Energy is a state that characterizes a body. Name the types of energy most relevant to biomechanics and describe how they differ.

- If someone were to get a wrench with a larger handle, would it be easier or harder for the individual to turn a bolt? Explain.

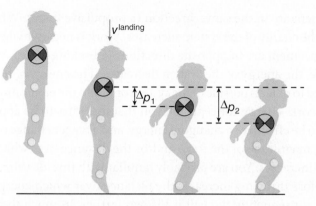

FIGURE 4-9 During landing, the kinetic energy must be absorbed by the body. A stiffer landing results in smaller displacement (Δp_1) and consequently higher forces. A softer landing results in a larger displacement (Δp_2) and less forces.

S. P. Flanagan. (2014). *Biomechanics: A case-based approach*. Burlington, MA: Jones & Bartlett Learning.

extension pattern
A multijoint pattern whereby two segments are rotating in opposite directions and the distance between the beginning and end of the chain is increasing.

flexion pattern
A multijoint pattern whereby two segments are rotating in opposite directions and the distance between the beginning and end of the chain is decreasing.

When you learned Newton's laws, you probably learned them for a single body, such as a ball or pendulum. The human body is not a single element (although it can sometimes be modeled that way), but is made up of many connected segments. For example, the "simple" act of reaching for something requires movement of both the upper arm and forearm, and throwing requires the coordinated activities of the lower extremities, trunk, and upper extremities. Some unique properties emerge when the body is examined as a system of interacting elements rather than as a single body (or by looking at the parts in isolation). The second set of rules acknowledges the multisegmented nature of the human body. Two multisegment principles we will examine in this chapter are choosing the correct movement pattern and the sequencing of joint motions.

The first multisegment principle is to use the correct movement pattern for a particular task. An **extension** or **flexion pattern** occurs when the segments in the chain are simultaneously rotating in opposite directions (**FIGURE 4-10**). When this occurs, the end effector (e.g., hand, foot, center of mass) has a more-or-less linear motion path. With an extension pattern, the distance between the origin of the chain and the end effector is increasing. With a flexion pattern, the distance between the origin of the chain and the end effector is decreasing. Collectively, these will be referred to as *flexion/extension patterns*.

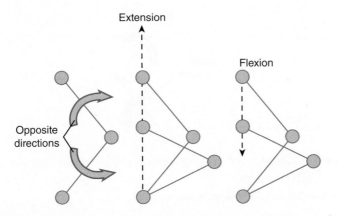

FIGURE 4-10 When the segments rotate in opposite directions, the endpoint moves in a linear path, extending when the origin and endpoint move further away and flexing when the origin and endpoint move closer together.

S. P. Flanagan. (2014). *Biomechanics: A case-based approach*. Burlington, MA: Jones & Bartlett Learning.

Because we usually think in terms of joint rather than segment motion, it is helpful to think about the joint motions associated with flexion and extension patterns. These are listed in **TABLE 4-1**. You have to be careful because nomenclature for the knee is different from that for the elbow: A clockwise rotation of the elbow is called *flexion*, whereas the same clockwise rotation of the knee is called *extension*.

TABLE 4-1 Anatomical Motions Associated with Flexion and Extension Patterns of the Upper and Lower Extremities

		Pattern	
Extremity	**Joint**	**Extension**	**Flexion**
Upper extremity	Shoulder	Flexing	Extending
	Elbow	Extending	Flexing
Lower extremity	Hip	Extending	Flexing
	Knee	Extending	Flexing

S. P. Flanagan. (2014). *Biomechanics: A case-based approach*. Burlington, MA: Jones & Bartlett Learning.

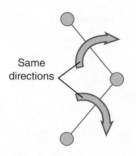

Same
directions

FIGURE 4-11   Rotation of the segments in the same direction result in a swing or whip type pattern.

S. P. Flanagan. (2014). *Biomechanics: A case-based approach.* Burlington, MA: Jones & Bartlett Learning.

swing pattern
Multijoint pattern whereby two segments are rotating in the same direction at submaximal speed.

whip pattern
Multijoint pattern whereby two segments are rotating in the same direction at maximal speed.

The opposite of a flexion/extension pattern occurs when the segments are rotating in the same direction (**FIGURE 4-11**). These patterns have been called throwlike patterns (Luttgens & Hamilton, 1997; Kreighbaum & Barthels, 1996), concurrent patterns, in-phase patterns, and rotations. Although *throwlike* seems like a good descriptor, this pattern is also seen with kicking. You may also throw something with an extension pattern. Here, when segments are rotating in the same direction, they will be called **swing patterns** if the movement speed is submaximal and **whip patterns** if the movement speed is maximal. Collectively, they will be referred to as *swing/ whip patterns*.

The two basic movement patterns have their advantages and disadvantages. To illustrate, let us compare throwing a baseball, a dart, and a shot put. Throwing a baseball is usually done with a whip pattern, whereas throwing a dart and a shot put are usually done with an extension pattern. Why?

In general, swing/whip patterns lead to a greater end-effector velocity than flexion/extension patterns. Although greater velocities are achieved with whip patterns, greater accuracy is achieved with flexion/extension patterns. With an extension pattern, the end effector is traveling along a rectilinear (i.e., straight line) path towards the target. Subsequently, there is more time to correct for errors (Kreighbaum & Barthels, 1996). With the whip pattern, the end effector is traveling a curvilinear path. If the whip pattern is used to throw an object, there are very few points where the ball can be released and hit the target. Greater precision is required; errors will be magnified if the angle of release is slightly off.

That is not to say that whip patterns cannot be accurate. Professional baseball players are highly accurate in their placement of the ball with whip patterns. They choose the whip pattern when throwing a baseball because they could not possibly achieve the high velocities necessary using an extension pattern. But it takes years of practice to skillfully place the ball. A dart is lighter than a ball, and the distance to the dartboard is much less than the distance from the mound to the plate. With a dart, you do not need to develop as high of a velocity. Of course, the bull's-eye is much smaller than the strike zone, and thus darts require a high degree of accuracy. That is why you are better off using an extension pattern for darts.

Which pattern do you think a field athlete uses for the shot put? A typical baseball weighs about 0.14 kg, whereas a shot put weighs 7.26 kg for men and 4 kg for women. The shot put used by men is 50 times heavier than a baseball. It is simply too heavy for the whipping pattern used to throw a baseball. Although the whipping pattern can generate a larger endpoint velocity, flexion/extension patterns can generate more force.

From a purely kinematic standpoint, to maximize endpoint velocity, all of the joints should reach their maximum velocity at the same time during swing/whip patterns (Putnam, 1993). But this does not happen with human movement for a number of reasons (Blazevich, 2007). Rather, joint rotations follow a particular sequence. When generating energy during the propulsive phase of a movement, joint movements follow a proximal (beginning of the chain) to distal (end of the chain) sequence: A more distal segment's maximal velocity occurs after the more proximal segment. When absorbing energy during the braking phase of a movement, the opposite sequencing occurs: Distal motions occur before more proximal ones.

This principle is easily illustrated by throwing a ball straight up in the air using an extension pattern with both your legs and arm (Alexander, 1991). To maximize the height of the ball, you would want to deliver as much energy to the ball as possible before it leaves your hand. This would require a precise timing between the legs and arm. If the arm reached full extension before the legs, then the ball would leave the hand before the legs could deliver all of their energy to the ball (hence the need for a proximal-to-distal sequence). However, you would not want too long of a delay between the proximal and distal joints: If too much time passed between extension of the legs and arm, then the arm would not be able to generate as much energy and deliver it to the ball either.

STOP AND THINK

- Name two multisegment principles, and apply them to familiar movements.

- Describe extension, flexion, swing, and whip patterns. Which multisegmented principle works best for maximal precision versus maximal velocity?

- How are swing and flexion movement patterns similar? Different?

This principle can also be illustrated within a limb. During the propulsive phase of a jump, the extension sequence is proximal to distal: hip, then knee, then ankle. If the ankle were to extend (plantar flex) before the other joints, the body would leave the ground before full extension of the other joints. This would limit the amount of energy the muscles around the hip and knee could generate, and the jump would not be as high as a result.

During landing, when you are absorbing energy, the sequence is distal to proximal. Imagine what would happen if the hips were to flex first. In addition to having a very awkward-looking landing, the joints would decrease the amount of energy they could absorb because they would be flexing before contact is made with the ground.

BIOLOGICAL PRINCIPLES

The third set of rules is based on the fact that we are not inanimate objects or machines. As a living being, you will not violate the laws of physics, but you do influence them in a particular way. This is where the "bio" portion of biomechanics comes in. For example, think about Newton's second law: $F = ma$, where force (F) is the product of mass (m) and acceleration (a). This law is one of the foundations of classical mechanics, and you are as affected by it as any other object on Earth. However, in many instances the source of the force in Newton's second law is your muscles or, more specifically, the **muscle–tendon complex** (MTC; Latash, 2008). So although the law will always apply, a rather large number of factors based on the anatomy and physiology of your muscles influences the production of force.

muscle–tendon complex
The muscle (belly) and all of the elastic components (tendon, fascial layers, etc.).

ACTIONS OF THE MTC

The fundamental principle of the MTC is that it can only pull, it cannot push. In other words, the force developed in the MTC attempts to bring the two insertion points closer together (**FIGURE 4-12**). Which end ultimately moves depends on the amount of resistance present at each segment to which the muscle attaches. However, even though the MTC can only develop force in this one direction, it is capable as acting as a motor, brake, spring, or strut (**FIGURE 4-13**) (Dickinson et al., 2000).

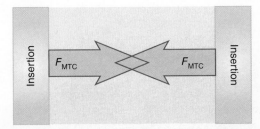

FIGURE 4-12   A muscle-tendon complex (MTC) can only develop force in one direction: towards the center of the MTC.

S. P. Flanagan. (2014). *Biomechanics: A case-based approach.* Burlington, MA: Jones & Bartlett Learning.

Consider the case where hopping is performed only in the vertical direction and the only movement occurs at the ankle joint. To really exaggerate the movement, imagine that you are on an incline facing upward. (At this point, it may be helpful for you to review some basic gross anatomy and kinesiology of this joint if you are not already familiar with it.) Your primary attention should be directed toward the muscles of the calf, which functionally are referred to as the *ankle plantar flexors.* You are going to examine two muscles in particular, the gastrocnemius and soleus (collectively known as the *triceps surae group*), which are connected to the foot via the Achilles tendon. These muscles will be considered a single MTC. For the purposes of this discussion, it is helpful to think of hopping as occurring in three distinct phases: (1) an upward (propulsive) phase from initiation of upward movement to the instant of takeoff, (2) a flight phase, and (3) a downward (braking) phase from the instant of landing to maximum dorsiflexion of the ankle.

During the propulsive phase, the ankle is plantar flexing and the MTC is shortening. Looking at **FIGURE 4-14**, notice how the two insertion points are further away in A and are closer together in B. During the braking phase, the opposite occurs. The ankle dorsiflexes, and the two insertion points move further away from each other (from B to A). Because the two insertion points are further apart, the MTC must be lengthening during the braking phase.

Now ask yourself, what is the function of the MTC? First, think about what happens during the propulsive phase. To move in the vertical direction and achieve liftoff, the energy of the body must be increasing. Where does that energy come from? It comes from the MTC. How does it do it? The force generated by the MTC and the displacement are in the same

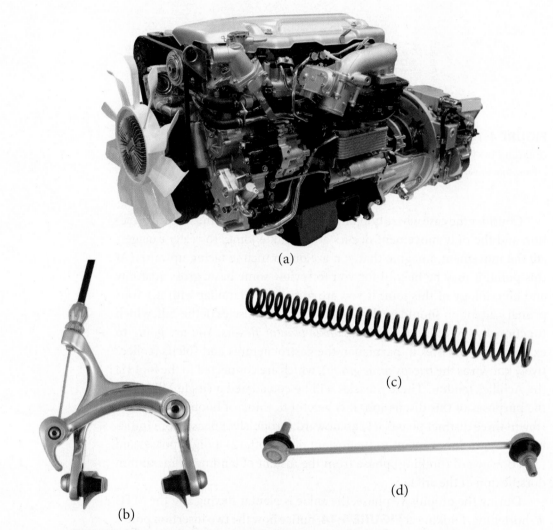

FIGURE 4-13   The MTC can act like a motor, brake, spring, or strut.

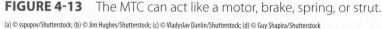

(a) © sspopov/Shutterstock; (b) © Jim Hughes/Shutterstock; (c) © Vladyslav Danlin/Shutterstock; (d) © Guy Shapira/Shutterstock

---

concentric action
Action whereby
the MTC length
is shortening and
generating energy.

direction, so the MTC is shortening and doing positive work. For the MTC to shorten, the force produced by the MTC must be larger than the external force acting on it. Such MTC actions are called **concentric actions**, and the energy that is generated by the MTC is delivered to the segments. During concentric actions, the MTC is acting as a motor.

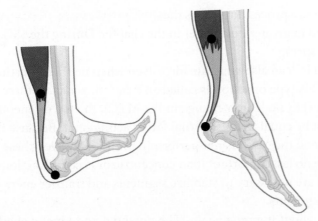

FIGURE 4-14   During plantar flexion (from A to B), the muscle-tendon complex is shortening. During dorsiflexion (from B to A), the muscle-tendon complex is lengthening.

During the braking phase, the body is losing energy. The energy has to go somewhere, and in this case the energy is going to the MTC. The MTC is still generating force, but it is also lengthening. The force and the displacement are in opposite directions. For this to occur, the external forces acting on the MTC must be greater than the force produced by it. This type of MTC action is called an **eccentric action**. When the force and displacement are in opposite directions, negative work is being performed by the MTC. Energy is moving from the segments to the MTC. During eccentric actions, the MTC is acting as a brake by absorbing energy.

Notice how the same MTC (the triceps surae) is controlling both the propulsive and the braking phases, albeit with different actions. During the propulsive phase, the ankle is plantar flexing and the MTC is acting concentrically. During the braking phase, the ankle is dorsiflexing and the MTC is acting eccentrically. If both the joint motion and MTC actions are opposite of each other (e.g., concentric plantar flexion, eccentric dorsiflexion), then the same MTC is controlling both phases of the movement.

During eccentric actions, the energy absorbed by the MTC can be briefly stored. If a concentric action immediately follows an eccentric action (as is the case during hopping), the energy stored can be added to the energy produced, enhancing the energy of the concentric muscle action.

eccentric action
Action whereby the MTC length is increasing and absorbing energy.

stretch-shortening cycle (SSC)
A concentric MTC action that is immediately preceded by an eccentric MTC action.

isometric action
Action whereby the length is not changing and the MTC is transferring energy.

This involves a process known as the **stretch-shortening cycle (SSC)**, which will be explored in greater detail later in the chapter. During the SSC, the MTC acts like a spring.

The MTC can also generate force even when neither insertion point is moving. This type of action is called an **isometric action**. If there is no displacement (i.e., no length change in the MTC), the force generated by the MTC must be equal to the external forces acting on it. Because there is no displacement, the MTC is not performing work. However, these isometric actions are no less important than concentric or eccentric actions. Isometric actions are necessary to stabilize segments and transfer energy between different segments.

Think about hopping again. The potential and kinetic energies of all segments are cyclically increasing and decreasing, but the only source of energy is the triceps surae. But what would happen if the triceps surae was the only MTC active during hopping? It would be very difficult to change the energies of all the segments if the other joints (such as the knee, hips, and spine) were not stabilized but were free to move around. In this case, even though movement is not occurring at these other joints, there is still a level of muscle activation at each of them. So while the action of the plantar flexors is changing the energy of all the segments in the body, isometric actions of MTCs at other joints are necessary to transfer the energy from the triceps surae to the other segments. The MTCs at the other joints are acting like struts.

The three actions of the MTC are reviewed in **FIGURE 4-15**). The MTC has four functions. Three of these functions correspond to three of the actions: (1) during concentric muscle actions the MTC acts like a motor, (2) during eccentric actions the MTC acts like a brake, and (3) during isometric actions the MTC acts like a strut. The fourth function is a combination of two actions: the MTC acts like a spring when an eccentric action is immediately followed by a concentric action. (This function will be explained in greater detail in the section on the stretch-shortening cycle.) By essentially developing force the same way, the MTC can perform these four functions to produce a wide array of movements.

STOP AND THINK

- Name several biological principles, and apply them to familiar movements.

- How many ways can the MTC develop force?

- List the three types of muscle actions. Describe how they differ and the type of displacement produced by each. Which type of action can produce the most force?

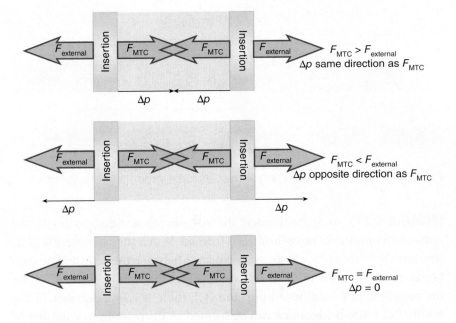

FIGURE 4-15 The three types of muscle actions: (A) When the force produced by the muscle-tendon complex (MTC) is greater than the external force acting on it, the MTC will shorten; (B) When the force produced by the MTC is less than the external force acting on it, the MTC will lengthen; (C) When the force produced by the MTC is equal to the external force acting on it, there is no displacement and no change in length of the MTC.

FACTORS AFFECTING MTC FORCE

Several factors affect how much force the MTC can produce (**FIGURE 4-16**). Here, we will concentrate on four of them: length, type of action, velocity, and the stretch-shortening cycle.

MTC LENGTH

The length of the MTC influences the amount of force it can produce. When considering MTC length, you must think in terms of sarcomere length, fiber length, and the length of the MTC as a whole. Sarcomere length is related to the number of actin–myosin cross-bridges that can be formed

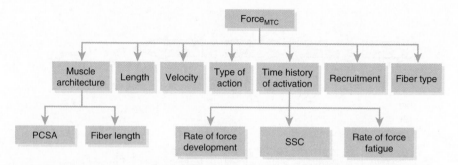

FIGURE 4-16 Factors affecting a muscle's force-producing capabilities.

(**FIGURE 4-17**). At approximately the sarcomere's resting length (B), the maximum number of cross-bridges is formed. When the sarcomere is in its shortened position (A), a large overlap occurs between the actin and myosin heads, decreasing the number of cross-bridges that can be formed. When the muscle is in a lengthened position (C), there is also a decrease in the number of cross-bridges that can be formed. A decrease in the number of cross-bridges corresponds to a decrease in the amount of force produced by the muscle fiber.

Do not assume that every sarcomere will operate through the entire range in Figure 4-17. Sarcomeres tend to operate in a more narrow range in vivo (i.e., in the living body), particularly if that MTC only crosses one joint. However, the length has important implications for MTCs that cross more than one joint. Consider the biarticular (i.e., crosses two joints) hamstring group. To stretch a biarticular MTC, you must lengthen the MTC across both ends (joints). For the hamstrings, this means that you would flex the hip while the knee is extended. If your knee were flexed, the distal end of the hamstrings would be slack, and you would not have an effective stretch. This is probably somewhat obvious.

What might not be as obvious is that to produce the most force with a biarticular MTC, you should lengthen the MTC at one end while it is shortening at another. This will allow the muscle to operate at close to its optimal length. Consider the hamstrings again. If you wanted to generate the greatest amount of torque in knee flexion, you would want to have the hip flexed. This would have the hamstrings in a lengthened position at the proximal end while shortening at the distal end. If the hip were extended, the muscle would be in a more shortened position and less able to generate force.

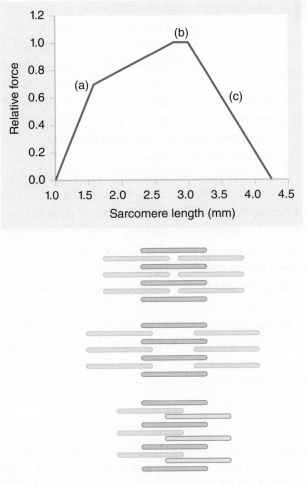

FIGURE 4-17   The force-length curve of an individual sarcomere: (A) the ascending curve, where the actin and myosin overlap too much; (B) the plateau region, where the number of actin-myosin interactions is optimal; (C) the descending limb, where the actin and myosin are too far apart.

MTC ACTION

The force produced by the MTC is also determined by its action. Eccentric actions can produce more force than isometric actions, which, in turn, can produce more force than concentric actions. These differences in force production due to MTC action must be viewed with respect to the elastic components (tendons) and the contraction dynamics. First, think about

STOP AND THINK

Use the reasoning presented in this section to make recommendations concerning proximal and distal joint positions when stretching or strengthening other biarticular muscles in the body.

why isometric muscle actions may produce more force than concentric muscle actions. For example, think about pulling a rope. After every pull (power stroke), one of your hands (the myosin heads) must let go of the rope before it reaches out and grabs another section of the rope. Do you think you can develop more tension on the rope if you just maintain both hands on the rope rather than alternating hand over hand? It is probably the same thing with the actin and myosin filaments.

If that is the case, why can you develop more force eccentrically than isometrically? It is important to remember that just because the MTC is lengthening, it does not mean that the muscle fibers themselves are lengthening. Evidence suggests that during eccentric actions the muscle fiber is acting isometrically and the tendons are lengthening. Forces developed passively by the tendons are added to the active force generated by the muscle itself, increasing the total force that can be produced.

Do not confuse the various MTC actions (i.e., concentric, isometric, eccentric) with the length–tension relations. An MTC can have an eccentric action in a shortened position, just as it can have a concentric action in a lengthened position.

VELOCITY

Velocity also affects the force an MTC can produce, but its effect is determined by both the type of action and the fiber length. The relation between force and velocity with the various types of actions is presented in **FIGURE 4-18**.

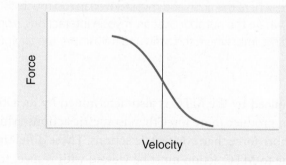

FIGURE 4-18 The force-velocity relation of a muscle-tendon complex.

You should first verify what was explained earlier: Eccentric actions can produce greater force than isometric actions, which, in turn, can produce greater force than concentric actions. Second, note that during concentric muscle action, a nonlinear, inverse relationship exists between force and velocity. As velocity increases, force decreases, and vice versa. You should recognize this from your everyday experience. The speed of movement decreases as you lift heavier objects. Third, notice that eccentric actions do not appear to be as affected by velocity as concentric muscle actions. The most likely reason for this relates to the force produced by the tendon. The tendon can act as a speed buffer.

THE STRETCH-SHORTENING CYCLE

Earlier, we mentioned that the MTC acts like a spring during the stretch-shortening cycle (SSC). Not all concentric actions preceded by an eccentric action involve a SSC. The SSC is only involved if the following three conditions are met (Komi & Gollhofer, 1997):

1. A well-timed preactivation of the muscle prior to the eccentric action
2. A short, rapid eccentric action
3. An immediate transition from the eccentric action to the concentric action (amortization phase)

It is well established that a properly used SSC can enhance the force produced by the MTC. You can see this for yourself. Try jumping as high as you can without flexing your knees before you jump. Because you did not move very far, you could not generate much energy, and your jump height was probably extremely small. If you squatted before you jumped, but held that bottom position before you jumped (a squat jump), then you would certainly jump higher than you could if you did not flex your knees. But this would not be the highest you could jump. If you rapidly squatted and immediately jumped (a countermovement jump), then you would jump the highest you could. That is because the countermovement jump takes advantage of the SSC, whereas the squat jump does not.

STOP AND THINK

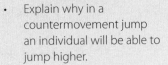

- Give an example of a typical movement, not previously mentioned, that utilizes the SSC.
- Explain why in a countermovement jump an individual will be able to jump higher.

What Can You Do With a Degree in Biomechanics?

CAREERS IN BIOMECHANICS

To be honest, relatively few jobs are available for the card-carrying biomechanists out there. Almost all of those jobs require an advanced degree, and most of those are either at a university or in a research lab. Some other areas where biomechanists are employed are identified in **TABLE 4-2**. However, just because there are few specific jobs in the field does not mean that you should not study it. That would be like saying that you do not need to know math because there are few jobs for pure mathematicians. You still use math every day; in many careers a thorough understanding of biomechanics is not only useful, but probably essential. Some of these careers are listed in **TABLE 4-3**.

BIOMECHANICS FOR EVERYONE

Because of the large and diverse number of careers listed in Table 4-3, we feel that it is important to discuss the steps that are involved in putting your knowledge of biomechanics to use. They include (Knudson & Morrison, 1997):

- Observation
- Evaluation and diagnosis
- Intervention

TABLE 4-2 Careers in Biomechanics

Area	Career
Sport and exercise biomechanics	Olympic Training Centers
	Professional sports teams
	Equipment manufacturers
Occupational biomechanics	Human factors
	Ergonomics
Forensic biomechanics	Accident investigations
	Expert witnesses
Clinical biomechanics	Orthotics and prosthetics
	Gait laboratories

TABLE 4-3 Careers that Require Knowledge of Biomechanics

Area	Career
Sport and exercise biomechanics	Physical educators
	Skill coaches
	Strength and conditioning coaches
	Personal trainers
	Dance instructors
Occupational biomechanics	Safety officers
Clinical biomechanics	Athletic trainers
	Physical therapists
	Occupational therapists
	Chiropractors
	Orthopedists
	Podiatrists

Let's look at each of these a little more closely.

OBSERVATION

If you want to improve the way someone moves, you have to observe them performing that movement. But observation is a little more complicated than just simply watching someone with your eyes. Although that is the most common method of observation, it suffers from the following limitations: You are unable to detect small changes, you can only see a movement once, and you might not catch things that are happening really fast (Knudson & Morrison, 1997). Because of these limitations, biomechanists record the movement for the next stage of the program. The recording device can be something as simple as a mobile device, tablet, or digital video recorder to a research-grade motion-analysis system costing tens of thousands of dollars. Regardless of the recording device, you want to ensure that you record the movement from multiple vantage points (to see movement in multiple planes) and record enough observations (usually 3–10) to capture not only the critical elements associated with the movement, but also the variability inherent within it.

EVALUATION AND DIAGNOSIS

After recording the movement, you must evaluate it. Depending on the sophistication of the recording device and software, the evaluation can be either qualitative or quantitative; it may include only kinematics or both kinematics and kinetics. As with recording devices, you could choose to simply look at the recording or analyze it with a special app or software.

Evaluation is all about comparing the recorded movement *to* something. That something could be normative data, models, results from experiments, some form of "expert" performance, or biomechanical principles (Lees, 2002). Because of the unique interactions of a person's capabilities and the environmental constraints, we advocate analyzing movement based on biomechanical principles, some of which we highlighted above.

Regardless of the criteria used, judgments are then made concerning the performance. The analysis of the movement will tell you that something is less than optimal, but it cannot identify the cause (Flanagan, 2012). Due to the multifactorial nature of the human body, several different causes could produce the same effect. So if you determine that someone could be moving better, you still have to determine what is limiting the performance. Such limitations are called **impairments**. Impairment in the range of motion, strength, power, or endurance of any of the joints involved in the movement could be a potential cause. Additionally, the coordination of those joints or the ability to respond to a disturbance during the movement (stability) may also be a factor. So you must also conduct a detailed analysis of the performer before you can create a targeted intervention. The diagnosis is then determining which impairments are limiting the performance. A quick word of caution here: Do not stop at the first impairment that you find. It might not be the only (or even the most important) impairment limiting performance.

impairment
Something that causes a limitation in performance, such as a deficit in range of motion, strength, power, endurance, etc.

INTERVENTION

With the intervention, you are attempting to correct impairments uncovered by your evaluation. If someone's strength is limiting his or her ability to complete the task, then you need to strengthen the muscles involved in the task. But if the impairment is with the range of motion at a particular joint, then all of the strength training in the world will not correct the impairment. You must match the intervention to the impairment, and this highlights the multidisciplinary nature of kinesiology: Correcting the impairment requires knowledge of anatomy, physiology, motor behavior, and psychology, in addition to biomechanics.

A program aimed at improving performance or reducing injury risk cannot stop there. First, you must ensure that your intervention was successful at addressing the impairment(s). If strength of the knee extensors was a limiting factor, you should determine that your program did, in fact, make the knee extensors stronger. But you must also make sure that the improved strength of the knee extensors transferred to improved performance of the task (Flanagan, 2012). This requires you to repeat the process and once again observe the performance. If the performance is less than optimal, then you are once again tasked with finding the impairment(s) limiting performance.

> ## STOP AND THINK
>
>
>
> - List the steps involved in a biomechanics intervention.
> - Choose a typical athletic movement, such as a squat or the swing of a bat or racquet. What would you be looking for? What would be the best way to evaluate this particular movement?

Areas of Research in Biomechanics

Research in the four areas of biomechanics (sport and exercise, occupational, forensic, and clinical) is carried out every day in labs all over the world. Regardless of the area, almost all investigations use one or a combination of three main methodological approaches (Quatman, Quatman, & Hewett, 2009): in vivo, in vitro, or in silico. All three approaches have the goal of improving our understanding of performance enhancement, injury prevention, or injury rehabilitation.

In vivo investigations use living, breathing people. The most common investigations involve either videotaping people performing an activity in their natural environment or conducting a more extensive (and expensive) motion analysis using digital optoelectrical cameras and force platforms. Other studies quantify muscle activity (electromyography [EMG]), strength and power (isokinetic dynamometry), joint laxity (arthrometers), bone health (dual-energy x-ray absorptiometry [DXA]), and/or other clinical measures (magnetic resonance imaging [MRI], ultrasound, questionnaires, etc.). With this method of research, investigators are trying to determine not only how people move, but why they are moving the way they are.

In order to understand injury mechanics better, it is necessary to see how various tissues and structures respond under load. These loads often

in vivo
An investigation of a living person.

need to be large enough to break, fracture, or tear bones, muscles, ligaments, tendons, etc. As you might imagine, there are probably not a lot of people lining up to volunteer to be subjects in those types of studies. This is where **in vitro** methods are used. Either animal or cadaveric specimens are put into specialized devices that can measure both the magnitude and direction of an applied load and the material's response to that load. These types of studies provide insights into the most injurious positions and loads for various structures in the body.

in vitro
An investigation using cadaveric or animal tissues.

Some things cannot be measured directly (such as muscle forces). Other measurements that we may wish to take would be so invasive that they would alter the way someone naturally moves. Still other things that we would like to know are either too impractical or too risky to perform experiments on living people, and cadavers typically do not run, jump, swim, or climb stairs. In these instances, computer simulation (**in silico**) studies can help fill the gaps in our understanding. With the gains in speed and power of desktop computers, these types of studies are being used with increasing frequency in biomechanics research.

in silico
An investigation using computer simulation.

It is important to note that no single approach (in vitro, in vivo, or in silico) can provide us with all of the answers. Each one complements and informs the others. Together, they can provide deeper insights into the way we move. Although we have learned much since the time of Aristotle, our understanding is not yet complete. It will be exciting to see what the future will bring. Will you be a part of it?

CHAPTER SUMMARY

Biomechanics is a branch of science that looks to uncover the rules that govern movement by applying the methods of mechanics to the study of the structure and function of biological systems. Currently, biomechanics has four broad areas: sport and exercise, occupational, forensic, and clinical. We began the chapter by providing a brief history of the field, outlining some of the pioneers who helped uncover those rules, starting with Aristotle and ending with the first half of the 20th century. We outlined the current understanding of three major categories of biomechanical principles (mechanical, multisegment, and biological) that are used to improve performance and prevent injury. Although there are few jobs specifically in biomechanics, we hoped to have impressed upon you the need to understand biomechanical principles in a number of careers (basically, any that involve people moving) and a three-step process for implementing them into a program.

We finished by explaining three methodological approaches to biomechanics research (in vivo, in vitro, and in silico), upon which the next chapter of biomechanics history will be written. We challenge you to have your name be one of them when that chapter is written.

DISCUSSION QUESTIONS

1. What is biomechanics, and why should you be interested in learning about biomechanics?
2. What are two major objectives within the study of biomechanics? Explain the importance of each.
3. From a biomechanical perspective, what are the steps in implementing a program to improve performance?
4. From a biomechanical perspective, what are the steps to reducing injury risk?

REFERENCES

Alexander, R. M. (1991). Optimum timing of muscle activation for simple-models of throwing. *Journal of Theoretical Biology, 150*(3), 349–372. doi:10.1016/s0022-5193(05)80434-5

Baker, R. (2007). The history of gait analysis before the advent of modern computers. *Gait & Posture, 26*(3), 331–342. doi:10.1016/j.gaitpost.2006.10.014

Blazevich, A. (2007). *Sports biomechanics. The basics: Optimising human performance*. London: A&C Black.

Braun, M., & Whitcombe, E. (1999). Marey, Muybridge, and Londe: The photography of pathological locomotion. *History of Photography, 23*(3), 218–224.

Dickinson, M. H., Farley, C. T., Full, R. J., Koehl, M. A. R., Kram, R., & Lehman, S. (2000). How animals move: An integrative view. [Review]. *Science, 288*(5463), 100–106. doi:10.1126/science.288.5463.100

Flanagan, S. P. (2012). Systems and principles of therapeutic exercise. In *Education and intervention for musculoskeletal injuries: A biomechanics approach* (pp. 1–30). Lacrosse, WI: APTA, Inc.

Hatze, H. (1974). The meaning of the term biomechanics. *Journal of Biomechanics, 7*(2), 189–190. doi: 10.1016/0021-9290(74)90060-8

Knudson, D. V., & Morrison, C. S. (1997). *Qualitative analysis of human movement*. Champaign, IL: Human Kinetics.

Komi, P. V., & Gollhofer, A. (1997). Stretch reflexes can have an important role in force enhancement during SSC exercise. *Journal of Applied Biomechanics, 13*(4), 451–460.

Kreighbaum, E., & Barthels, K. M. (1996). *Biomechanics: A qualitative approach for studying human movement* (4th ed.). Boston: Allyn and Bacon.

Latash, M. L. (2008). *Synergy*. Oxford: Oxford University Press.

Lees, A. (2002). Technique analysis in sports: A critical review. *Journal of Sports Sciences, 20*(10), 813–828. doi:10.1080/026404102320675657

Luttgens, K., & Hamilton, N. (1997). *Kinesiology: Scientific basis of human motion* (9th ed.). Boston: WCB McGraw-Hill.

Martin, R. B. (1999). A genealogy of biomechanics. Retrieved from http://www.asbweb.org/html/biomechanics/genealogy/genealogy.htm

Pope, M. H. (2005). Giovanni Alfonso Borelli—The father of biomechanics. *Spine, 30*(20), 2350–2355. doi:10.1097/01.brs.0000182314.49515.d8

Putnam, C. A. (1993). Sequential motions of body segments in striking and throwing skills: Descriptions and explanations. *Journal of Biomechanics, 26,* 125–135. doi:10.1016/0021-9290(93)90084-r

Quatman, C. E., Quatman, C. C., & Hewett, T. E. (2009). Prediction and prevention of musculoskeletal injury: A paradigm shift in methodology. *British Journal of Sports Medicine, 43*(14), 1100–1107. doi:10.1136/bjsm.2009.065482

Thurston, A. J. (1999). Giovanni Borelli and the study of human movement: An historical review. *Australian and New Zealand Journal of Surgery, 69*(4), 276–288. doi:10.1046/j.1440-1622.1999.01558.x

Watson, D. (2011). Energy (definition). Retrieved from http://www.ftexploring.com/energy/energy-1.htm

CHAPTER 5

Exercise and Sport Psychology

ASHLEY A. SAMSON

LEARNING OBJECTIVES

1. Define *sport psychology*.
2. Describe the evolution of the field of sport psychology.
3. Explain how one becomes a sport psychology professional.
4. Describe what a sport psychology consultant does on a day-to-day basis.
5. Describe the basic orientations/approaches in sport psychology.
6. Identify and describe some of the current major topics in the field of sport psychology.
7. Describe how the principles of sport psychology can be applied to other fields.

KEY TERMS

achievement goal theory
attribution theory
clinical sport psychology
cognitive-behavioral orientation
cohesion
educational sport psychology
exercise psychology

extrinsic motivation
group norms
group roles
intrinsic motivation
mental toughness
motivation
psychological skills development (PSD)

psychophysiological orientation   social-psychological orientation
qualitative measures   sport psychology
quantitative measures   sport psychology consulting
social cognitive theory

What Is Sport Psychology?

sport psychology
The study of the
psychological
factors that come
into play before,
during, and after
sport performance
situations and the
application of that
knowledge.

exercise psychology
The application
of psychological
principles in
exercise settings,
usually not involving
competition.

When most people hear the term *sport psychology*, they immediately think,
"Oh, that sounds interesting. What is that?" Broadly defined, **sport psychology**
is the study of the psychological factors that come into play before, during,
and after sport performance situations and the application of that knowledge (Gill & Williams, 2008). These factors include such things as anxiety,
team dynamics, and motivation. The field of sport psychology has two main
objectives: (1) to understand how these factors can affect sport performance
and (2) to understand how best to manipulate these factors to create more
positive sport performance outcomes. Related to sport psychology is **exercise psychology**, which is very similar to sport psychology except that its
main focus is not on sport performance, but rather on exercise behaviors
of people in the general population (i.e., nonathletes). Although the purpose of this chapter is to introduce you to the field of sport psychology, it
is important to mention exercise psychology because the two fields are so
closely related. In the field of exercise psychology, researchers and practitioners study the psychological factors that influence exercise behaviors and
the psychological outcomes of participating in physical activity. For example, someone who studies exercise psychology might be interested in how
personality can influence the type of exercise someone might enjoy or the
effects of exercise on self-esteem. See **TABLE 5-1** for more information on
the differences between sport and exercise psychology.

History of Sport Psychology

Although it is only in the last 10 years or so that sport psychology has become
better known in mainstream culture, the field of sport psychology has been
around since the late 1800s. One of the more famous early studies in sport
psychology is Norman Triplett's 1898 investigation of social effects on performance in cyclists. He noticed that cyclists rode faster when they rode
in groups than when they rode alone and conducted several experimental

TABLE 5-1 Comparison of Sport and Exercise Psychology

Aspect	Sport Psychology	Exercise Psychology
Focus	Athletes and performance outcomes	General population (i.e., nonathletes) and their exercise behaviors
Main goal	To manipulate psychological factors in order to enhance performance	To understand the factors that influence individuals' exercise behaviors to increase adoption and adherence
Areas of interest	Performance enhancement techniques to increase consistency and accuracy and improve athletic performance (e.g., energy management, attentional focus, positive self-talk, confidence)	Psychological factors that influence whether an individual participates in exercise (e.g., self-esteem, motivation, confidence, effects of exercise on depression or anxiety)

studies that enabled him to predict when cyclists would be more likely to perform better (Davis, Huss, & Becker, 1995). Around the same time, E. W. Scripture explored the effects of reaction time and muscle movement activation on performance of sport tasks. Scripture and his graduate students conducted a number of laboratory experiments to examine how the brain's ability to think and act quickly could affect sport performance (Kornspan, 2007). Scripture also was the first researcher to discuss how sport participation could lead to the development of good character. His early conclusions are still accepted today.

STOP AND THINK

If an athlete becomes proficient in self-regulation of emotions and responses to competition, what are some areas in which these self-regulatory skills may come into play later in life?

Moving into the early 20th century, a period in sport psychology history emerged that is now known as the "Griffith era," due to the numerous contributions to the field by Coleman Griffith, who became known as the "father of sport psychology" in North America (Kroll & Lewis, 1970). During his most productive years, Griffith established the first laboratory in sport psychology at the University of Illinois, created a coaching program that provided training for coaches to become stronger leaders who would better understand the psychology of their athletes, and wrote two classic books in the field: *Psychology of Coaching* (1926) and *Psychology and Athletics* (1928). Additionally, he was a pioneer in applied work, conducting studies on the Chicago Cubs, consulting with Notre Dame football coaches, and interviewing famous athletes such as Red Grange.

Sport psychology began to grow in popularity, and several other researchers emerged, such as Franklin Henry, who established a lab for sport psychology and a graduate program at the University of California at Berkeley
in 1938; and Dorothy Yates, one of the first women in the sport psychology
field, who studied the effects of relaxation on boxers in 1943 (Gill, 1995;
Vealey, 2009). Following the establishment of Henry's program at Berkeley,
programs were developed at other universities, and the idea of sport psychology as a field of study began to take form. Researchers such as Warren
Johnson and Arthur Slater-Hammel were instrumental in this process as
they helped to develop curriculum and coursework paths in the field.

During the 1960s, sport psychology really began to grow as an academic
discipline. The first World Congress of Sport Psychology was held in Rome
in 1965, marking the first time that scientists and practitioners from around
the world came together to share ideas. Two years later, the North American
Society for the Psychology of Sport and Physical Activity (NASPSPA) held
its first conference and the field continued to advance. Also, applied work
was becoming more common during this time, with Dr. Bruce Ogilvie's
(**FIGURE 5-1**) work with the San Francisco 49ers and his publishing of
several books about applied sport psychology (Vealey, 2009).

Since the 1970s, the field has continued to grow in popularity and respect,
both in North America and internationally. Several scientific journals have been

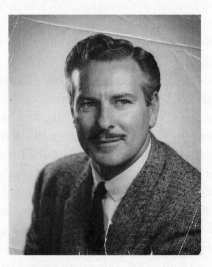

FIGURE 5-1   Dr. Bruce Ogilvie.
Courtesy of the family of Bruce Ogilvie

established (e.g., *Journal of Sport Psychology* in 1979 and the *Journal of Applied Sport Psychology* is 1989) so that knowledge gained from research and applied work can be communicated to other scientists. The U.S. Olympic Committee (USOC) began to hire sport psychologists in 1985, and sport psychology's main organization, the Association for Applied Sport Psychology (AASP), was established in 1986. Today in the United States, hundreds of undergraduate and graduate programs focus on the study of sport psychology, and there are many established research programs around the world for both scientific and applied work in the field. It is also fairly common to hear professional athletes and teams talking about the importance of the "mental side" of their performance and their work with sport psychology professionals/consultants.

What Do Sport Psychologists Do?

Usually, after someone asks what sport psychology is, his or her next question is, "What do you do with that, do you counsel crazy athletes?" After explaining, "That's not what sport psychologists typically do," I then explain what sport psychology professionals actually do in their professional work. Most sport psychology professionals practice in three areas: research, consulting, or teaching. Many professionals in sport psychology are involved in all three areas on some level, although it will vary by individual and specific career characteristics.

RESEARCH

One of the primary responsibilities of members of an academic or scholarly field is to help advance knowledge; thus the research component of sport psychology is very important (Weinberg & Gould, 2011). Most sport psychologists conduct research in a university setting and are usually associated with an undergraduate or graduate program in sport psychology that allows students to be involved in their studies. Some examples of this work might be in a lab setting where, for example, a research team might explore the effects of an autocratic versus democratic leader on the effectiveness of a team or the effects of music/no music on perceived exertion during a sport task. A research program in a nonlab setting might look at the effects of team dynamics on performance during practice or explore the influence of a preshot routine on free-throw shooting in a basketball gym.

TEACHING

Many sport psychologists are employed as university professors and instructors, thus another component of their job usually includes teaching courses in sport psychology. Through educating others about the principles and major research findings in sport psychology, this is an additional way to advance knowledge in the field. Courses taught by sport psychologists might include a basic foundations of sport psychology course, applied sport psychology, advanced sport psychology, or social psychology of sport. Depending on the focus and depth of the program, sport psychologists might teach more specific courses, such as personality psychology in sport, team dynamics in sport, or developmental psychology in sport.

CONSULTING

Sport psychology consulting is what most people think of when they picture what a sport psychologist does. In this role, psychologists apply principles learned from research, and perhaps personal experience, to help individual athletes, teams, coaches, and sport organizations develop the psychological skills necessary to be successful in their endeavors. As the field has become more familiar and respected, more consultants are being sought to employ their skills and impart their knowledge. Many universities and professional sport organizations now hire full-time sport psychologists as part of their staff, and the USOC has full-time sport psychologists who are part of their training programs and travel with the Olympic teams. Just as it is important to have a strength and conditioning coach as part of an athletic team staff, people are now recognizing the importance of having professional help in addressing mental skill development as well.

How Does One Become a Sport Psychologist?

Most sport psychology professionals take one of two possible paths to becoming a sport psychologist: **clinical sport psychology** or **educational sport psychology**. Both paths typically require a doctoral degree (Ph.D.) or at least a master's degree and some level of applied experience, but the focus of each is slightly different.

---

sport psychology consulting
Role where sport psychologists apply principles learned from research, and perhaps personal experience, to help individual athletes, teams, coaches, and sport organizations develop the psychological skills necessary to be successful in their endeavors.

---

clinical sport psychology
Branch of sport psychology that focuses on personality factors that influence performance and/or team interactions.

---

educational sport psychology
Branch of sport psychology that focuses primarily on cognitive factors in performance enhancement.

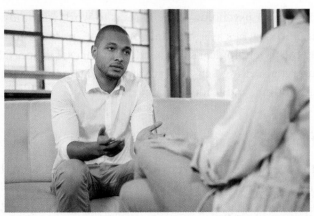

© Wavebreak Premium/Shutterstock

CLINICAL SPORT PSYCHOLOGY

Clinical sport psychologists are typically licensed psychologists who have extensive training and knowledge regarding clinical issues and are trained and qualified to diagnose and treat severe emotional disorders (e.g., depression, anxiety, etc.). Typically, these professionals are licensed in general clinical psychology, and then they specialize in working with athletes. Often they will work with people in the general population, as well as athletes. Clinical sport psychologists are invaluable in helping athletes with severe emotional disorders; it is important for athletes to have someone who understands their disorder as well as the sport/athlete factors involved (Hays, 1995). For example, eating disorders in athletes is an area in which a clinical sport psychologist might specialize.

STOP AND THINK

It is important to realize that all three of these roles are equally important and completely interrelated. Without research, problems are never resolved nor understood. The lessons from research inform both consulting in the world of performance and in the preparation of new cohorts of teachers, coaches, and sport psychology professionals.

EDUCATIONAL SPORT PSYCHOLOGY

Educational sport psychology professionals typically have an extensive background in kinesiology or exercise science and additional training in counseling and the psychology of physical activity and/or sport. These individuals are not licensed psychologists, and thus are not trained to diagnose or treat individuals with severe emotional disorders. The primary focus of educational sport psychology specialists is to work with individual athletes, teams, and coaches as a "mental consultant" in order to understand and develop the psychological skills needed for success in sport. Such skills might include goal-setting, self-talk, anxiety management, communication, confidence-building, and leadership development.

Orientations in Sport Psychology

Although the overall goal in sport psychology is to understand the psychological factors that impact sport performance, several different "orientations" (or explanations) have emerged for how these psychological factors are believed to influence behaviors and subsequent performance. The three most commonly adopted orientations are psychophysiological, social-psychological, and cognitive-behavioral.

PSYCHOPHYSIOLOGICAL ORIENTATION

psychophysiological orientation
Sport psychology approach that posits that the best explanation for sport and exercise behavior lies within the physiological processes that are happening within the brain and body.

Sport psychologists who adopt a psychophysiological orientation posit that the best explanation for sport and exercise behavior lies within the physiological processes that are happening within the brain and body (Weinberg & Gould, 2011). They examine physiological phenomena in the body such as heart rate, brain activity, and muscle activation to better understand how those functions affect sport performance behaviors. An example of what someone might study under this orientation would be the relationship between heart rate and anxiety levels and whether an athlete could be taught to control heart rate in an attempt to quell pregame anxiety.

SOCIAL-PSYCHOLOGICAL ORIENTATION

social-psychological orientation
Sport psychology approach that posits that behaviors are the result of an interaction between environmental and personal factors.

Professionals in sport psychology who adopt the social-psychological orientation to studying behavior believe that behaviors are the result of an interaction between environmental and personal factors (Weinberg & Gould, 2011). Researchers and practitioners operating under this orientation seek to understand how the social environment influences individuals' behaviors and also how their behaviors influence the environment. For example, someone under this orientation might be interested in team dynamics, the effect of home-field advantage, or leadership styles.

COGNITIVE-BEHAVIORAL

Sport psychology professionals who adopt the **cognitive-behavioral orienta-tion** argue that behaviors stem from individuals' thoughts and beliefs (i.e., cognitions). They examine variables such as self-perception, motivation, and locus of control (sense of control over situations). An example of a research project under this orientation would be an exploration of burnout and per-formance in young soccer players.

cognitive-behavioral orientation
Sport psychology approach that posits that behaviors stem from individuals' thoughts and beliefs (i.e., cognitions).

Major Topics in Sport Psychology

Now that you have a good understanding of what sport psychology is, where it came from, and the major research orientations, it is time for you to explore some of the major topics in this field. Therefore, the purpose of this section of the chapter is to provide an overview of some of the main areas of research and practice within sport psychology. Although there are numerous areas of research focus, the most widely studied domains in sport psychology include motivation, psychological skill development, and team dynamics.

MOTIVATION

Motivation can best be defined as the direction and intensity of effort, and it can be influenced by many different internal and external factors (Vealey, 2009). Motivation is an essential characteristic needed for success in both the sport domain and in everyday life! Several theories are used to explain motivation and how we might increase motivation to create better perfor-mance outcomes, but at its most basic level motivation can be broken down into two types: intrinsic and extrinsic.

motivation
The direction and intensity of effort.

Intrinsic motivation is motivation that comes from within the individual. For example, an athlete might play her sport because she enjoys it, it makes her feel good, and perhaps she experiences a sense of accomplishment when participating. In contrast, **extrinsic motivation** comes from external factors outside of the individual. For example, an athlete might participate in his sport because of the money or recognition it brings or run extra miles so that his coach doesn't yell at him.

intrinsic motivation
Motivation that comes from within the individual.

extrinsic motivation
Motivation that comes from external factors outside of the individual.

In terms of which type of motivation seems to be stronger, the research points to intrinsic motivation. Although the influence of extrinsic motiva-tion can be very strong, its effects are usually contingent on the external factors present, and thus when the external rewards go away, so does the motivation. In other words, if we refer back to our earlier examples, the athlete who plays for money and recognition will not be as motivated when the money and fame go away or won't run if the coach isn't making him do it. In contrast, because intrinsic motivation comes from within, it is not going to "go away," and thus leads to long-term commitment and enjoyment for the activity. Therefore, an important question in the sport psychology field is, "How do we increase motivation, specifically intrinsic motivation, in our athletes?" Several different motivational theories have been developed, and a few of the major ones will now be briefly discussed.

SOCIAL COGNITIVE THEORY

social cognitive theory
Theory of motivation developed by Alfred Bandura that views behavior as being influenced by the combination of personal, environmental, and behavioral factors.

Social cognitive theory was developed by Alfred Bandura (1977, 1986), and it is still one of the most prominent theories of motivation used today (**FIGURE 5-2**). According to Bandura, behaviors are influenced by the combination of personal, environmental, and behavioral factors. In other words, the likelihood that a person will choose to engage in a behavior and how he or she performs in the behavior is influenced by the person's personal characteristics, his or her environment, and the characteristics of the behavior in which he or she is engaging. For example, if an athlete is asked to perform a skill that she is familiar with (behavioral characteristic) in an environment that she is comfortable in (environmental characteristic), she will

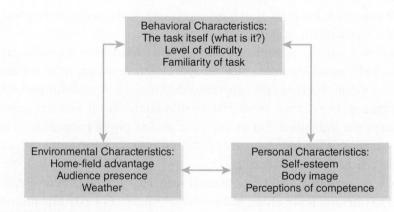

FIGURE 5-2   Social cognitive theory.

most likely have high self-confidence to perform the skill (personal characteristic), and thus be motivated to perform well.

ACHIEVEMENT GOAL THEORY

According to the **achievement goal theory**, individuals tend to create their own goals based on either task or ego orientations, which subsequently influence motivation (Dweck, 1986; Duda, 1989; Nicholls, 1984). People who adopt a task (or mastery) orientation base their success on their own performance relative to their past performance. In other words, they are not focused on what others are doing; they are only worried about their own personal improvement. An example of this could be a runner who runs her personal best in the mile race, but does not care that she came in fifth place. In contrast, those who adopt an ego (or performance) orientation base their perceptions of success on how they compare to others around them. For example, an athlete may not care if she ran her best time in the mile, just so long as she won the race and beat everyone.

So which one is "better" in terms of motivation? Most of the research reports that a task (mastery) orientation leads to a stronger work ethic, persistence in the face of failure, and optimal performance (Duda, 1989; Weinberg & Gould, 2011). Researchers argue that this orientation places the focus on something that the athlete can control (i.e., their own performance) rather than something they cannot control (i.e., the performance of others), and thus it can protect them from disappointment, frustration, and decreases in motivation when others happen to perform better than they do (Weinberg & Gould, 2011). Additionally, those who adopt a task orientation tend to choose more challenging (but realistic) goals and opponents.

> **achievement goal theory** Theory of motivation that states that individuals tend to create their own goals based on either task or ego orientations, which subsequently influence motivation.

ATTRIBUTION THEORY

Attribution theory focuses on the factors that individuals use to explain their successes and failures (Heider, 1958; Weiner, 1985, 1986). Adherents of this theory believe that successes and failures can be attributed to three main categories of factors: (1) stability (whether the issue causing the success/failure is permanent), (2) locus of causality (whether the issue is internal or external to the individual), and (3) locus of control (whether the issue is under a person's control). In general, researchers have concluded that attributions are important because they can influence emotional reactions to

> **attribution theory** Theory of motivation that focuses on the factors that individuals use to explain their successes and failures.

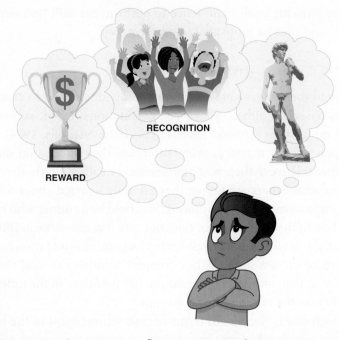

FIGURE 5-3   Attributions can influence emotional reactions to success and failure.

success and failure and shape future motivation and expectations of success (**FIGURE 5-3**). Oftentimes, individuals are affected by successes and failures that they attribute to stable, internal, and controllable factors rather than unstable, external, and uncontrollable ones.

Although these three theories of motivation are by no means the only ones, they are some of the most well-established ones in sport psychology. Hopefully, these will give you a small understanding of how complicated motivation can be and the various factors that may influence it. **TABLE 5-2** provides a few tips for increasing motivation based on sport psychology research.

PSYCHOLOGICAL SKILL DEVELOPMENT

Because one of the major responsibilities of a sport psychologist is consulting with athletes, teams, and coaches for the development of psychological skills, it is important to discuss some of the research and issues within this area. Although there is not enough room in this chapter to discuss all of the psychological skills and techniques that exist, it is the aim of this section to

TABLE 5-2   Five Tips for Increasing Motivation

1. Recognize that both situations and personality characteristics can influence motivation.
2. Remember that sometimes people can have multiple reasons behind their motivation.
3. Sometimes changing the environment or the situation can influence motivation in athletes.
4. Remember that leaders can play a large role in impacting motivation.
5. Set goals so that individuals can see what they are working towards.

provide you with an overview of the major principles that guide psychological skill development and discuss a few of the major psychological skills.

According to Weinberg and Gould (2011), **psychological skill development (PSD)** is the systematic and consistent practice of mental/psychological skills for the purpose of enhancing performance, increasing enjoyment, or achieving greater sport and physical activity self-satisfaction. One of the major outcome goals of PSD is a concept called mental toughness. **Mental toughness** can be defined as being motivated, dealing with pressure, having confidence, and maintaining concentration (Jones, Hanton, & Connaughton, 2007). It is believed that by developing their psychological skills, athletes can increase their mental toughness, leading to better performance outcomes (Kaiseler, Polman, & Nicholls, 2009).

MYTHS ABOUT PSYCHOLOGICAL SKILL DEVELOPMENT

Many myths surround the development and improvement of psychological skills that prevent many athletes and coaches from recognizing the value of the "mental side" of sport and how to train it. The following are some common myths regarding PSD:

- PSD is only for "problem" athletes.
- PSD is only for elite athletes.
- PSD provides "quick fix" solutions.
- PSD is not useful, it just makes you feel warm and fuzzy for a while.

Although some of these myths may seem silly, they are beliefs that are still held by a large portion of individuals who are not yet educated on the potential benefits of PSD. It is hoped that these myths will continue to fade as

psychological skill development (PSD) The systematic and consistent practice of mental/psychological skills for the purpose of enhancing performance, increasing enjoyment, or achieving greater sport and physical activity self-satisfaction.

mental toughness Being motivated, dealing with pressure, having confidence, and maintaining concentration.

more people learn about what sport psychology is and how it can help them to improve performance.

DELIVERY OF PSD PROGRAMS

Numerous books are available that seek to educate coaches and sport psychologists on how to develop psychological skills within their athletes. Jean Williams (1993) wrote one of the first of these books in the early 1990s. Although these books vary in their approaches, a commonality across all of them is that the first step in delivering a program aimed at improving psychological skills is to get a baseline on what skills the athletes (or team) currently use, their perceptions on psychological skills, and their openness to try new interventions aimed at PSD. In order to answer the first question (what skills are currently being used), several questionnaires have been developed to assess psychological skills use. One example of this type of survey is the Test of Performance Strategies, or TOPS (Thomas, Murphy, & Hardy, 1999). In order to answer the second two questions (perceptions of PSD and openness to change), the sport psychologist typically will simply ask the athlete his or her views during an intake interview.

Once the sport psychologist has the baseline information, it is time to implement the program. Deciding what skills to include, and in what order, will vary by individual athlete and depend on what has and has not been tried in the past. An example of a hierarchy of psychological skills can be seen in **FIGURE 5-4**. Using this example, a sport psychology professional might start with anxiety/arousal management, and then slowly work up the pyramid to end with the creation of a pregame routine for the athlete to utilize before practice and competition. As with any program aimed at improving something, an important component to integrate throughout the program is evaluation of effectiveness and making changes, if necessary. Just as a strength and conditioning coach might do a maximal lift test to evaluate a weight-training program, it is important to regularly evaluate the PSD program to make sure progress is actually happening.

TEAM/GROUP DYNAMICS

Group and team issues are important for sport psychologists because of the amount of time athletes typically spend in group settings. Additionally, it is important for sport psychologists to understand how the dynamics of

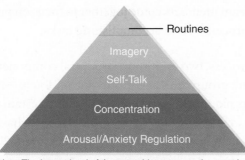

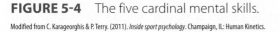

Note. The lowest level of the pyramid represents the most basic and foundational skills, while the peak of the pyramid (routines) represents the integration of all lower levels.

FIGURE 5-4   The five cardinal mental skills.

Modified from C. Karageorghis & P. Terry. (2011). *Inside sport psychology*. Champaign, IL: Human Kinetics.

a group can influence individual athletes and, in turn, can influence the performance of the whole team.

FORMATION OF GROUPS

Although most individual athletes are placed together on a team through a default method such as tryouts, a draft, or age groupings, it is important to recognize that there is a difference between a group of individuals placed on a team and an actual cohesive team "unit." Sport groups (or teams) are characterized by a collective sense of identity, distinctive roles, structured modes of communication, and norms (Weinberg & Gould, 2011). Researchers have identified four main stages that individuals go through when forming a cohesive unit (Tuckman, 1965):

1. *Forming*: Team members familiarize themselves with other team members, engage in social comparisons, and assess the strengths and weaknesses of other team members.
2. *Storming*: Characterized by resistance to leaders and interpersonal conflict (who is going to lead, where are we headed, how will be get there?).
3. *Norming*: Hostility is replaced by cooperation; consensus on the above questions is reached.

group role
The set of expected behaviors required of someone occupying a certain position within the team.

group norms
Levels of performance, behavior patterns, or the belief systems held by the group.

cohesion
The total field of forces that act on members to remain in a group.

4. *Performing*: Team members come together to focus on problem-solving, using group processes, and accomplishing tasks.

During this process, two important structural components of the group are also established: group roles and group norms. **Group roles** are the set of expected behaviors required of someone occupying a certain position within the team. **Group norms** refer to levels of performance, behavior patterns, or the belief systems held by the group (Weinberg & Gould, 2011).

FACTORS INFLUENCING TEAM PERFORMANCE

Once a group is functioning as a unit, it would be easy to assume that performance automatically follows, but that is not always the case. One of the main factors that influences team performance is team cohesion (**FIGURE 5-5**). **Cohesion** is the total field of forces that act on members to remain in a group (Festinger, Schacter, & Back, 1950). The two main types of cohesion are task and social. *Task cohesion* refers to the degree to which group members work together to achieve common goals and objectives (i.e., how productive they are), whereas *social cohesion* reflects the interpersonal attraction among group members (i.e., how much they like each other).

The relationship between cohesion and performance is complex, but, in general, task cohesion is more closely related to performance than is social cohesion, and cohesion is more important for interactive sports (i.e., sports where team members interact directly with each other during competitions such as soccer and basketball; Weinberg & Gould, 2011). The relationship between cohesion and performance also appears to be circular, with performance success leading to increased cohesion, which, in turn, leads back to increased performance. Additionally, cohesion is positively related to group member satisfaction, conformity, social support, group goals, and stability. Furthermore, research has shown that teams with higher cohesion scores can better deal with disruption than teams lower in cohesion. Teams that stay together tend to be more cohesive, which leads to improvements in performance (Beal, Cohen, Burke, & McLendon, 2003; Weinberg & Gould, 2011).

Several factors have been found to influence team cohesion, including the environment (team size, scholarships), personal factors (motivation,

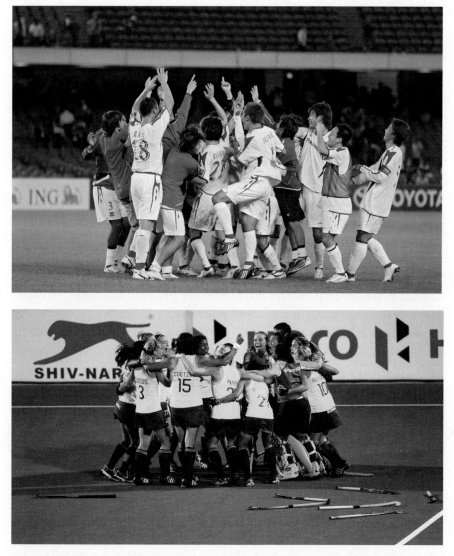

FIGURE 5-5 Cohesion is one of the main factors that influences team performance.

© FlashStudio/Shutterstock © epa european pressphoto agency b.v. / Alamy Stock Photo

social background), team factors (team norms, team stability), and leadership (the leader's style or goals). To build cohesion, coaches and leaders should communicate effectively, explain individual roles to team members, develop pride within smaller subgroups within the team (e.g., offense and defense), set challenging group goals (that group members have a say in), encourage group identity, avoid formation of social cliques, prevent excessive turnover, conduct periodic team meetings, know the team climate, and attempt to know something personal about each group member (Weinberg & Gould, 2011).

Research Methods in Sport Psychology

As was mentioned earlier, one of the primary responsibilities of those in the field of sport psychology is to advance the knowledge base through research. How do sport psychologists do that? A variety of research methods are available to researchers, and the choice of which method to use depends on the research question. At the most basic level, research can be divided into two types: quantitative and qualitative.

quantitative research
Research that generates numerical data and seeks to establish causal relationships between two or more variables by using statistical methods to test the strength and significance of the relationships.

With **quantitative research**, the researcher uses methods to explore human behavior that can be quantified, or put into numbers. In other words, a researcher might give an athlete a pregame anxiety questionnaire to assess the athlete's anxiety score, which gives an indication of how he is feeling. With **qualitative research**, the researcher explores behaviors and phenomena through methods that do not involve numbers in order to gain a more in-depth look at what is happening. In keeping with an earlier example, a researcher might decide to interview the athlete about his pregame anxiety rather than just giving a questionnaire. This approach allows researchers to examine the how and why behind behaviors rather than only obtaining a score that tells the level of a psychological factor.

qualitative research
Data collected and analyzed are expressed in the form of words or images to examine how people make sense of their world and the experience they have in the world.

Beyond the quantitative and qualitative distinctions in research, many different methods can be used to obtain information about the influence of psychological factors on sport performance. See **TABLE 5-3** to learn more about a few of the many methods that exist for conducting research.

Exercise psychology is a relatively new aspect of the field, but one that is evolving rapidly due to its life-enhancing promise among mainstream citizens not engaged in competitive sport and especially the aging. See **Boxes 5-1** and **5-2** for expert commentary on the future of exercise psychology.

TABLE 5-3   Research Methods Used by Sport Psychologists

Method	Description	Types of Research Questions Addressed	Examples
Questionnaires	Survey instruments that can assess demographic data and/or various psychological phenomena Psychological inventories	What is the athlete's level of confidence going into this competition? How do athletes rate their coach on communication?	Sport confidence inventories Pregame anxiety questionnaires Self-efficacy surveys
Interviews	Questions that allow a researcher to explore a psychological issue more deeply May be structured or unstructured	What is the experience of a rookie player like during his first year? How does burnout affect an athlete's motivation to go to practice?	Pre- and postgame interviews to capture the competition experience Preseason interviews with athletes to assess their perceptions of their teammates
Observations	Allow the researcher to observe a phenomenon without interfering with what is happening	What are the communication strategies used by team members during competition?	Coach behavioral observation checklists Communication assessments Aggression counts Positive and negative reinforcement tallies (counts)
Physiological measures	Usually done in a lab setting, allows the researchers to measure physiological processes that are happening	How does anxiety affect heart rate and sweat response?	Heart rate and blood pressure measures (e.g., EKGs, EEGs) Galvanic skin response (sweat rate) Neurotransmitter levels (e.g., serotonin, dopamine)
Content analysis	Researchers analyze large quantities of material from various sources, such as television, written media, or social media, in order to examine larger trends and patterns	What types of aggression are being displayed during NFL games? What are the types of coverage for female and male athletes?	Analysis of television content, magazine content, pictures, and/or social media traffic

Box 5-1 Exercise Psychology: Looking Toward the Future

Bonnie G. Berger

The exciting field of exercise psychology continues to grow as practitioners and researchers develop new directions and build on current ones. Many future directions in exercise psychology will result from a perplexing dilemma: there are so many benefits of exercise, and yet so few participants. We know that exercise is a major contributor to health, and yet a relatively small portion of the population exercises at the recommended level of 150 minutes/week of moderate-intensity exercise (American College of Sports Medicine, 2014). Resolving this dilemma of physical inactivity is a key initiative in exercise psychology and will continue to be an important goal into the future. More specifically, how can exercise psychologists, as well as physicians, physical therapists, exercise physiologists, athletic trainers, and teachers of physical education, successfully encourage more individuals to exercise on a regular basis to reap the benefits of physical activity?

Discovering the Joys of Exercise: The Hedonic Experience

In the future, a major focus of exercise psychology will be on discovering the joys of exercise, identifying the factors that contribute to making exercise meaningful, and encouraging diverse segments of the world's population to be physically active. By employing the theoretical approach of positive, or hedonic, psychology, which focuses on well-being rather than illness, exercise psychologists will lead clients in developing exercise programs that facilitate desirable experiences. The benefits of exercise include the ability to self-regulate mood, enhance the "feel good" sensation, promote enjoyment of the exercise experience, cherish peak moments and flow in exercise, and experience peak performances. Other hedonic exercise experiences include enhanced self-efficacy, feelings of competency, and self-esteem.

Another focus within exercise psychology will be to assist people to be successful in building on positive, hedonic exercise experiences to facilitate exercise adoption, participation, and adherence throughout the life span. Exercise psychologists will offer their expertise to diverse segments of the population, including all age groups, starting with toddlers and preschool-aged children, through the teen and young adult years, to mid-life adults and seniors. Additional segments of the population with whom exercise psychologists will work include underserved populations, such as underserved ethnic groups, and individuals who have illnesses such as heart disease, cancer, diabetes, osteoporosis, and clinical levels of depression and anxiety.

Educational Backgrounds of Specialists in Exercise Psychology

Specialists in exercise psychology primarily will employ positive psychology to help clients discover the hedonic contributions of exercise for their subjective well-being, health, and overall quality of life. To reach these lofty goals, specialists will approach the field from a variety of academic specialties. A few examples are listed below.

Kinesiology/Exercise Science

The academic areas of kinesiology and exercise science include courses in exercise psychology and diverse movement specialties. Examples of these courses include exercise physiology, biomechanics, motor development and learning, athletic training, and physical education teacher education. Integration of exercise psychology research and applied experiences with these movement specialties offers exercise psychologists a wonderful opportunity to coordinate body–mind processes within a somatopsychic approach. This somatopsychic approach emphasizes the influence of the body and exercise (*somato*) on the mind (*psychic*). Exercise psychology specialists with backgrounds in kinesiology and exercise science conduct research to further develop the field, and they also work with clients from the general population. Some exercise psychologists will be personal trainers in private practice and will facilitate mood alteration, stress management, and the enhancement of psychological well-being, resilience, flourishing, and overall quality of life in their clients.

Clinical and Health Psychology

The psychology specializations of clinical and health psychology enable psychologists to develop expertise in using exercise within a counseling or therapeutic setting, whether within independent practice or among clients within a hospital or clinic setting. Students in these psychology specializations develop skills for individual and group counseling and also conduct research concerning the mental benefits of physical activity. Characteristics of potential clients might include those with clinical levels of anxiety, depression, bipolar disorder, weight and body disturbances, and other psychological concerns. Diverse psychological approaches foster the incorporation of exercise in treating clinical and broad health concerns such as the role of

(continued)

exercise in the treatment and management of eating disorders, substance abuse, smoking cessation, overtraining, and exercise addiction.

Gerontology

The entire field of health sciences, and especially the subarea of gerontology, is another area of specialization that develops practitioners and researchers within exercise psychology. As the population ages, the importance of habitual exercise participation becomes more and more evident. Exercise can be used to enhance the quality of life in multiple segments of the older population by strengthening key movement abilities such as balance, strength, and cardiovascular endurance for activities of daily living as well as enhancing psychological well-being.

Conclusion

Exercise psychology is a rapidly expanding area of study that enables practitioners and researchers to have challenging and rewarding professional directions. In choosing this specialty, students can be a part of a movement that encourages more segments of the population to discover the joy of exercise throughout their life spans.

Reference

American College of Sports Medicine. (2014). *ACSM's guidelines for exercise testing and prescription* (9th ed.). Philadelphia, PA: Lippincott, Williams & Wilkins.

Box 5-2 Exercise Psychology: Where Are We Going as a Field?

Justine J. Reel and Robert A. Bucciere

The Future of Exercise Psychology

The critical area of exercise's influence on mental health will be central to the future of exercise psychology. Exercise psychologists need to move out of the lab and into the field so that they can be practitioners as well as researchers. One of the most significant specialty areas within the field of exercise psychology is the ability of physical activity to move the needle with respect to decreasing depression and anxiety and having a positive impact on mood. In the future, it will be important for exercise psychologists to join the treatment team of healthcare professionals that already includes a physician and mental health professional. We offer the following recommendations for advancing exercise psychology as a field.

Clinical Training

Currently, exercise psychologists are not adequately trained or equipped to deal with intense and complex mental health issues. Clinical depression should not be considered lightly. Exercise may be an adjunct form of treatment, but sometimes medication is necessary to reduce symptoms. Some individuals have symptoms of mania as well as depressed mood. Therefore, it is imperative that exercise psychologists acquire further training before entering into the clinical setting.

Exercise psychologists could bring an extremely useful perspective to the mental health field, given that exercise is beneficial and does not carry any negative side effects. However, exercise psychology students of 2016 and beyond need to have coursework in psychopathology and have an understanding of the current criteria of the *Diagnostic and Statistical Manual of Mental Disorders,* 5th edition (DSM-5; American Psychiatric Association, 2013). Coursework on ethics and on developing a supportive relationship with a client would also be helpful for preparing exercise psychology students for treatment teams.

Move out of the Lab and into Hospitals and Clinics

In the future, exercise psychologists will continue to be prominent researchers, but they will also practice in hospital and outpatient settings. The exercise psychologist could represent a new member of the treatment team, whose focus would be on promoting positive and recommended amounts of physical activity among clients. For certain individuals, such as those suffering from eating disorders, exercise may not be viewed in a positive way. In these cases, one's relationship with exercise may need to be retooled and modified to be healthy and sustainable.

Physical Activity Needs of Both Healthy and Disease Populations

Exercise psychology as a field has broad implications for the general population in promoting a healthy lifestyle and quality of life. Exercise has been shown to prevent many diseases as well as to assist with better sleep and enhanced mood. Exercise psychologists understand the research behind the motivations people cite to engage in physical activity as well as the need for an individualized approach that addresses each person based on willingness to engage in behavior change.

(continued)

For disease populations, exercise interventions have the potential to become a common "standard of care," just like a medication as part of the treatment plan. For example, when individuals are diagnosed with cancer or cardiac disease, they should be prescribed an individualized plan for exercise that meets their needs, ability level, and preferences. The monitoring of physical activity should be part of the therapeutic process in the way that medication supervision has been for traditional medicine. We are hopeful that using exercise as an evidence-based practice will help all individuals.

Interprofessional Education for Exercise Psychology Students

Physical activity has been shown to have a positive effect on both physical and mental health outcomes. Unfortunately, there continues to be a large chasm between the research and laboratory setting and applying findings to practice. Academic programs have inadequately prepared students to enter clinical settings when they graduate, but with the push for more interprofessional education (teaching students how to operate within interdisciplinary healthcare teams) this will likely change. Future students will have the ability to remain nimble. They will readily adapt from controlled research settings to applying those findings to individuals who are suffering from a variety of conditions. In summary, the medical field could truly benefit from having exercise psychologists serve as a regular presence on treatment teams.

Reference

American Psychiatric Association. (2013). *Diagnostic and statistical manual of mental disorders* (5th ed.). Arlington, VA: American Psychiatric Publishing.

CHAPTER SUMMARY

In this chapter, you have learned about the field of sport psychology: What it is, where it came from, how research is conducted, and an overview of the major topics within the field. As the field grows in knowledge and awareness, it is hoped that more and more individuals, teams, and coaches will take advantage of the vast knowledge that exists to help improve performance, both on and off the field. On that note, it is important to recognize that although it is called "sport" psychology, the principles can be applied in a variety of settings within the kinesiology field. See **Table 5-4** to see how you might use some of the techniques and/or knowledge from the field of sport psychology in your future career.

TABLE 5-4   Application of Sport Psychology Concepts by Field or Occupation

Field or Occupation	Application
Physical/occupational therapy	• Using motivational techniques to encourage clients to stick to therapy programs
Athletic training	• Using relaxation techniques to help an athlete get through a tough rehab exercise • Goal-setting
Coaching	• Understanding and applying knowledge about leadership, communication, and the use of a reward system to motivate athletes
Physical education	• Creating environments that are motivating to children for participating in activities • Using group dynamics principles to make sure students have a positive experience in their physical education class
Medicine (doctor, nurse, etc.)	• Applying relaxation and concentration techniques to be more precise in providing treatments/conducting surgeries • Communication techniques for speaking with patients
Fitness/wellness settings	• Using the theories of motivation when developing exercise programs

DISCUSSION QUESTIONS

1. Before sport psychology developed as a field, the only technique athletes and coaches had to fall back on was trial-and-error approaches. Do you think athletic performances would be at the level they are today without sport psychology knowledge?
2. Do you think that all three of these approaches are mutually exclusive? Can you think of any ways that at least two of the approaches could be utilized simultaneously by a coach or consultant in working with athletes, teams, or fitness participants?
3. Identify at least four different things that a coach or athlete could do or say to let the sport psychology consultant know that he or she believes the "myths" and does not have any belief that the PSD program will be a benefit. What are some steps you could take to offer assurance to the skeptical participant?

REFERENCES

Bandura, A. (1977). Self-efficacy: Toward a unifying theory of behavioral change. *Psychological Review, 84,* 191–215.

Bandura, A. (1986). *Social foundations of thought and actions: A social cognitive theory.* Englewood Cliffs, NJ: Prentice Hall.

Beal, D. J., Cohen, R. R., Burke, M. J., & McLendon, C. L. (2003). Cohesion and performance in groups: A meta-analytic clarification of construct relations. *Journal of Applied Psychology*, *88*(6), 989–1004.

Davis, S. F., Huss, M. T., & Becker, A. H. (1995). Norman Triplett and the dawning of sport psychology. *The Sport Psychologist*, *9*(4), 366–375.

Duda, J. L. (1989). Relationship between task and ego orientation and the perceived purpose of sport among high school athletes. *Journal of Sport & Exercise Psychology*, *11*(3), 313–335.

Dweck, C. S. (1986). Motivational processes affecting learning. *American Psychologist*, *41*, 1040–1048.

Festinger, L., Schachter, S., & Back, K. (1950). *Social pressures in informal groups: A study of human factors in housing.* Palo Alto, CA: Stanford University Press.

Gill, D. L. (1995). Women's place in the history of sport psychology. *The Sport Psychologist*, *9*, 418–433.

Gill, D., & Williams, L. (2008). *Psychological dynamics of sport and exercise* (3rd ed.). Champaign, IL: Human Kinetics.

Griffith, C. R. (1926). *Psychology of coaching: A study of coaching from the point of psychology.* New York: Scribner's.

Griffith, C. R. (1928). *Psychology and athletics: A general survey for athletes and coaches.* New York: Scribner's.

Hays, K. F. (1995). Putting sport psychology into (your) practice. *Professional Psychology: Research and Practice*, *26*(1), 33–40.

Heider, F. (1958). *The psychology of interpersonal relations.* New York: Wiley.

Jones, G., Hanton, S., & Connaughton, D. (2007). A framework of mental toughness in the world's best performers. *The Sport Psychologist*, *21*, 243–264.

Kaiseler, M., Polman, R., & Nicholls, A. (2009). Mental toughness, stress, stress appraisal, coping, and coping effectiveness in sport. *Personality and Individual Differences*, *47*(7), 728–733.

Karageorghis, C. I., & Terry, P. C. (2011). *Inside sport psychology.* Champaign, IL: Human Kinetics.

Kornspan, A. S. (2007). E.W. Scripture and the Yale Psychology Laboratory: Studies related to athletes and physical activity. *Sport Psychologist*, *21*(2), 152–169.

Kroll, W., & Lewis, G. (1970). America's first sport psychologist. *Quest*, *13*, 1–4.

Nicholls, J. (1984). Concepts of ability and achievement motivation. In C. Ames & R. Ames (Eds.), *Research on motivation in education: Student motivation.* (Vol. 1, pp. 39–73). New York: Academic Press.

Thomas, P. R., Murphy, S. M., & Hardy, L. (1999). Test of performance strategies: Development and preliminary validation of a comprehensive measure of athletes' psychological skills. *Journal of Sport Sciences*, *17*(9), 697–711.

Tuckman, B. W. (1965). Developmental sequence in small groups. *Psychological Bulletin*, *63*, 384–399.

Vealey, R. (2009). Sport and exercise psychology. In S. J. Hoffman (Ed.), *Introduction to kinesiology: Studying physical activity* (3rd ed.). Champaign, IL: Human Kinetics.

Weinberg, R. S., & Gould, D. (2011). *Foundations of sport and exercise psychology* (5th ed.). Champaign: Human Kinetics.

Weiner, B. (1985). An attribution theory of achievement motivation and emotion. *Psychological Review, 92,* 548–573.

Williams, J. M. E. (1993). *Applied sport psychology: Personal growth to peak performance.* Houston, TX: Mayfield Publishing.

CHAPTER 6

Exercise and Sport Physiology

KIM HENIGE

LEARNING OBJECTIVES

1. Describe the general scope of the field of exercise and sport physiology.
2. Describe the general history and major events of the field of exercise physiology in the United States.
3. Describe the importance of exercise physiology as a component of the kinesiology educational curriculum.
4. Define key terminology within exercise physiology.
5. Explain the general principles that form the basis of exercise physiology.
6. Describe and provide examples of the health- and skill-related components of physical fitness.
7. List and explain the principles of exercise training.
8. Identify careers related to exercise physiology.

KEY TERMS

activities of daily living (ADLs)
acute exercise effects
acute physiological responses
adenosine triphosphate (ATP)

chronic exercise effects
demand
exercise
exercise physiology

exercise physiology
The study of how the body responds and adapts to physical stress.

sport physiology
The application of exercise physiology principles to guide training and enhance sport performance.

acute exercise effects
Sudden and immediate responses to exercise.

chronic exercise effects
Gradual and long-term responses to exercise.

health-related components of physical fitness
instrumental activities of daily living (IADLs)
physical activity (PA)
physical fitness
physiological mechanisms
physiological training adaptations
principle of overload

principle of progression
principle of reversibility
principles of exercise training
skill-related components of physical fitness
sport physiology
stress
supply
supply equals demand

What Is Exercise and Sport Physiology?

Exercise physiology is the study of how the body responds and adapts to physical stress. Sport physiology is the application of exercise physiology principles to guide training and enhance sport performance. Exercise and sport physiology overlap significantly, and therefore are generally considered together. For the remainder of this chapter, the term *exercise physiology* will be used to encompass the areas of both exercise and sport physiology. Exercise is an intentional physical stress placed upon the body, producing both acute and chronic effects that can be studied. Acute exercise effects are sudden and immediate, whereas chronic exercise effects are gradual and long term. When you start jogging, the systems in your body (cardiovascular, respiratory, nervous, endocrine, etc.) immediately respond with acute changes (e.g., increased heart rate and breathing rate) that permit your body to meet the demands of the stress and perform the processes necessary for you to jog. If you jog regularly, the stress is placed upon the body chronically, and the body's systems respond over time with long-term physiological adaptations. Physiological adaptations result in less stress on the body's systems, greater efficiency of the systems, and improved physical performance during exercise and other types of physical activity.

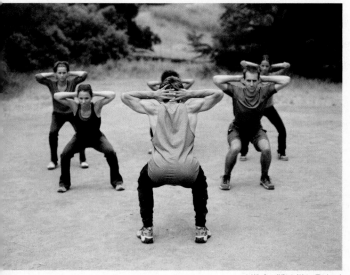
© Mike Powell/Digital Vision/Thinkstock

The History of Exercise Physiology in the United States

STOP AND THINK

How do you think exercise physiology relates to your specific career area of interest?

Exercise physiology is relatively new as a formal discipline; however, evidence suggests that individuals have been studying the physiological responses to physical activity as far back as ancient Greece. This historical review is a capsule summary and will focus on the modern history of exercise physiology, which first became formalized in the United States in the early 1800s when physiology textbooks began to appear.

In the earliest years of the field in the United States, one of the first texts published was *The Principles of Physiology Applied to the Preservation of Health and to the Improvement of Physical and Mental Education* by A. Combe in 1843. It included a limited amount of information on exercise. In 1855, William H. Byford published the first research paper on the physiology of exercise. In 1861, Edward Hitchcock at Amherst College was the first to collect anthropometric data before and after physical training.

Arguably one of the most significant years in the history of exercise physiology was the year 1886, when the American Association for the Advancement of Physical Education was founded. In the years following, exercise physiology began to enter the college curriculum at a number of colleges and universities. In the 1890s, Thomas Wood at Stanford University established a 4-year degree program in physical training and hygiene, which included exercise physiology as a major component. Around the same time, students majoring in physical education at Harvard, Stanford, and Oberlin were required to take exercise physiology courses.

In 1891, George W. Fitz at Harvard University was the first to establish a formal research laboratory for physical education in the United States. The name of the department was *Anatomy, Physiology, and Physical Training*. Part of the Lawrence Scientific School, it offered a 4-year Bachelor of Science (B.S.) degree and included both lecture and laboratory courses in exercise physiology. In 1900, the title of the department was changed to *Anatomy and Physiology*, and the focus shifted away from exercise physiology.

In 1898, the first edition of the *American Journal of Physiology* was published. In the early 1900s, several researchers began exploring exercise physiology and publishing information in the field. Exercise physiology labs began to open around the country, such as those founded at the

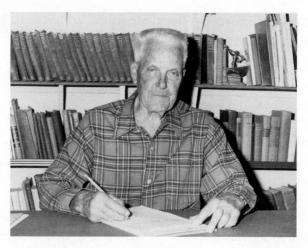

FIGURE 6-1   This is David Bruce ("DB") Dill. He was the founding director of Harvard's Fatigue Laboratory and he served as President of the American Physiological Society (APS).

© Elton and Madeline Garrett photo collection [Collection MSS 93–40 Photo Number 0265 0420]. Special Collections, University Libraries, University of Nevada, Las Vegas

University of Illinois, Springfield College, and Williams College. Exercise physiology established itself firmly as an academic discipline in 1927 when L. J. Henderson and G. E. Mayo established the Harvard Fatigue Laboratory (**FIGURE 6-1**) and named David Bruce "D.B." Dill the director. This lab became prominent and productive, publishing 50 papers in 20 years. Arguably, no lab since has obtained the same level of prestige. In the 1930s, several exercise physiology textbooks and the first issue of the physical education journal *Research Quarterly* were published.

The years from 1946 to 1962 have been termed the "embryonic years" of the exercise physiology discipline (Massengale & Swanson, 1997). As evidence of this growth, in 1946 there were 14 exercise/exertion citations in 5 professional journals and manuscripts, and by 1962 there were 128 citations in 51 professional journals and manuscripts. And as evidence of the increasing rigor and scientific basis of the field, in 1946 the Federation of American Societies for Experimental Biology (FASEB) national conference had a session dedicated to exercise physiology.

STOP AND THINK

What were some of the significant events that occurred during the early years of exercise physiology?

In 1947, the Harvard Fatigue Laboratory was closed because the president of the university, James B. Conant, felt that the lab would lose its value after the end of World War II. Many of the professors, staff, and graduate students from the lab went on to establish new exercise physiology labs across the United States. This event resulted in the expansion of exercise physiology labs across the country. The increase in the number of labs led to more research, and thus the need for new journals. In 1948, the American Physiological Society (APS) began publishing the *Journal of Applied Physiology*.

During this period, physical fitness emerged as a national concern. Thomas K. Cureton from Springfield College established the Physical Fitness Research Laboratory at the University of Illinois. Many of Cureton's graduates went on to research and leadership positions in physical education departments across the United States. Largely due to Cureton and his graduates, exercise physiology was recognized for its potential contribution to fitness.

George Williams College in Illinois and Springfield College in Massachusetts became known for their emphasis on exercise physiology in physical education and for their preparation of students for careers in the YMCA. Many graduates of these colleges went on to become important leaders in university and state organizations, significantly impacting exercise physiology as an academic discipline.

In 1954, the American College of Sports Medicine (ACSM) was established. The 11 founding members were physical educators and physicians, including A. H. Steinhaus from George Williams College and P. V. Karpovich from Springfield College, and one woman, Josephine L. Rathbone from Teachers College, Columbia University. ACSM was, and continues to be, instrumental in increasing the visibility and growth of the discipline of exercise physiology.

In 1956, the President's Council on Youth Fitness was established by President Dwight D. Eisenhower when it was discovered that 57% of American children had failed fitness tests. The name of the council has

STOP AND THINK

- Based on the events from 1946 to 1962, why do you think this period has been referred to as the "embryonic years"?

- What do you think was the most significant event of this time period? Why?

been changed several times over the years, most recently by President Barack Obama, who changed the name to the President's Council on Fitness, Sports & Nutrition in 2010 to reflect the expansion of the council's mission to include nutrition.

In 1960, the first exercise physiology textbook for graduate students, *Science and Medicine of Exercise and Sport*, was published. In 1961, the first exercise physiology project was funded by the National Institutes of Health (NIH). The project was entitled "Human Adaptation to Environmental and Exercise Stress."

The years from 1963 to 1976 have been termed the "formative years" (Massengale & Swanson, 1997). During this period, the visibility and credibility of exercise physiology continued to improve, and the number of textbooks, journals, and journal articles related to exercise physiology increased significantly.

In 1963, J. B. Conant published the Conant Report. The former president of Harvard University was critical of teacher training in the United States. In particular, he singled out physical education for its lack of academic rigor. In 1964, programs at large universities in the Pac-10 and Big 10 (and Penn State) began to implement more rigorous graduate programs and added exercise physiology emphases. Physical education departments began to collaborate with other science departments, and joint appointments for faculty were established. The academic credibility and recognition of exercise physiology improved significantly. However, immediate changes were not made to the curricula of undergraduate programs, and as a result, students were forced to take several science courses, not yet required by the undergraduate major, in order to qualify for graduate admission to exercise physiology programs.

Also in 1964, the NIH established the Applied Physiology Study Section to accommodate the increasing number of proposals for funding of physical fitness and exercise physiology research. Funding subsequently increased, which resulted in increased financial support for graduate students in exercise physiology. In 1969, the ACSM established a journal entitled, *Medicine and Science in Sports and Exercise*. The majority of the articles in this journal were to be related to exercise physiology.

In the early 1970s, physical education departments began changing their names (e.g., to kinesiology or exercise science) to better define their objectives and highlight the increasing emphasis on science-related courses and activities.

The years from 1977 to the present have been termed the "recognition years" (Massengale & Swanson, 1997). In 1977, the APS established a membership section for exercise physiologists. In 1983, it published a handbook of physiology dedicated to muscle physiology, and in 1996 it published a handbook of exercise physiology.

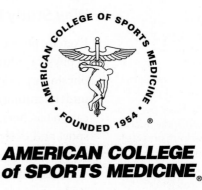

AMERICAN COLLEGE of SPORTS MEDICINE®

Courtesy of ACSM

Several new organizations related to exercise physiology were also established during this period. In 1978, the National Strength and Conditioning Association (NSCA) was established. In 1985, the American Association of Cardiovascular and Pulmonary Rehabilitation (AACVPR) was founded. In 1997, the American Society of Exercise Physiologists (ASEP) was established. Reflecting the field's rigor and focus on experimentation, in 2005 the ACSM was admitted into the Federation of American Societies for Experimental Biology (FASEB).

Women also began to take on more leadership roles in the field. In 1988, the ACSM elected its first female president, Barbara Drinkwater, from the Department of Medicine at Pacific Medical Center in Seattle, Washington. In 2002, the APS elected its first female president, Barbara Horwitz, from the University of California, Davis.

> ## STOP AND THINK
>
> - Based on the events from 1963 to 1976, why do you think this period has been referred to as the "formative years"?
>
> - What do you think was the most significant event of this period? Why?

In 2007, ACSM spearheaded its Exercise Is Medicine (EIM) initiative, based on the efforts of two physicians, Robert Sallis and Ronald Davis. The objective of EIM is "To make physical activity and exercise a standard part of a global disease prevention and treatment medical paradigm" (ACSM | EIM, n.d.). This initiative has resulted in a significant increase in the mainstream appreciation and attention given to the benefits of physical activity and the application of the principles of exercise physiology.

physical activity (PA)
Any type of bodily
movement.

**activities of daily
living (ADLs)**
The basic personal
tasks individuals
perform on a daily
basis.

**instrumental
activities of daily
living (IADLs)**
Daily activities
involved in
maintaining a
household.

exercise
A specific type of
physical activity
that is planned and
structured with the
explicit purpose of
improving physical
fitness.

Why Study Exercise Physiology?

Exercise physiology is one of many topics traditionally taught within the core of physical education, Kinesiology, and exercise science programs. Exercise physiology is an essential part of the curriculum because knowledge and understanding of the principles of exercise physiology enable physical education teachers, athletes, coaches, dance teachers, fitness trainers, and other sport and exercise science professionals to enhance physical performance and health through the application of the principles.

It is important to note that exercise physiology is not limited to the study of exercise and sport; it includes the study of the effects of any type of physical activity on the systems of the body. **Physical activity (PA)** includes any type of bodily movement, including **activities of daily living (ADLs)** and **instrumental activities of daily living (IADLs)**. ADLs are the basic personal tasks individuals perform on a daily basis, including dressing, bathing, grooming, using the toilet, eating, and moving around (**FIGURE 6-2**). IADLs are the daily activities involved in maintaining a household, including cooking, cleaning, and shopping (**FIGURE 6-3**). **Exercise**, a subset of physical activity, is planned and structured physical activity with the explicit purpose of improving physical fitness. Exercise physiology is not limited to improving performance during sport and exercise; it is also used to help individuals attain and maintain optimal health and independence through the life stages.

The American Society of Exercise Physiologists (ASEP, n.d.) classifies the scope of responsibilities of professional exercise physiologists into four

STOP AND THINK

- Based on the events of 1977 to the present, why do you think this period has been referred to as the "recognition years"?

- What do you think was the most significant event of this period? Why?

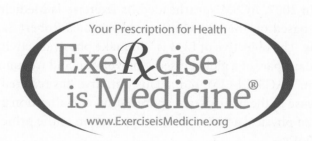

Your Prescription for Health

www.ExerciseisMedicine.org

Courtesy of Exercise is Medicine

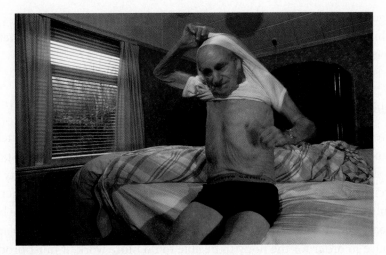

FIGURE 6-2   Getting dressed requires a certain amount of strength and flexibility.

© Clynt Garnham Lifestyle / Alamy Stock Photo

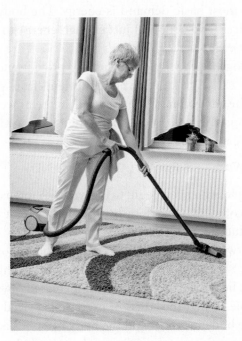

FIGURE 6-3   Housework requires a certain amount of muscle endurance and aerobic capacity.

© Piotr Marcinski/Shutterstock

categories: (1) to promote health and wellness, (2) to prevent illness and disability, (3) to restore health, and (4) to help athletes reach their potential in sports training and performance.

The Principles of Exercise Physiology

There are many sources of stress on the body, referred to as *stressors*, including anxiety, physical trauma, illness, and disease. **Stress** is the body's response to a stressor that interferes with normal physiology. Physical activity and exercise are also stressors on the body. When the body performs increasing intensities of physical activity, the stress level and demands on the body increase because it must do more work. The normal physiology is disrupted because in order for the body to be able to do more work, it must produce and use more energy:

$$\uparrow PA \rightarrow \uparrow Work \rightarrow \uparrow Energy\ (ATP)\ DEMAND$$

The body's most basic demand is energy. The body is efficient, and therefore produces (and supplies) just enough energy to meet the current demand (**supply equals demand**). **Supply** and **demand** are central themes in exercise physiology. The fuel the body uses to provide energy to do work is called **adenosine triphosphate (ATP)**. Food nutrients from your diet and oxygen (O_2) from the environment are used within the processes that produce most of the ATP used by your body. Therefore, as demand for ATP increases, demand for oxygen also increases:

$$\uparrow PA \rightarrow \uparrow Work \rightarrow \uparrow Energy\ (ATP)\ DEMAND \rightarrow \uparrow O_2\ DEMAND$$

As an example, when you begin to jog, your PA intensity level increases and the amount of work being done by the body increases. Therefore, your body must produce more ATP by using more oxygen.

One of the two major areas within exercise physiology is the study of the specific **acute physiological responses** that occur within the body's systems in order to help meet the demands of increased physical activity. The concept is simple. When the stress of exercise is placed on the body, the demands on the body increase, and the body responds acutely to increase the supply to meet the increased demand (i.e., supply = demand). During exercise, the greatest increase in demand is on the skeletal muscles (the muscles that cause bone and limb movement). For example, when you

---

stress
Response of the body to a stressor that interferes with normal physiology.

supply equals demand
When the amount of resources needed are matched by the amount made available; for example, when the amount of ATP needed is matched by the amount of ATP produced.

supply
Amount of resources made available; for example, the production of ATP.

demand
Amount of resources needed; for example, the need for ATP to do the required work.

adenosine triphosphate (ATP)
The body's fuel source.

acute physiological responses
The immediate effects on the body's systems in response to the stress of exercise.

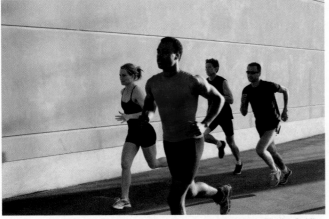

© Cultura Creative (RF) / Alamy Stock Photo

STOP AND THINK

- Why is knowledge and understanding of exercise physiology important for different careers? Provide specific examples.

- What is the difference between physical activity (PA) and exercise? Provide an example of each.

- How do activities of daily living (ADLs) and instrumental activities of daily living (IADLs) differ? Provide an example of each.

- According to the ASEP, what are the four items in the scope of responsibility of professional exercise physiologists? Why do you think ASEP chose each of these items?

start to jog, your breathing and heart rates increase. Did you ever stop to wonder why? One purpose of the increased breathing rate is to bring more oxygen into your lungs, and one purpose of the increased heart rate is to deliver the oxygen (carried in your blood) to the muscles at a faster rate (oxygen supply). Faster supply of oxygen to the muscles allows them to produce and use (supply) ATP at a faster rate in order to meet the higher demand for ATP so that the muscles can do more work:

$\uparrow$ PA $\rightarrow$ $\uparrow$ Work $\rightarrow$ $\uparrow$ Energy (ATP) DEMAND $\rightarrow$ $\uparrow$ O_2 DEMAND
$\uparrow$ Breathing Rate $\rightarrow$ $\uparrow$ O_2 Intake into Lungs
$\uparrow$ Heart Rate $\rightarrow$ $\uparrow$ O_2 Delivery to Muscles
$\uparrow$ O_2 Intake & Delivery $\rightarrow$ $\uparrow$ O_2 SUPPLY $\rightarrow$ $\uparrow$ ATP Production & Usage $\rightarrow$ $\uparrow$ ATP SUPPLY
SUPPLY = DEMAND

Exercise physiology explains why the breathing and heart rates increase during exercise, the **physiological mechanisms** the body uses to cause these increases, and the mechanisms the body uses to precisely match supply with demand.

The second major area of study in exercise physiology is how the body responds to repeated stress through chronic physiological adaptations. The body resists stress, so when a stress becomes chronic, as with regular exercise, the body finds ways to resist the stress. Stress resistance is accomplished with physiological changes within the systems; these changes are referred to

physiological mechanisms
Interacting processes within the body that bring about one or more effects.

physiological training adaptations
Long-term changes within the systems of the body in response to the stress of exercise.

as *physiological adaptations*. After these adaptations occur, the body's systems experience less stress in response to the stressor (i.e., physical activity). In exercise physiology, **physiological training adaptations** are those adaptations that occur in response to the stress of exercise. Returning to our previous example, your heart rate increases when you start to jog. One reason the heart rate increases is to increase the delivery rate of oxygen to the muscles so they can make and use more ATP (increased supply to meet the increased demand). An increased heart rate stresses the cardiovascular system. If you jog on a regular basis, adaptations within the cardiovascular system result in a lower heart rate while jogging at the same intensity. This means that the body is able to meet the same demand (i.e., same jogging intensity, same demand for ATP and oxygen) with less stress. The lower heart rate means that there is less stress on the cardiovascular system, and therefore the body has accomplished its goal, which was to reduce the stress caused by the stressor. Exercise physiology explains the mechanisms the body's systems use to respond to chronic stress with physiological adaptations that resist future stress.

Physiological training adaptations occur because the body resists stress. The adaptations do, in fact, reduce stress on the body systems, but they also have other positive side effects. As a result of training adaptations, the body becomes more efficient, which means it can perform the same amount of work with less energy. Training adaptations, including better efficiency result in an increased ability to perform physical activity, which can improve an athlete's performance in his or her sport or an older adult's ability to carry his or her own groceries. In addition, exercise adaptations strengthen the body's systems, making them more resistant to illness and disease, resulting in a lower risk for many diseases and better general overall health.

STOP AND THINK

- Use complete sentences to explain the following relationships:

  $\uparrow$ PA $\rightarrow$ $\uparrow$ Work $\rightarrow$ $\uparrow$ Energy (ATP) DEMAND $\rightarrow$ $\uparrow$ O_2 DEMAND

  $\uparrow$ Breathing Rate $\rightarrow$ $\uparrow$ O_2 Intake into Lungs

  $\uparrow$ Heart Rate $\rightarrow$ $\uparrow$ O_2 Delivery to Muscles

  $\uparrow$ O_2 Intake & Delivery $\rightarrow$ $\uparrow$ O_2 SUPPLY $\rightarrow$ $\uparrow$ ATP Production & Usage $\rightarrow$ $\uparrow$ ATP SUPPLY

  SUPPLY = DEMAND

- What is adenosine triphosphate (ATP)? What is its role in enabling physical activity?

- When PA intensity level increases, what happens to the demand for ATP? Why?

- When PA intensity level increases, what happens to the demand for oxygen (O_2)? Why?

- What are some of the acute physiological responses within the body that contribute to an increased supply of O_2?

- Define and explain *physiological mechanisms*.

- What are physiological training adaptations?

- Why does the body adapt? What are the benefits to the body?

The Components of Physical Fitness

When you exercise, probably without realizing it, you intentionally place stress on your body, hoping that it will respond and adapt. When you say you want to become more "fit," you are usually expressing your desire to improve one or more of your health-related components of fitness through physiological adaptation. **Physical fitness** is a set of physiological attributes that reflect the ability of the systems of the body to support physical activity. The **health-related components of physical fitness** are those components that have been shown to have a relationship with good physical health and the prevention of many types of disease (**TABLE 6-1**).

Another category of fitness components that generally receive less consideration in a general exercise program, but that are still affected by physiological adaptation, are the **skill-related components of physical fitness** (**TABLE 6-2**). The skill-related components of physical fitness are related to sport and motor-skill performance.

physical fitness
Physiological attributes that reflect the ability of the systems of the body to support physical activity.

health-related components of physical fitness
The components of physical fitness that are associated with good physical health, including body composition, muscular strength, muscular endurance, aerobic capacity, and flexibility.

TABLE 6-1   Health-Related Components of Physical Fitness

Component	Description
Aerobic capacity	The ability to perform prolonged, large-muscle, dynamic exercise at moderate to high levels of intensity
Body composition	The proportion of total body weight made up of fat mass and fat-free mass
Flexibility	The ability of the joints to move freely through their normal range of motion
Muscular endurance	The ability of skeletal muscles to repeatedly generate force
Muscular strength	The ability of skeletal muscles to generate force

TABLE 6-2   Skill-Related Components of Physical Fitness

Component	Description
Agility	The ability to change body position quickly and accurately
Balance	The ability to maintain steady body posture
Coordination	The ability to perform physical tasks smoothly and accurately
Power	The ability of the muscles to generate force quickly
Reaction time	The ability to respond to a stimulus quickly
Speed	The ability to move quickly

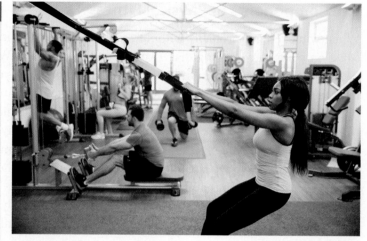

© Monkey Business Images/Shutterstock

skill-related components of physical fitness The components of physical fitness that are associated with good sport and motor-skill performance.

principles of exercise training Foundational guidelines for planning an exercise program that successfully leads to the desired physiological adaptations without causing undo stress and/or injury.

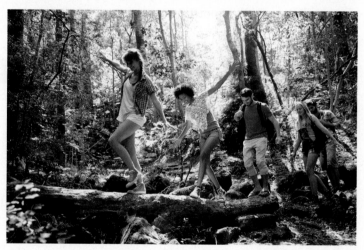

© Monkey Business Images/Shutterstock

The Principles of Exercise Training

As stated previously, one of the reasons people exercise is to improve their physical fitness. The **principles of exercise training** are the foundational guidelines for planning an exercise program so that it successfully leads to the desired improvements without causing undue stress and/or injury. The principles of exercise training have been established from evidence-based scientific knowledge of the stimuli and physiological responses that lead to physiological adaptations, and therefore improvements in fitness. Whether you are a physical education teacher, sport coach, strength and conditioning coach, dance teacher, fitness trainer, or fitness instructor, knowledge, understanding, and application of these principles are essential for your professional success.

The primary, overarching principle of exercise training is the **principle of overload**, which states that the body must be stressed to a level beyond which it is normally accustomed in order to stimulate physiological training adaptations. Overload is essentially the stress that we discussed earlier. The body is stressed when it is forced to do something that it is not accustomed to. When the body and its systems are stressed regularly, the body detects the pattern of stress and responds by making physiological changes (adaptations) to resist the stress. For each fitness component, tests can be used to measure physiological adaptations to exercise. For example, one test of cardiorespiratory endurance is the step test. During the step test, we measure the heart rate response to stepping up and down for 3 minutes. When you first start a jogging program, the cardiovascular system is overloaded because it is forced to deliver oxygen at a rate that is higher than it is accustomed to. Part of the overload in this situation is that the heart has to contract (beat) faster. The high heart rate puts stress on the heart, and if the heart rate is raised long and often enough, the cardiovascular system will respond with physiological adaptations that result in a lower heart rate when jogging at the same intensity. This training adaptation can be measured by performing the step test again, after several weeks of training.

It is important to note that not all physical activity causes overload, because your body is "accustomed" to activities you do often. For example, if you walk 1–2 miles around campus every day, walking this distance will not overload your body and stimulate physiological changes. However, if someone is sedentary and moves around very little each day, walking 1–2 miles will likely cause an overload, and if done regularly will result in adaptations. If you want your exercise program to result in training adaptations, it must consist of physical activity that your body is not accustomed to. In addition, as you exercise regularly over time, your body adapts, plateaus, and eventually becomes "accustomed" to the exercise. When that occurs you must increase the intensity of the exercise stress such that it, again, becomes a physical activity that your body is not accustomed to. This is called the

principle of overload
The body must be stressed to a level beyond that to which it is normally accustomed in order to stimulate physiological training adaptations.

principle of progression
As the body adapts to exercise, the exercise intensity must be increased in order to continue to stimulate physiological training adaptations.

principle of reversibility
When an exercise stress is removed, the physiological training adaptations to that stress are lost.

principle of progression. You must progress the overload as your body adapts. For example, the stress of jogging can be increased many ways, including increasing the speed, grade (run up hills), duration (more minutes per session), or frequency (more sessions per week).

Just as the body recognizes a pattern of stress and subsequently adapts, it also recognizes when that stress has been removed. If you jog regularly over time, adapt, lowering your exercise heart rate, and then stop your jogging routine, your body will reverse its adaptations. As mentioned earlier, the body adapts to resist tress, but if the stress is no longer present, the physiological systems no longer maintain the adaptations, and therefore they are lost. Because it strives for efficiency, the body will not exert its energy and resources to maintain an unnecessary physiological adaptation. This is called the **principle of reversibility**, which is sometimes referred to by the saying "use it or lose it."

Other exercise training principles exist, but they are beyond the scope of this chapter. In other courses, you will learn more about the principles explained above, as well as other principles, such as the principles of specificity, individuality, and overtraining. All of these principles come from evidence-based scientific data about the physiological responses to exercise.

What Can You Do with a Degree in Exercise Physiology?

Students typically struggle in their quest to discover career options related to exercise physiology because job titles are rarely labeled "exercise physiologist." However, exercise physiology concepts make up the basis for understanding the human body and how it responds to the stresses of life, including exercise and disease. Therefore, individuals with a degree in exercise physiology are employed in a wide variety of career areas that can be categorized as clinical, fitness, research, sport, and teaching. See **TABLE 6-3** for a list of some of these careers and **TABLE 6-4** for a list of research areas related to exercise physiology.

Although there are many exercise physiology–related careers, many of the career paths require additional schooling and/or certification beyond

TABLE 6-3   Career Areas Related to Exercise Physiology

Career Area	Career
Clinical	Athletic trainer
	Cardiac rehabilitation specialist
	Chiropractor
	Massage therapist
	Medical doctor/osteopathic doctor
	Nurse/nurse practitioner
	Occupational therapist
	Occupational therapy assistant
	Physical therapist
	Physical therapy assistant
	Physician assistant
	Podiatrist
	Pulmonary rehabilitation specialist
	Recreational therapist
Fitness	Adapted physical activity specialist
	Business owner/entrepreneur
	Community physical activity specialist
	Corporate fitness specialist
	Director of wellness and health promotion
	Fitness consultant
	Fitness writer
	Group fitness trainer
	Master trainer
	Personal trainer
	Public health physical activity specialist
	Senior fitness specialist
	Wellness coach
	Wellness director
Research	Academia
	Military
	Olympic Training Center
	Pharmaceuticals
	Sports equipment companies

(continues)

TABLE 6-3   Career Areas Related to Exercise Physiology (*continued*)

Career Area	Career
Sport	Athlete
	Coach
	Dance teacher
	Sports nutritionist
	Strength and conditioning specialist
Teaching	College
	Fitness workshop presenter
	Health educator
	High school teacher

a bachelor's degree. Students should research the various career options early (as freshmen and sophomores) to evaluate practicality and feasibility in terms of personal interest and strengths. Early preparation also provides time to plan appropriately for graduate schooling and certification, if necessary.

STOP AND THINK

- For each career area in Table 6-3, choose one specific career you think you would enjoy the most and explain why.

- For each career area in Table 6-3, choose one specific career that you think you would be most successful at and explain why.

- Can you think of any other careers related to exercise physiology that are not listed in Table 6-3?

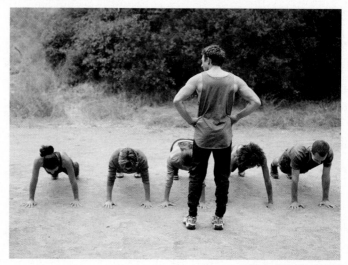

© Mike Powell/Digital Vision/Thinkstock

Areas of Research in Exercise Physiology

TABLE 6-4   Areas of Research in Exercise Physiology

Area of Research	Example Research Topics
Exercise testing	Fitness assessment Performance assessment Physical activity assessment
Exercise training	Aerobic training Anaerobic training Athletic performance training Exercise prescription Flexibility training Muscular endurance training Muscular strength training
Bioenergetics and muscle metabolism	Carbohydrate metabolism Energy expenditure Lipid metabolism
Body composition	Energy balance Obesity Weight control
Clinical exercise physiology	Clinical exercise prescription Clinical exercise testing Exercise epidemiology Exercise immunology
Disease	Alzheimer's disease Arthritis Cancer Depression Heart disease Hypertension Stroke Type II diabetes
Environmental physiology	Altitude Diving Space travel Thermoregulation

(continues)

TABLE 6-4   Areas of Research in Exercise Physiology *(continued)*

Area of Research	Example Research Topics
Fatigue	Central nervous system fatigue Muscular fatigue Neuromuscular fatigue
Gender differences	Performance differences Training differences
Lifespan	Senior fitness and aging Youth fitness and development
Occupational physiology	Fire and rescue Law enforcement Military
Physical activity and health promotion	Community health Public health Schools Workplace health
Rehabilitation	Cardiac rehabilitation Occupational therapy Physical therapy Respiratory therapy
Sports nutrition	Ergogenic aids In-competition nutrition Precompetition nutrition Recovery nutrition Supplements
Systems exercise physiology	Bone and connective tissue physiology Cardiovascular physiology Cellular and molecular physiology Endocrine physiology Neural physiology Respiratory physiology Skeletal muscle physiology

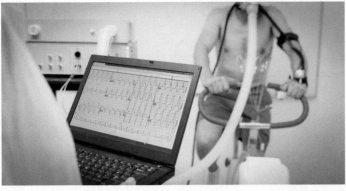

© wavebreakmedia/Shutterstock

STOP AND THINK

- For each area of research in Table 6-4, what are some specific issues related to exercise physiology that may be studied?

- Can you think of any other research areas related to exercise physiology that are not listed in Table 6-4?

CHAPTER SUMMARY

In this chapter, you have learned that exercise physiology is the study of how the body responds and adapts to physical stress. Exercise is an intentional physical stress placed upon the body. Within the field, both acute and chronic exercise effects are studied. Although exercise physiology is relatively new as a formal discipline, it has likely been studied as far back as the ancient Greeks. Currently, exercise physiology is one of many topics traditionally taught within the core of physical education, kinesiology, and exercise science programs. Exercise physiology is an essential part of the curriculum because knowledge and understanding of it permits physical education teachers, athletes, coaches, dance teachers, fitness trainers, and other sport and exercise science professionals to enhance physical performance and health through the application of exercise physiology principles. Some of the core principles that form the basis of exercise physiology include stress and supply and demand as they relate to physical activity, energy (ATP) use, and physiological training adaptations. The principles of exercise are the foundational guidelines, based on evidence-based science, for planning a successful exercise program. The principles of overload, progression, and reversibility were also discussed in this chapter. Individuals with a degree in exercise physiology are employed in a wide variety of career areas that can be categorized as clinical, fitness, research, sport, and teaching.

DISCUSSION QUESTIONS

1. Describe the study of exercise physiology and explain how it differs from sport physiology.
2. Briefly explain the evolution of exercise physiology as a discipline in the United States.

3. Why is exercise physiology a core curricular component of most kinesiology programs?
4. Explain the terms stress, demand, supply, response, mechanism, and adaptation as they relate to the basic underlying principles of exercise physiology.
5. What is the difference between acute and chronic exercise effects?
6. What is the difference between the health- and skill-related components of physical fitness?
7. What is the purpose of the principles of exercise training?
8. For each career area in Table 6-3, randomly choose a specific career and describe the characteristics you think an individual must have in order to be successful in that career and explain why you think those characteristics are important.
9. Why do you think it is important to both enjoy and be good at your career? What would be some of the consequences if you did not like your career or were not good at it? Consider the consequences for you, your coworkers, your patients/clients, and your family.

REFERENCES

ACSM | EIM. Exercise is Medicine®: A global health initiative. Retrieved 31 August 2016, from http://exerciseismedicine.org

American Society of Exercise Physiologists. (n.d.) Standards of practice. Retrieved from https://www.asep.org/index.php/organization/practice/

Massengale, J. D., & Swanson, R. A. (eds.). (1997). *The history of exercise and sport science.* Champaign, IL: Human Kinetics.

OTHER RESOURCES

www.acsm.org
www.asep.org
www.healthinaging.org/resources/resource:eldercare-at-home-problems-of-daily-living/
www.nsca.org
www.the-aps.org

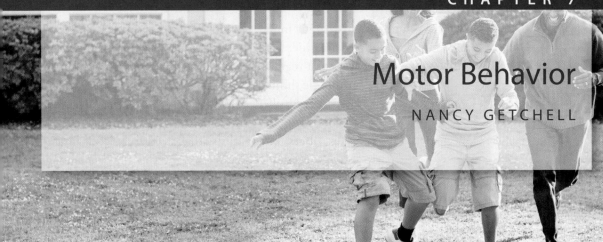

CHAPTER 7

Motor Behavior

NANCY GETCHELL

LEARNING OBJECTIVES

1. Explain the general scope of the field of motor behavior.
2. Outline the contemporary history of motor behavior.
3. Identify the subdisciplines within motor behavior.
4. Describe the theoretical perspectives within motor behavior.
5. Explain how researchers study motor behavior.
6. List some of the careers related to motor behavior.

KEY TERMS

Fitts's law
information processing
longitudinal study
motor behavior
motor control

motor development
motor learning
motor performance
nature versus nurture

What Is Motor Behavior?

Every day, and often without much thought, people face many different movement challenges. Consider this simple example: In order to lift a cup of coffee to your lips, you must regulate 23 arm and 25 hand muscles. Within each muscle, hundreds of muscle fibers and motor units need to be controlled. Quickly, a simple task becomes complex when you consider all the separate elements (limbs, muscles, fibers, motor units) that need to be coordinated to move successfully. Yet, day in and day out, we manage these everyday movements remarkably well. One of the most fundamental aspects of the human body is its ability to move effectively in a frequently changing environment. Humans move constantly, whether consciously (e.g., to eat, type a text message, walk) or unconsciously (e.g., to breathe, maintain upright balance, blink). When you think about it, the fact that we move successfully most of the time is remarkable! Understanding how people move—how they control their bodies, how they learn new skills or relearn lost ones, and how their movement changes from infancy through older adulthood—is the purpose of the field of study known as **motor behavior** (Magill, 2013).

BASIC BUILDING BLOCKS OF THE STUDY OF MOTOR BEHAVIOR

Motor behavior, as a field of study, relates to the different ways in which humans control their movement. These include both psychological and physiological processes, which require different research methods. We call movement **motor performance**, which simply means observable actions that humans make when trying to accomplish a task (Schmidt & Lee, 2014). For example, when you walk to class, your walk is your motor performance. In motor behavior, we study the conscious decision making that goes into that walk as well as the neuroanatomy used to move the body.

Motor behavior also is an umbrella term used to describe a group of related subdisciplines. All the subdisciplines focus on human movement control, but do so in different time frames. **Motor control** is primarily related to motor performance at a given point in time (Schmidt & Lee, 2014). Going back to our coffee cup example, the way in which the coffee drinker

---

STOP AND THINK

For the following, think about your family and friends.

- Is there any time, in daily life, that they seem aware of the complexity of the movement activity in which they are engaged?

- Do you see differences and similarities between family and friends in how they are aware of the complexity of movement?

- Does it matter whether they have this awareness?

---

motor behavior
Study of how humans move, including control, acquisition of skills, and change throughout the lifespan.

motor performance
Observable actions that humans make when performing a task.

motor control
Study of motor performance at a given point in time.

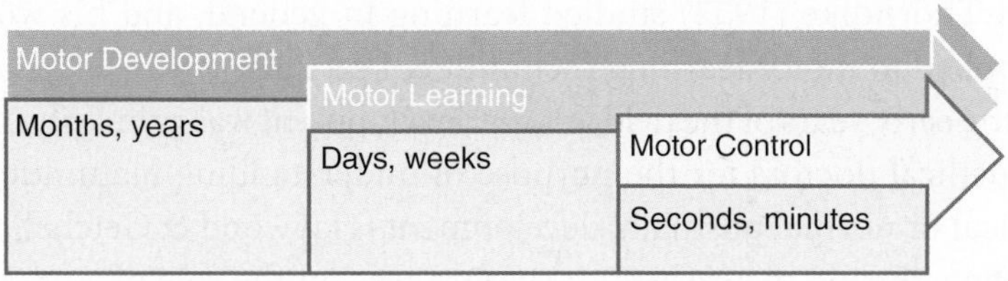

FIGURE 7-1   The different time frames of the motor behavior subdisciplines.

controls hand, wrist, arm, and trunk movements to successfully lift the cup to the lips falls under the domain of motor control. Another important area of study involves how people learn to move effectively. This process takes time (e.g., days, weeks, months) and practice. The subdiscipline focused on these processes is called **motor learning** (Magill, 2013). Finally, **motor development** involves changes in motor performance over longer time periods (e.g., months or years), and includes processes in addition to practice, such as growth and maturation (Haywood & Getchell, 2014). In sum, the three subdisciplines are tied together in that they relate to how humans control movements, but differ with regards to the time frame over which motor performance is observed (**FIGURE 7-1**). We will discuss the specific subdisciplines in detail later in the chapter.

motor learning
Study of the acquisition of skills for effective movement over time and with practice.

motor development
Study of the change of performance over time, including growth and development factors as well as practice.

Contemporary History of Motor Behavior as an Area of Inquiry

Because effective motor performance is essential for human survival, motor behavior has been a topic of informal study throughout history. Researchers began studying motor behavior as a formal area of inquiry more recently, early in the 20th century. Charles Sherrington, an early researcher in the field, was interested in understanding the nervous system. In 1906, he published a book titled *The Integrative Action of the Nervous System*, in which he described the action of reflexes and how they help to create coordinated movement. His work represented a landmark in the physiological study of motor control, and it is still referenced today. With regards to the psychology of motor behavior, experimental psychologists such as R. A. Woodworth (1899) began to examine the behavioral aspects of motor control, such as how movement speed and accuracy of motor performance are interactive.

Edward Thorndike (1932) studied learning in general, and his work has been applied to motor learning (Schmidt & Lee, 2011).

In the early years of the field, motor development was primarily of interest to medical doctors for the purpose of understanding maturation during typical or normal postnatal development (Haywood & Getchell, 2014). One debate during the early 20th century was on the role of **nature versus nurture** (i.e., genes versus environment and upbringing) in human development. Researchers found a clever way to study the impact of nature and nurture: They examined twins in so-called co-twin control studies. Identical twins were considered to have identical genes, so researchers could determine the impact of the environment by altering the experiences of one of the twins. In these studies, the performance of each twin was measured prior to beginning the research, then one twin received specific training (thus enhancing the environment) over some time period. Performance was then measured at the end of the study. Any differences in the twins' performance were then attributed to the environment (Clark & Whitall, 1989). Arnold Gesell (Gesell & Thompson, 1934) and Myrtle McGraw (McGraw, 1943) were two leaders in the study of twins. You may be wondering how this relates to motor development, which is understandable! Remember, interest was in early development, and motor development provides a window into overall development during the first 3 or so years of life, before young children can speak.

World War II (1939–1945) marked the beginning of motor behavior research on a large scale. During the war, military analysts were interested in finding ways to determine who would perform best in different military positions (e.g., pilots, gunners, strategists) and how these servicemen could be better trained. Fatigue was of particular concern, given the long hours and strenuous task demands on military personnel. Aircraft were used extensively during the war, and questions related to the motor performance of pilots, such as who would make the best pilot and what was the most effective flight training, became critically important (Edwards, 2010).

After World War II, the different subdisciplines began to come together under the umbrella term *motor behavior*. Interest in motor performance grew beyond military needs, and the range of research broadened substantially into sport, work, and rehabilitation. For example, Paul Fitts (1954) studied the relationship between speed and accuracy in aiming tasks, a relationship so robust it is known as **Fitts's law**.

nature versus nurture
Study of the effects of genetic predisposition on performance versus the effects of environmental factors.

Fitts's law
The label for the observed, and exceedingly robust, relationship between speed and accuracy in motor tasks.

Franklin Henry, from the University of California at Berkeley, often receives credit as one of the founders of the field of motor behavior (Schmidt & Lee, 2011). Researchers in the fields of kinesiology, physical education, and sport sciences were becoming increasingly interested in the study of motor behavior. Henry believed that kinesiology and physical education had to be based on empirically derived facts and scientific knowledge, leading to the creation of many research areas we know today, such as biomechanics, exercise physiology, and motor behavior. During the 1950s and 1960s, physical educators such as G. Lawrence Rarick and Anna Espenscade (both of Berkeley) studied motor performance changes during childhood and adolescence, and Ruth Glassow used biomechanics to study developmental change in motor performance (Haywood & Getchell, 2014). Interest grew in theories of motor control and learning. In 1971, Jack Adams proposed his closed-loop theory of motor learning, which Dick Schmidt expanded upon in 1975 in his schema theory. The intricacies of these elegant theories will be covered in detail in later courses you may take in kinesiology.

> ### STOP AND THINK
>
> A great deal of our movements in daily life go completely unrecognized. This changes dramatically when a person loses a limb or has other impairments in body function as a result of an accident or military action. Reflect on the likely increase in motor behavior personnel in hospitals and veterans' treatment contexts during the past decade.

During a period of the 1970s, the **information processing** perspective drove much of the research in motor behavior. In a nutshell, this theory proposes that humans act like computers, and heavily emphasizes the role of the brain and central nervous system (CNS) in controlling movements (Magill, 2014). Researchers used this analogy to understand motor performance and examined the impact of sensory input, decision making, the number of choices, and the like on the speed, efficiency, and accuracy of movements. Not all researchers followed this perspective. The Russian scientist Nicholas Bernstein, a neurophysiologist, questioned the role of the CNS as the dominant control structure in coordinated movement. His work, published in English posthumously in 1967, sparked a theoretical debate, which resulted in an alternative theoretical perspective known as the dynamic pattern perspective. This perspective uses the mathematics of complex systems as well as an ecological-psychological approach to examine motor performance. Researchers such as Michael Turvey (1980) of Yale University and J. Scott Kelso (1995) of Florida Atlantic University have spent their careers studying the coordination and control of movement using this perspective.

information processing
A focus on the brain and nervous system in the control of movement; views the brain as a computer.

Major Topics in Motor Behavior and Research Approaches

Today, researchers continue to use experimental methods along with other approaches to better understand how humans develop, learn, and move on a day-to-day basis. There is no one correct way to study motor behavior, and in fact the different perspectives have helped push the field forward not only in understanding of movement, but also in creating effective interventions for developing and learning motor skills. In general, motor behavior research starts with movement as its fundamental level of analysis; that is, researchers start with the movement, and then attempt to describe something about the movement using a psychological or physiological basis for their explanation. This approach could be described as "outside-in." Compare this to a more neurophysiological approach, which may start "in" at the level of the anatomical structures, such as neurons or muscle spindles, and work "out" to the movement (**FIGURE 7-2**).

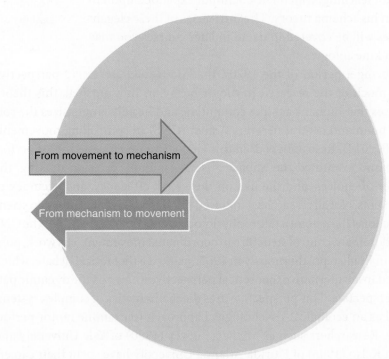

FIGURE 7-2   The outside-in approach.

As mentioned earlier, the three primary subdisciplines of motor behavior are motor control, learning, and development. The differences between these subdisciplines are related to the time frames addressed, which then translate into different types of research questions. Researchers interested in motor control tend to focus on motor performance at one time or over a period of seconds or minutes. Those who study motor learning focus on longer time periods, such as hours, days, and weeks. For example, participants in a study may be given an intervention, such as feedback and/or instruction, to facilitate learning. Motor development research focuses on longer time periods, often months or years. For example, a motor development study may focus on the development of throwing skills in children from 2 to 12 years old. Clearly, the subdisciplines have some overlap among them, which is why the umbrella term *motor behavior* is helpful in identifying the overall area of study.

STOP AND THINK

For each subdiscipline (motor development, motor learning, and motor control), devise a way to study the motion of pitching a baseball or softball.

MOTOR CONTROL

Motor control research often begins with a movement of interest and then focuses on some key aspect of how that movement is regulated (Haywood, Roberton, & Getchell, 2012). The movement can be an activity of daily living, such as reaching for and grasping an object; or a sport skill, such as a throw. It can also occur in populations with and without disabilities or diseases. For example, a researcher might ask, "When a person picks up a beverage can, how does he determine the optimal grip force so that he doesn't crush the can?" Another question might be, "What is the optimal relationship between club velocity and arm force in a golf putt?" Other important questions can relate to the process of coordinating different limbs to produce a complex movement such as running. Research tools vary widely, and often overlap into other areas of study. For example, a motor control researcher may use electromyography, motion analysis, or force platforms as methods of explaining motor control. Frequently, researchers will use mathematical models to describe relationships among different variables related to movement.

Another important aspect of motor control research is neurophysiology, particularly when researchers examine different patient populations who have suffered CNS damage. Researchers may investigate deficits in motor control when certain structures are damaged. By comparing these to "normal" movements, researchers can learn a lot about the function of the damaged structure.

MOTOR LEARNING

In motor learning studies, the researcher's interest lies not in motor performance per se, but what lies behind the change in motor performance over practice or training sessions (Schmidt & Lee, 2014). Motor learning can be described as a change in the capability for motor performance as a result of practice or experience. Oftentimes, researchers look to the brain and the CNS as being responsible for this change; the change should be relatively permanent. Many motor learning studies involve some sort of intervention that occurs over a period of time. For example, researchers might examine the impact of different practice schedules on learning, asking the question, "Is learning facilitated by practicing the same skill over and over in a block?" or "Will a novice basketball player benefit from varying shot position on the floor?" Other researchers might examine the type or amount of feedback that the learner gets, asking "Is it better to know the success or failure of your movement or how you move?" Again, research methods often involve tools used in other disciplines, such as biomechanics, sport psychology, or exercise physiology. Motor learning research can involve people of all ages, including children. However, motor learning research that uses children as participants isn't the same as motor development research, because it focuses on shorter time periods as well as on experience and practice.

MOTOR DEVELOPMENT

Motor development research focuses on change in motor performance over time and the factors that underlie that change (Haywood & Getchell, 2014). As compared to motor learning, motor development research tends to be focused on the "bigger" picture, factoring in growth, maturation, and other factors into the long-term change. Recently, focus has been placed on the interaction of individuals, environments, and tasks in driving motor development. For example, a question asked by a researcher who studies motor development might be "What changes in muscular strength can be associated with the onset of walking in infants?" or "Will changing the size of objects in the environment change the way an infant crawls?" Motor development research is not focused exclusively on infancy; in fact, these types of studies can involve people of all ages. The gold standard for motor development research is the **longitudinal study**, where several individuals are followed for long periods of time, either months or years. These types of studies enable researchers to track the impact of different variables related to individual, task, or environment in different participants over time. Research tools from other disciplines are often used, just as with motor control and learning research.

longitudinal study
Observational research method where data are gathered from the same subjects repeatedly over a long period of time.

How Can You Use Motor Behavior in Your Career?

Anyone who has an interest in the effectiveness and efficiency of motor performance can use motor behavior principles and practices in their profession. Knowledge of general motor behavior principles will give practitioners some specific rules about how people move. A great example of this is Fitts's law, which states (in general) that as movement speed increases, accuracy decreases, and vice versa. This information can be used to help athletes find a balance between moving fast and moving accurately. Those interested in youth sport or pediatric rehabilitation can examine children's motor behaviors and compare them to age norms to look for motor delays. Essentially, anyone who wants to affect movement efficiency and performance quality can benefit from understanding motor behavior.

COACHING

Most coaches have a limited amount of time to work with their athletes on a one-to-one basis. Therefore, optimizing that time is critical. For any given motor performance skill, knowing the different mechanisms responsible can help coaches target where they will focus their instruction. Knowledge of the different stages of motor learning can help coaches tailor their instruction (both what they say and how they say it) to the level of their athletes. Acknowledging the unique contributions of environment and task to motor performance can open new avenues for changing movements over time, and in time lead to changes in individual performance. Information from motor behavior research informs coaches on the best ways to structure their practice environments to facilitate motor learning and performance. Coaches can modify feedback, increase rest, or make other changes based on evidence-based practice emerging from motor behavior studies. Athletes can use this information as well to ensure peak performance.

PHYSICAL EDUCATION

Teaching physical education requires a fundamental understanding of motor development, because children of different ages generally have different developmental statuses. A first-grade class will not have the motor performance capability of a third- or even a second-grade class. This is not simply because they have not practiced the skills as much, but also because their nervous systems (among others) have not matured to the level of that found in older children. Physical educators can use their knowledge of motor behavior to modify skills to match developmental levels. Physical educators are also faced with severe time restrictions, and thus will be well served by motor behavior research in optimizing learning environments to get the most out of the time they have. They can use tests such at the Test of Gross Motor Development-2 (TGMD-2) to assess motor skill performance in their classes and age-based norms to see how their students perform in comparison to other children of the same age.

PHYSICAL OR OCCUPATIONAL THERAPY

It is hard to imagine a physical or occupational therapist who does not use motor behavior as a foundation for their practice! For example, the study of motor control provides us with both psychological and physiological information on how people without injury or disability move their bodies. Therapists can use this knowledge of typical movement and compare it to that of their patients so that they can better understand their clients' movement deficits. This can be a starting point for developing a plan of action to help patients recover their lost function, learn compensatory strategies, or even acquire new movements that accomplish the task in a different way. Motor behavior provides a framework from which practitioners can examine motor performance. This gives them a feel for what their patients are doing well and what could be improved. By using motor learning principles, these health professionals can create an environment that facilitates motor learning for each individual. Because individuals are at different stages of learning and different levels of impairment, therapists must carefully consider how these interact and impact motor learning for each of their patients.

Career Opportunities in Motor Behavior

In general, students study motor behavior as one or two classes within a kinesiology or exercise science baccalaureate major rather than as a standalone major or concentration. This is most likely by design. Although the knowledge of motor behavior can enhance performance in a wide array of careers, there are few employment opportunities that require a skill set that solely consists of motor behavior. For example, to be an exceptional exercise specialist, a person should have a foundation in motor behavior as part of a well-rounded knowledge base that includes biomechanics, exercise physiology, and psychology. Physical educators need motor development in order to understand the developmental progression of motor performance. This provides physical educators with a road map (e.g., how the children moved previously, how they move now, and how they should move in the future), which allows for the targeting of specific movements, actions, or skills for instructional intervention. Certainly, physical and occupational therapists use motor behavior information all the time. All of these professions, however, require further education as part of a bachelor's degree program, such as physical education, or continuing on in a professional program, such as physical or occupational therapy. For those who find the study of motor behavior fascinating, numerous graduate programs around the country provide masters and doctoral degrees in motor behavior or in the subdisciplines of motor control, motor learning, or motor development. With these degrees, a person could become a consultant within industry, working in human factors or ergonomics, or they may find positions within the healthcare system, such as a technician in a gait lab at a children's hospital or clinic. Of course, those who truly love motor behavior may decide to share their knowledge with undergraduate students, and become a professor!

STOP AND THINK

A situation has emerged in a physical education class in which three students (two boys and one girl) are acting out and negatively affecting the class. It emerges that all three seem developmentally delayed in motor performance. Whenever they cannot perform, they become targets of ridicule for the other children. The problems rapidly escalate from there.

Based on their knowledge of motor behavior that they gained in their professional training, what are some possible solutions that a physical educator, a coach, an adapted physical education specialist, or a sport psychology consultant would develop to address this situation?

CHAPTER SUMMARY

In this chapter, the broad and general scope of the study of motor behavior was presented, as well as a brief history of the development of the field. Special attention was given to concerns arising out of the military actions of World War II. The three subareas of motor behavior—motor control, motor learning, and motor development—were defined, and descriptions of the typical research approaches of each were presented. The chapter concluded with a discussion of how knowledge of motor behavior can be useful in one's career.

DISCUSSION QUESTIONS

1. In small groups, reflect on the following question; in two very distinct and different environments (Military and Elementary Education) how would motor control, motor learning and motor development be applied? Share your best ideas with the rest of the class.
2. Discuss the differences and similarities between motor development, motor learning, and motor control with two other classmates.
3. In small groups, talk about how motor behavior would apply to your anticipated profession (e.g., personal trainer, dance instructor).
4. How would the study of motor behavior improve your own physical activity performance?

REFERENCES

Adams, J. A. (1971). A closed loop theory of motor learning. *Journal of Motor Behavior, 3*, 111–150.

Bernstein, N. A. (1967). *The co-ordination and regulation of movement.* Oxford: Pergamon Press.

Clark, J. E., & Whitall, J. (1989). What is motor development? The lessons of history. *Quest, 41*, 183–202.

Edwards, W. H. (2010). *Motor learning and control: From theory to practice.* Belmont, CA: Wadsworth.

Fitts, P. M. (1954). The information capacity of the human motor system in controlling amplitude of movement. *Journal of Experimental Psychology, 47*(6), 381–391.

Gesell, A., & Thompson, H. (1934). *Infant behavior: Its genesis and growth.* New York: McGraw-Hill.

Haywood, K., & Getchell, N. (2014). *Lifespan motor development* (6th ed.). Champaign, IL: Human Kinetics.

Haywood, K., Roberton, M. A., & Getchell, N. (2012). *Advanced analysis of motor development.* Champaign IL: Human Kinetics.

Kelso, J. A. S. (1995). *Dynamic patterns: The self-organization of brain and behavior.* Cambridge: MIT Press.

Magill, R. A. (2013). *Motor learning and control: concepts and applications* (10th ed.). New York: McGraw-Hill.

McGraw, M. B. (1943). *The neuromuscular maturation of the human infant.* New York: Colombia University Press.

Schmidt, R. A. (1975). A schema theory of discrete motor skill learning. *Psychological Review, 82,* 225–260.

Schmidt, R., & Lee, T. (2011). *Motor control and learning: A behavioral emphasis* (5th ed.). Champaign, IL: Human Kinetics.

Schmidt, R., & Lee, T. (2014). *Motor learning and performance: From principle to application* (5th ed.). Champaign, IL: Human Kinetics.

Sherrington, C. S. (1906). *The integrative action of the nervous system.* New Haven, CT: Yale University Press.

Thorndike, E. (1932). *The fundamentals of learning.* New York: AMS Press.

Turvey, M. T. (1980). Clues from the organization of motor systems. In U. Bellugi & M. Studdert-Kennedy (Eds.), *Signed and spoken language: Biological constraints on linguistic form.* Weinheim: Verlag Chemie.

Woodworth, R. S. (1899). The accuracy of voluntary movement. *Psychological Review, 3,* 1–114.

CHAPTER 8

Philosophy of Kinesiology

DOUGLAS W. McLAUGHLIN

LEARNING OBJECTIVES

1. Explain the philosophy of kinesiology and describe its methods.

2. Discuss what makes philosophical arguments more or less compelling.

3. Identify the different types of philosophical inquiry, and provide examples of each from kinesiology.

4. Describe how the different types of philosophical inquiry inform the field of kinesiology.

5. Understand how philosophical insights impact personal and professional practices.

KEY TERMS

aesthetics	experience
axiology	fair play
conceptual clarity	game
critical inquiry	good life
dualistic interpretation of a person	holistic interpretation of a person
epistemology	intrinsic reasons
equality	knowing how
ethics	knowing that

materialistic interpretation of a person

metaphysics

philosophy of kinesiology

physical culture

play

reflective scrutiny

sound philosophical arguments

sport

Introduction

Although often referred to as *philosophy of sport* or *sport philosophy*, it is important to recognize that the insights of philosophy pertain to all aspects of kinesiology. This shift to **philosophy of kinesiology** has been more than just a name change for the subdiscipline. Although the application of philosophy to the study of sport continues to provide new and greater depth of understanding about sport (McNamee & Morgan, 2015, Reid, 2012, and Torres, 2014), a broadening of philosophical investigations into health and fitness would strengthen its value as a core kinesiology subdiscipline. In this chapter, we will look at the philosophy of kinesiology, examine the types of questions asked, and discuss how the philosophy of kinesiology can be implemented to provide new insights into the field of kinesiology more generally.

philosophy of kinesiology
The subdiscipline of kinesiology that uses philosophical methods to examine various aspects of kinesiology.

critical inquiry
The use of sound reasoning and clear arguments to identify concepts and principles.

conceptual clarity
When concepts are presented in a coherent, intelligible, and straightforward manner to support deeper insight.

play
An activity that is pursued intrinsically and for its own sake.

What Is the Philosophy of Kinesiology?

Philosophy means the "love of wisdom." Although this is true, it is unhelpful. Many of your professors are doctors of philosophy (Ph.D.), and professors from every subdiscipline of kinesiology care deeply about the wisdom their respective subdisciplines provide for the field of kinesiology more generally. Although philosophy does not have a privileged position that allows it to claim wisdom for itself, it does rely on **critical inquiry** based on sound reasoning and argumentation to identify concepts and principles about our world. Philosophers of kinesiology apply these methods when answering a broad array of questions related to kinesiology.

An important contribution of philosophy to kinesiology is the **conceptual clarity** it provides. Unlike most of the other kinesiology subdisciplines, philosophy does not fundamentally rely on facts. Philosophers rely on theories and interpretations that cannot merely be reduced to, or derived from, empirical evidence. **Play** is a valued form of human behavior (Huizinga, 1934).

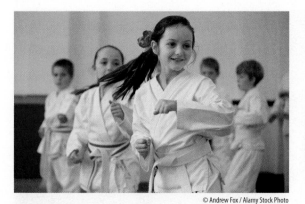
© Andrew Fox / Alamy Stock Photo

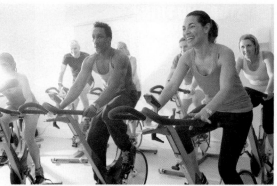
© ableimages / Alamy Stock Photo

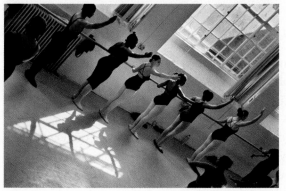
© Marwood jenkins / Alamy Stock Photo

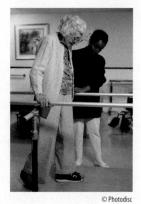
© Photodisc

But what exactly is play? Despite being fundamental to our lives, it is quite difficult to provide a clear and concise interpretation of this particular kind of human behavior. Philosophy provides tools so that we can better understand the concept of play. **Fair play** is an ethical concept about appropriate behaviors in sport (Simon et al, 2015). But for most of us it is only a vague notion that we are unable to explain in precise detail. Philosophical resources aid in our efforts to clearly articulate what fair play is and informs our efforts at encouraging or discouraging certain types of behaviors and practices in sport. As kinesiologists, we wish to promote a **good life** that incorporates physical activity (Anderson, 2001). But if we are unable to express physical activity's role in experiencing a life most worth living, then the task is left to others who might not fully appreciate or understand the value of physical activity to the good life. Philosophy provides theories that explain why

fair play
Appropriate behaviors in sport that respect the rules and opponents.

good life
A form of living that consists of personal well-being, fulfillment, and meaning.

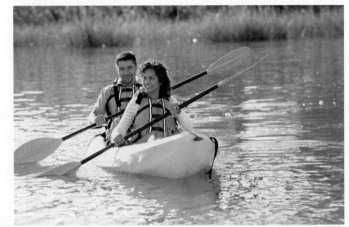

© Blend Images / Alamy Stock Photo

experience
Knowledge, skills, and mastery of an activity that is developed through participation.

sound philosophical arguments
Statements that present consistent and impartial reasons for accepting a conclusion.

reflective scrutiny
Critical analysis of a position to determine if it is supported by compelling arguments and reasons that are consistent and unbiased.

physical activity is a fundamental human right and helps us achieve a good life. Facts about play, fair play, and the good life are not irrelevant, but some theoretical and interpretative analysis is needed in order to achieve conceptual clarity on these topics.

Another contribution of philosophy is its examination of our **experience**. Philosophy of kinesiology provides insight into how our experiences of and through physical activity can promote meaningful lives (Hochstetler, 2015). It helps us explain why we incorporate, and why we should incorporate, physical activity into our lives. It helps us identify how and why some physical activity experiences are more likely to develop into meaningful practices than others.

Philosophy provides insights into a variety of issues concerning kinesiology, some of which will be presented in the next section. But it is important to realize that philosophy can be done well or poorly. **Sound philosophical arguments** must be consistent and impartial. Logical inconsistencies or errors of judgment compromise the validity of philosophical conclusions. Biased perspectives can lead to unfairness and injustice. When consistent and impartial, philosophical reasoning is much more likely to hold up to **reflective scrutiny**. When challenged, our philosophical positions must be defended with compelling arguments and reasons. Although there may be some details that people cannot agree on, a willingness to engage in honest intellectual exchange should lead to a modest consensus on relevant factors.

When asking philosophical questions, sound arguments often lead to more compelling answers. But it is important to realize that not all philosophical answers are the same. In some cases, philosophical conclusions are more a matter of right or wrong, correct or incorrect, or valid or invalid. An athlete cannot cheat and play fairly at the same time. To think otherwise is to be confused about the concept of cheating and/or the concept of fair play. It

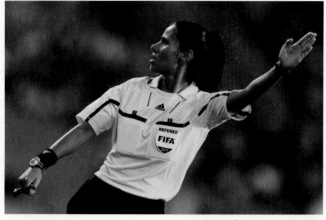

© Jonathan Larsen/Diadem Images / Alamy Stock Photo

would be incorrect to label an action as an example of both cheating and fair play because these terms refer to behaviors that are logically distinct. But in other cases, philosophical conclusions are more a matter of stronger or weaker or more compelling or less compelling. Should the pursuit of excellence be promoted in sports? While the demonstration of excellence is what makes **sport** such a cherished activity, our answer to the question cannot be an unqualified yes. In elite sport, the pursuit of excellence can be vigorously defended. But in youth sport, other values, such as participation and development of skills, may be more important. The extent to which we pursue excellence depends on a host of factors; thus the context is important. An argument for the promotion of the pursuit of excellence is

sport
Games that test and contest physical skills and abilities.

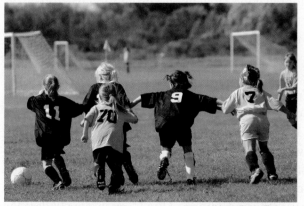

© Lorraine Swanson/Shutterstock

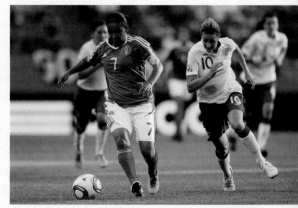

© Jonathan Larsen/Diadem Images / Alamy Stock Photo

STOP AND THINK

Philosophical reasoning can be done well or done poorly. Philosophical arguments can be persuasive or implausible.

- Can you identify an example of a viewpoint in the field of kinesiology that is supported by compelling philosophical insights?

- Can you identify an example of a viewpoint that is supported by unsubstantiated philosophical arguments?

physical culture
A social, organized way of life that promotes the physical development in persons.

much stronger at elite levels than it is in more recreational and educational levels of sport.

A Brief History of the Philosophy of Kinesiology

While the philosophy of kinesiology is a relatively new field, the origins of philosophical ideas pertaining to physical activity are often attributed to ancient Greece. The role of the *agon*, the competitive spirit, and *arête*, the virtues commonly associated with competitive practices, are viewed as positive legacies of sport in ancient Greece, as seen, in part, by the moral underpinnings of the modern Olympic Games. But the ancient Greeks also introduced prizes for victory in athletic competition, a practice that underpins many of our harshest criticisms of modern sport. Although the ancient Greeks considered a sound curriculum to necessarily include athletics in order to develop a balanced life, some ancient Greek scholars were critical of the overemphasis that was placed on athletic training.

While the seeds of the philosophy of kinesiology were there from the beginning, and philosophical ideas about physical culture can be identified throughout human history, it was not until recently that the philosophy of sport became a distinct subdiscipline. Since the mid-1800s, a number of concerns have been raised about the role and importance of physical education. Philosophical justifications have been based on concerns of the state, such as developing good citizens and promoting patriotism, as well as concerns of virtue, such as building character or pursuing excellence. Values have permeated the development and delivery of physical training.

It was not until the late 1960s that the philosophy of sport came into its own. The work of philosophers Paul Weiss and Bernard Suits established sport as a topic of serious philosophical study. Warren Fraleigh, Dean of the Faculty of Physical Education and Recreation at the State University of New York, Brockport, was instrumental in the rise of the subdiscipline. In 1973, after two symposiums on the philosophy of sport, Brockport was the site of the first annual conference of the Philosophic Society for the Study of Sport. The following year the first edition of the *Journal of the Philosophy of Sport* was published. A significant proportion of the early research dealt with foundational questions such as defining the nature of sport, play, and games; discerning the relationship between sport and art; and gaining clarity about ethical concepts such as cheating and sportsmanship.

Starting in the 1980s, new scholarship began to focus on ethical issues pertaining to the use of performance-enhancing drugs, and in the 1990s questions of gender inequality, violence in sport, and character development emerged. In the 2000s, more philosophical traditions were used to explore issues related to sport. Perhaps most significant were the debates as to how theories of sport inform ethical issues. Broad internalism, the idea that sport has its own internal gratuitous logic that provides a reasoned and critical basis for ethical deliberation, has been adopted by many philosophers as the best theory of sport.

In 1999, the Philosophical Society for the Study of Sport changed its name to the International Association for the Philosophy of Sport. This change better reflected the global interest and participation in the philosophy of sport that continues to grow to this day. One concern is that the field has been too narrowly focused on sport. The advent of the British Philosophy of Sport Association introduced in 2007 the publication of a new journal, *Sport, Ethics, and Philosophy*. The editor Mike McNamee took a more inclusive and comprehensive approach to philosophical issues impacting kinesiology. Although many interesting philosophical investigations pertaining exclusively to sport remain, the future of philosophy for our field is one that identifies as and explores issues of the philosophy of kinesiology. With this brief introduction to the philosophy of kinesiology, we can now turn to an examination of the core topics that philosophy addresses related to the field of kinesiology.

Major Topics in the Philosophy of Kinesiology

Philosophers of kinesiology can ask a variety of questions regarding different aspects of our world and experience. The questions are not exclusively academic questions for philosophers of kinesiology, and the answers often have practical implications for a range of kinesiology professionals.

Metaphysics is the branch of philosophy that is concerned with the nature of things. Understanding the nature of the person and making distinctions among the forms of physical activity are two important metaphysical

metaphysics
The branch of philosophy that is concerned with the nature of things.

epistemology
The branch of philosophy that is concerned with the nature of knowledge.

axiology
The branch of philosophy that is concerned about the nature of values or the good.

ethics
The branch of philosophy that is concerned about the nature of right and wrong conduct.

aesthetics
The branch of philosophy that is concerned with the nature and appreciation of beauty.

considerations for the field of kinesiology. **Epistemology** is the branch of philosophy that is concerned with the nature of knowledge. The distinction between different types of knowing ("knowing how" and "knowing that") and the nature of intelligence are two important epistemological considerations for the field of kinesiology.

Axiology is the branch of philosophy that is concerned about the nature of values or the good. Why and how we value physical activity are important axiological considerations for the field of kinesiology. Two important subsets of value theory are ethics and aesthetics. **Ethics** is the branch of philosophy that is concerned with the nature of right and wrong conduct. Fair play and equality are important ethical considerations for the field of kinesiology. **Aesthetics** is the branch of philosophy that is concerned with the nature and appreciation of beauty. Our lived experiences of physical activity and the role of physical activity in the good life are important aesthetic considerations.

Although these different philosophical approaches can be considered independent of one another, it is important to recognize the interplay that exists between them. For example, metaphysical considerations can inform our ethical deliberations. How we define sport is an important factor in determining what behaviors we deem right or wrong in sport. Rules have a constitutive function because they determine what actions are allowed or disallowed in the course of play. In establishing what is permitted and prohibited in sport, rules also serve as a basis for making ethical judgments. Another example is how epistemological considerations inform axiological and aesthetic considerations. The extent to which people value physical activity is impacted greatly by the quality of their experiences with physical activity. Knowing that physical activity promotes health is very different than the lived experience of being healthier through participating in regular physical activity. People are likely to value physical activity more deeply when they know it

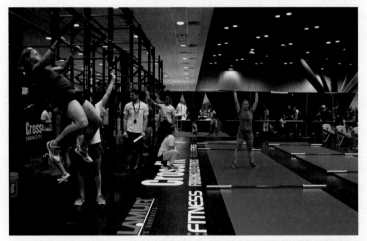
© Mike Roach/Zuffa LLC / Getty Images

through personal experience rather than as an impersonal prescription for health. Our aesthetic judgments are also enriched when we have firsthand experiences of the challenges presented by a particular activity and have developed skills to overcome them.

STOP AND THINK

Identify another example of two or more types of philosophy informing an issue pertaining to kinesiology.

Metaphysics

At its core, kinesiology is primarily concerned about human movement. But what do we mean by "human" and what do we mean by "movement." Different theories about the nature of persons and the nature of physical activity exist. The theories we rely on have implications for everything else we do related to physical activity. So, the metaphysical questions about the nature of persons and the nature of physical activity are fundamental questions that every student of kinesiology should examine carefully.

The nature of a person can be understood from many different perspectives. A **materialistic interpretation of a person** reduces a person to physical matter. Physics and chemistry are the only necessary disciplines to fully understand the nature of persons. Although this mechanistic view of the person has provided much insight into the role of physical activity for improving health and performance, it does not fully capture the breadth or depth of our physical activity experiences.

A **dualistic interpretation of a person** divides a person into two parts: the mind and the body. While the benefit of a materialistic concern for the body is maintained, the dualistic perspective also takes seriously the mental aspects of our existence. Dualism provides the opportunity to consider moods, motivation, values, and ethics that materialism has difficulty explaining. However, the dualistic approach has two problems. First, the strong delineation between the mental and the physical does not accurately reflect the nature of persons. Because human experience is fully integrated, a concept of the person that makes a sharp distinction between the two parts is fundamentally flawed. The other problem is more practical. Dualistic theories of the person have generally favored the mind and mental aspects over the body and the physical aspects of a person, a bias that leads to an undervaluing of the importance of physical activity in our lives.

A **holistic interpretation of a person** takes seriously our lived experience from an integrated perspective. Holism recognizes that the mental and

materialistic interpretation of a person
The viewpoint that people are reducible to physical matter and can be fully understood through the disciplines of physics and chemistry.

dualistic interpretation of a person
The view that body and mind are separate and distinct parts of human beings and that we can isolate one aspect from the other within a person.

holistic interpretation of a person
The view that we must take seriously and account for all aspects of a person's experience, realizing that mind, body, and spirit are interconnected.

physical are not distinct from one another but fully at work in all that we do. Unlike the dualistic interpretation, a holistic approach is not concerned with distinguishing parts of people, but rather in accurately describing their experiences and behavior. For dualism, the hallmark of intelligence involves the extent to which the mind is employed. For holism, the hallmark of intelligence involves the quality of behavior (Kretchmar, 2005). From a holistic perspective, exceptional performances in dance and sport demonstrate profound intelligence just as much as exceptional performances in science and math.

These different interpretations of the nature of persons have important implications. Materialistic interpretations of a person diminish the importance of our subjective experiences, our desires and values, and the role of ethics. Dualistic interpretations of a person at best have difficulty explaining how parts of people are integrated and at worst diminish the value of human behavior that kinesiologists care most deeply about.

Holistic interpretations of a person address the concerns of materialism and dualism with the added benefit of giving clear direction on how to interact with people. Imagine that two people have the exact same knee injury in terms of severity. Should the injury be treated the same? From a strict materialistic perspective, the answer is too often "yes." From a holistic perspective, we would want to know details about both people, including the ways they value and regularly participate in physical activity to better determine how they are impacted by the knee injury. If the one person is sedentary, a "couch potato," then the treatment efforts may require significant

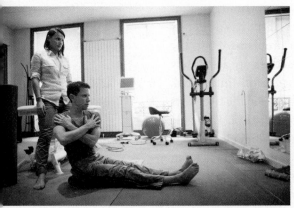
© BSIP SA / Alamy Stock Photo

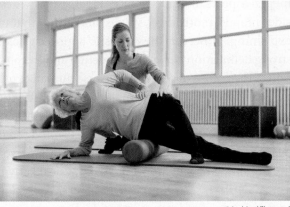
© Jacob Lund/Shutterstock

motivational efforts in order for the person to fully recover. If the other person is a competitive athlete, then it may be necessary to encourage patience so the person does not risk additional injury by trying to come back too soon. Same injury, very different approaches. A holistic account of a person helps us see that more clearly than a materialistic account.

What place should physical education have in our curriculum? A dualist may appreciate physical education but consider it as less important than core subjects such as math, science, and English. A holist, appreciating the range of behaviors that can lead to human flourishing, would advocate for a more comprehensive curriculum that educates people for a full array of behaviors. Recognizing that our conceptual understanding of the nature of a person impacts the field of kinesiology in a variety of important ways, we can now turn to the nature of physical activity.

People move in all sorts of ways, and it is important for kinesiologists to consider the general and specific ways in which people move. Most kinesiologists are not concerned with common movements such as brushing teeth or using a spoon, but these movements can become central to those working in certain therapeutic settings. Many kinesiologists are interested in promoting active lifestyles, but do not consider what forms of physical activity best promote such lifestyles. It is important to have some conceptual clarity regarding the types of physical activity in order to best achieve the aims and goals we may pursue in particular settings.

One modestly helpful distinction is between movement that is work and movement that is play. Physical activity that is work is undertaken for extrinsic reasons, such as promoting health. Physical activity that is play is undertaken for **intrinsic reasons**, such as pursuing enjoyment. These categories are only modestly helpful because one person's play may be another person's work. Also, a person may pursue physical activity for both intrinsic and extrinsic reasons. However, it is important to recognize that the reasons why people engage in physical activity and how they experience it as meaningful in their lives are important considerations. Although a few people may be inclined to engage in physical activity as work, most people are more inclined to engage in physical activity that they experience as play. If very few people enjoy running on a treadmill, then trying to promote an

STOP AND THINK

- Identify one way that dualistic or materialistic interpretations on the nature of persons can limit how kinesiology promotes physical activity.

- Identify one way that a holistic interpretation can improve how kinesiology promotes physical activity.

intrinsic reasons
Explanations or justifications that rely on the thing itself rather than on something else.

active lifestyle by encouraging people to run on a treadmill is not an effective strategy. If we want people to develop an enduring relationship with physical activity, then we need to help them develop an intrinsic passion for some form of physical activity.

Historically, the major forms of physical activity have been identified as sport, exercise, and dance. Play is often associated with sport and work with exercise. But if we focus on the intrinsic and extrinsic reasons for participating in physical activity, then we must recognize that all three forms can be pursued as play or work. How do we maintain the playful nature of sport so that it does not become work? In some settings, we may want to emphasize competition, whereas in others we may want to provide noncompetitive sports. Can we make exercise playful? Some people experience exercise, even running on a treadmill, as a fun, playful experience. But there are other ways to enliven exercise so that people develop an intrinsic relationship with it. Although the intensity may not be appropriate for everyone, and it is important to seek out qualified, trained instructors, high-intensity exercise programs such as CrossFit provide a structure that, for some people, makes "working out" a passionate pursuit. Because of a lack of familiarity, many people are not confident in pursuing dance. They believe they cannot dance. But introducing dance in a way that does not focus too much on getting the moves right but rather on learning to express and experience the lived body can encourage people to pursue and develop dance intrinsically.

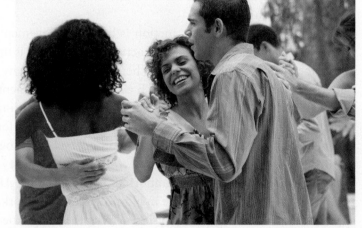

© Blend Images / Alamy Stock Photo

STOP AND THINK

Identify three different careers in the field of kinesiology. Describe how professionals can promote an intrinsic pursuit of physical activity.

A final metaphysical consideration of physical activity is the nature of games. Bernard Suits (1978) defines playing a **game** as "the voluntary attempt to overcome unnecessary obstacles" (p. 40). This involves two central features: games involve (1) problem-solving that is (2) intrinsically valued. This is interesting given Suits's analysis related to the nature of a good life. For Suits, a good life consists of activities that we choose to do rather than we have to do. But those activities must present some sort of challenge, otherwise they would become boring. Therefore, a good life consists of intrinsically valued problem-solving. That means that playing games is the central activity of a good life.

This is a profound insight that should be carefully considered. How might we reform and implement physical education programs and promote physical activity with the understanding that we are preparing people for a good life? For Suits, games are a much broader concept that entail much more than play and sports. Many examples of exercise and dance are pursued as intrinsically valued problem-solving.

Suits (1967) offers the maxim "Life is a game. Live accordingly" (p. 213). Such a simple maxim cannot in itself address concerns about chronic inactivity. But we must do more than promote physical activity. Levels of physical activity will improve if we make an effort to cultivate people's experiences of physical activity as intrinsically valued problem-solving.

> **game**
> A voluntary attempt to overcome unnecessary obstacles that is a form of intrinsically valued problem-solving.

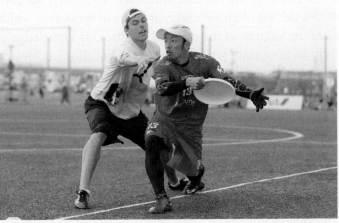

© Aflo Co. Ltd. / Alamy Stock Photo

STOP AND THINK

Do you find the claim that physical activity is central to a good life compelling? Why or why not? Explain what you think the relationship between physical activity and a good life should be.

Epistemology

knowing that
Propositional knowledge that is demonstrated through abstractions and theories.

knowing how
Practical knowledge that is demonstrated through application and performance.

What do we know when we are skilled movers? How do we know it? A problem that arises from dualism is the distinction between "**knowing that**" and "**knowing how**." "Knowing that" refers to propositional or theoretical knowledge, whereas "knowing how" refers to practical or applied knowledge. What sort of "knowing" do we want to promote? Dualistic approaches often have a bias for theoretical "knowing that" over the practical "knowing how."

It certainly seems valuable to understand the underlying theories that determine the ways we should move. But if we are unable to perform the skill, then how useful is the theory? Forced to choose, most people would prefer being able to move well than know about how to move well. Although we can identify different types of knowledge, perhaps we are making too much of these distinctions. A holistic understanding of a person suggests that skilled behavior, whether applied to solving scientific, health, or sporting problems, requires a critical application of knowledge. When too much is made of the distinction between "knowing how" and "knowing that," it only serves to reinforce a dualistic interpretation of the person rather than provide an accurate account of human intelligence.

Another interesting epistemological question pertains to what we know through participating in competitive sport. How do we assess the results of competition? How valid is that knowledge? The purpose of competitive sport is to determine the relative abilities of the competitors. This is often thought of in the binary terms of winners and losers. But sometimes the competitors' performances do not result in any relevant difference. Therefore, the contest should result in a tie. Yet often we make an effort to break ties, which in effect diminishes the validity of the original results. Our knowledge of relative abilities is in an important sense hampered by not allowing for ties.

But there are also important things to learn from winning and losing. Sometimes results are convincing, but sometimes they are not. A team can play poorly and win or play exceptionally well and lose. Rather than looking at the final score as an objective measure of relative abilities, it is important to take an interpretative lens to make sense of the results. In victory or defeat, the process provides valuable information on how to improve skills for future performances. These epistemological insights are valuable because they help situate the role of competition in educational and developmental contexts. Shying away from competition in educational settings because it divides participants into winners and losers misses the point. Participants can gain self-knowledge through participation, win or lose, that can inform valuable information about how they can improve going forward. The education of participants entails not only the knowledge of relative abilities gained through competition but also knowledge related to the significance of results and how to respond in victory or defeat.

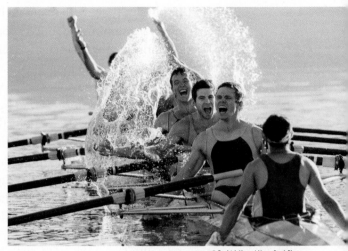

© Fredrick Kippe / Alamy Stock Photo

Values

Historically, the core values of kinesiology have been health, knowledge, fun, and skill (Kretchmar, 2005). It is important to clearly determine what we mean by these respective values, because how we define them impacts how we try to pursue, promote, and prioritize them. It is also important to recognize that we have to make difficult choices between

these values when a conflict arises between them. For elite sport, skill may be valued more highly. In rehabilitative settings, health may be valued more highly. For educators, knowledge may be valued more highly. For recreational sport leaders, fun may be valued most highly. This is why context matters.

It is also important to recognize how values are experienced as intrinsic or extrinsic. Intrinsic values are generally more powerful than extrinsic values in motivating us. When we value something intrinsically, we value it for its own sake, but when we value something extrinsically, we value it for the sake of some other end. When we value something intrinsically, we are unlikely to find the same value from some other source, but when we value something extrinsically, we may not only be able to find the same value from another source but are also likely to pursue other means if they make experiencing the ultimate end more easily attainable. If we value physical activity exclusively for its health benefits, then we value it extrinsically. If someday there is a pharmaceutical option, a "health pill," that eliminates the need for people to be physically active to maintain health, then the value of physical activity will be greatly diminished. But if people value the pleasure experienced from participating in physical activity itself, then they will likely continue participating even when it is no longer necessary for achieving health benefits. Someone may claim that she values beach volleyball because it is a "great workout." Not to diminish the effort exerted by elite beach volleyball players, but there are many forms of physical activity that have been or could be developed that are more challenging than playing beach volleyball. But creating a list of alternative workouts misses an important point. Even if there were no need to work out, many beach volleyball enthusiasts would still intrinsically value pursuing beach volleyball for the challenges and skills that are central to the game.

It is also important to consider how values promote a coherent, satisfying life. Although health is an important value for experiencing a coherent, satisfying life, for most people it is an extrinsic value that merely facilitates that life. Skill, in contrast, is often an intrinsic value that not only facilitates a coherent,

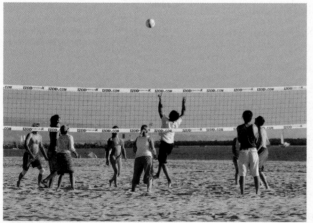

© Ellen Isaacs / Alamy Stock Photo

satisfying life but is also the very fulfillment of that life. When someone derives great value from dancing and organizes and budgets her life around her participation in dance, then it stands to reason that her dance skills and abilities will bring her deep satisfaction. It is from those skills that she identifies and expresses her sense of self, at least her best self.

It is important to understand how our values impact our lives and how they can be utilized to motivate others. When we help people learn to experience physical activity in intrinsically valued ways, we are promoting choices that will lead to physical activity becoming part of a more coherent, satisfying life.

STOP AND THINK

- Why do you value physical activity?
- What steps can you take to help others develop deeply valued experiences of physical activity?

Ethics

As mentioned earlier, ethics is concerned with values related to right and wrong. Ethical considerations are often related to issues of fairness and justice (Fraleigh, 1984, Loland, 2002,

McNamee, 2010, and Morgan, 2007). Some ethical issues, such as the use of performance-enhancing drugs in sport, receive frequent media coverage. Other ethical issues do not receive as much media coverage but still deserve our careful consideration.

Sensational media coverage and widespread condemnation have seemingly little effect on curbing athletes' unethical behaviors. Is this due to a lack of ethical awareness on the part of the athletes, or are other forces at play? Perhaps it is a bit of both. Being able to distinguish right from wrong actions in a given situation does not mean that a person will act in the right way. Actually, developing good moral habits may be more important than developing moral awareness. Not only must coaches and parents teach young athletes about what the moral standards are in sport, but they must also teach them why they are important and hold them accountable to that standard if they expect them to grow up to be virtuous athletes. Although it is important to forgive when someone has a moral lapse, it is equally important that we do not become too permissive. In a lax environment where the reward for being successful is greater than the punishment for getting caught, athletes who lack sound moral habits are more likely to risk the small chance of being caught for the increased potential for success.

This is why ethical decision-making needs to be understood in the larger cultural context. If athletes are not prepared to morally engage new ethical issues, then something must be done. For example, the potential development in the foreseeable future of the use of genetic modifications to enhance performance raises significant ethical concerns. What role do scientists, coaches, medical staff, and philosophers have in educating and preparing athletes to make sound moral decisions regarding such a complex moral issue? Furthermore, how can we condemn athletes for using performance-enhancing drugs when the general population has become so eager to use performance-enhancing drugs in their daily lives? A decrease in testosterone levels is part of the normal aging process of males. But it has recently been branded and marketed as a medical condition that requires testosterone replacement therapy. Ethical investigations into moral issues such as the use of performance-enhancing drugs must take into account the complex social and cultural forces at work.

Another ethical concern relates to equality and access. The American sporting tradition highlights certain landmarks in **equality**: Jackie Robinson

equality
A concern for the equal rights, access, and opportunities of all people.

breaking the color line in Major League Baseball; Title IX promoting gender equity in school sport; and the Paralympic Games partnering with the Olympic Games. But despite the celebrations related to race, gender, and disability, the contemporary sporting scene still deals with a vast amount of inequality. Although great strides have been made in women's sport, it is disappointing to find persisting inequalities in intercollegiate athletics and minimal professional opportunities for elite women athletes. Despite Oscar Pistorius, a double amputee, participating in the 2012 Olympic Games, there was still minimal coverage of the 2012 Paralympic Games. In 2013, professional basketball player Jason Collins disclosed that he was gay. In 2014, football player Michael Sam disclosed that he also was gay. Despite these revelations, gay athletes still face a number of barriers. From an ethical perspective, access to participation in elite sport should be determined on criteria related to sporting abilities. But nonrelevant factors such as race, gender, sexuality, disability, and ethnicity continue to impact people's prospects to participate in sport. These factors, as well as economic factors, impact the opportunities for those who are participating in physical activity at a recreational level. But it is important that all people have access to meaningful physical activity experiences independent of these factors.

Aesthetics

Aesthetics, a subset of axiology, is concerned with the nature and appreciation of beauty. Physical activity can be an aesthetic experience in itself (Best, 1978). The sensation of buoyancy experienced when diving into a body of water can draw swimmers back to the water time and time again. The exhilaration of hurdling down a ridge trail can draw mountain bikers back to the trail time and time again. But aesthetics can also refer to the narrative structure of many forms of physical activity, such as the thrill of striving for victory or the struggle to choreograph a dance performance that evokes a certain response. These issues give rise to interesting considerations about the aesthetics of being a spectator (Mumford, 2012).

Although rules are often thought as determining the structure of games, it is interesting to consider how games and rules are informed by aesthetic sensibilities. When crafting rules, it is important to make the game not too hard and not too easy. In an interactive game, it is important that there is a balance between the offensive and defensive competitors. If the rules are too restrictive to the defense, then the offense will not be challenged. If the rules are too permissive to the defense, then the offense will face too difficult a challenge. Establishing rules that ensure a balance between offensive and defensive players is, in part, an aesthetic judgment. When the rules are drawn just right, it makes the contest exhilarating and exciting. An important consideration for physical educators is to have students not only learn the rules of the game, but also learn to appreciate through firsthand experience how those rules establish the just-right problems that make games so enjoyable in the first place.

But aesthetics can also pertain to general experiences of physical activity. When Suits (1978) argued that playing games is the central activity of the good life, he recognizes that more insightful and better games will be developed to fulfill that prospect. How can we develop physical activity experiences that promote aesthetic experiences? Can we enhance the likelihood that people will have just-right experiences that lead to a harmonious and exhilarating relationship with physical activity? Too often, physical activity is approached from a pragmatic perspective, such as how it can address the obesity epidemic. Running on the treadmill at a high intensity may burn many more calories than going on a hike, but if the treadmill holds no aesthetic appeal and the wilderness trail does, then there is much more long-term benefit in promoting hiking. Persistence is foundational to lifelong physical activity and requires that we promote forms of physical activity that are

STOP AND THINK

- How have aesthetic perceptions and judgments impacted your physical activity experiences?

- In what ways have they encouraged participation and developed meaningful experiences?

- In what ways have they discouraged participation and inhibited meaningful experiences?

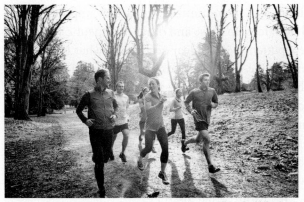

© Thomas Barwick/Getty Images

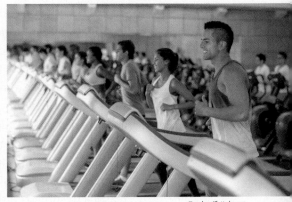

© andresr/Getty Images

personally and culturally significant. Aesthetic experiences should play a significant role in helping people decide what types of physical activity they want to adopt in their effort to pursue an active, good life.

What Can You Do with a Degree in the Philosophy of Kinesiology?

Careers in philosophy of kinesiology are very limited. The International Association for the Philosophy of Sport has fewer than 200 members around the world. Although people interested in philosophy take positons related to sport administration and leadership, most professionals who self-identify as philosophers of sport and kinesiology are professors in either departments of kinesiology or departments of philosophy. However, limited professional opportunities do not mean that the philosophy of kinesiology will not be important to consider in your own professional career.

The types of philosophical inquiry introduced in this chapter suggest several ways that the insights of philosophy benefit your pursuit of kinesiology. Whatever your professional aspirations are, if you are perceptive enough you will be able to identify philosophical issues related to your career choices. Physical therapists do not fix bodies, but help people heal and recover. Therefore, it is important to recognize a patient's values, interests, and fears in order to make appropriate programing accommodations that can go a long way toward facilitating the recovery process. An athletic trainer must recognize that his or her primary responsibility is to provide quality care to the athletes. The ethics related to returning athletes to play are often straightforward, but having the courage to act on them is another issue. Potential ethical issues can be minimized, in part, by improving professional standards and practices. In these and other therapeutic settings, it is important to provide a patient with a clear account of what the therapy and recovery process will be like. This epistemological grounding can help put people at ease and better contextualize the struggles they endure.

Coaches have to identify what values will guide their efforts. Some coaches rely on questionable motivational techniques. Is it ethical to yell at your athletes? Coaches also need to decide whether winning or skill development is more important. Should a coach's efforts be focused on the best athletes or more evenly distributed among all participants? Are there valid reasons to support either decision? What are they?

Physical educators need to provide opportunities for a diverse student population. Diversity relates not only to social factors such as gender, race, ethnicity, and class, but also to differences in personal factors such as experience, skill level, and confidence. How are decisions made to provide a variety of activities that maximize participation given social and personal differences? Should some noncompetitive activities be incorporated? Are competitive activities accompanied with lessons about the meaning of winning and losing? Are students merely introduced to a variety of activities, or do they have an opportunity to cultivate a meaningful relationship with a particular activity?

Fitness directors and recreational leaders need to provide sound programs based on current science. But aesthetic considerations may also come into play. CrossFit provides a narrative structure to intense workouts that has captured people's imaginations. Some recent research suggests that participating in yoga is no more effective than stretching in terms of health benefits. But how do we explain the rise of yoga studios across the nation without a comparable rise in stretching studios? A concern for aesthetics provides a means to develop physical activity opportunities that will engage more people.

Researchers must consider the implications of their findings. There is no best way to work out, because people participate in physical activity for a variety of different reasons. Even if a program could be identified that maximized strength gains, would it make it the best program? Only if maximizing muscular strength was the only performance goal. But if the program requires too much time it could take away from other performance goals. If the risks of injury are too great, then it may be contraindicated for most participants. Research questions may be reframed when taking a more holistic account of what people's goals are. It is important to contextualize research questions into the contemporary social and cultural fabric.

These are just a few examples. Philosophical insights are present in every area of kinesiology. Asking interesting philosophical questions is the first step. Crafting critical arguments that can hold up to scrutiny will lead to compelling philosophical answers.

As you pursue your kinesiology degree, it is important to consider how philosophy is not a specific class that you may or may not be required to take. Rather, you should try to identify the philosophical questions that arise in your classes. What concepts and theories can you identify? What assumptions are made without empirical evidence? What ethical considerations are

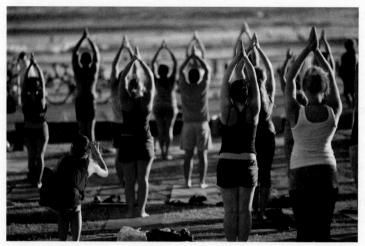

© Tony Potts/Getty Images

Identify a professional career in kinesiology that you are interested in pursuing, and describe five ways that philosophy can inform that profession.

present? What interpretation of the nature of the person is assumed? How do aesthetic values complement other course material? What values are emphasized? What values are deemphasized? Just as physiological, anatomical, and psychological influences are always at work in our lives, so are philosophical influences. It is just a matter of being attuned to their significance.

CHAPTER SUMMARY

In this chapter, we explored the philosophy of kinesiology. We learned how it is useful for developing critical evaluations, improving conceptual clarity, and engaging in meaningful narratives. We also learned that philosophy can be done well or poorly. In order for our philosophical arguments to be compelling and persuasive, they must be impartial and consistent, otherwise they will not hold up to scrutiny. Given this general overview, we identified the major types of philosophical investigations. Metaphysics is concerned about the nature of things. Epistemology is concerned about theories of knowledge. Axiology focuses on the nature of values and includes ethics and aesthetics. Ethical questions address the nature of right and wrong conduct, whereas aesthetic questions address the nature and appreciation of beauty. These types of philosophical questions are often integrated in a variety of ways, such as our metaphysical claims that the nature of competition has ethical implications about fair play and cheating. Although very few kinesiology majors will go on be philosophers of kinesiology, philosophical concerns impact all of us. It is important to identify what assumptions you are making and hold up your beliefs to scrutiny so that your philosophical commitments will be justified.

DISCUSSION QUESTIONS

1. How can philosophy inform your personal experiences related to kinesiology? Identify at least three different examples.
2. How can philosophy inform your professional experiences related to kinesiology? Identify at least three different examples.
3. What are the most important ethical issues facing the field of kinesiology today? Identify at least seven important issues, and describe how they will impact the future of kinesiology.

REFERENCES

Anderson, D. (2001). Recovering humanity: Movement, sport, and nature. *Journal of the Philosophy of Sport, 28*(2), 140–150.

Best, D. N. (1978). *Philosophy and human movement.* London: Allen and Unwin.

Fraleigh, W. P. (1984). *Right actions in sport: Ethics for contestants.* Champaign, IL: Human Kinetics.

Hochstetler, D. (2015). Narratives, identity, and transformation. *Quest, 67,* 161–172.

Huizinga, J. (1934). *Homo ludens: A study of the play element in culture.* London: Paladin.

Kretchmar, R. S. (2005). *Practical philosophy of sport and physical activity* (2nd ed.). Champagne, IL: Human Kinetics.

Loland, S. (2002). *Fair play in sport: A moral norm system.* London: Routledge.

McNamee, M. J. (ed.). (2010). *The ethics of sport: A reader.* Abingdon: Routledge.

McNamee, M. J., & Morgan, W. J. (eds.). (2015). *Routledge handbook of the philosophy of sport.* New York: Routledge.

Morgan, W. J. (ed.). (2007). *Ethics in sport* (2nd ed.). Champaign, IL: Human Kinetics.

Mumford, S. (2012). *Watching sport: Aesthetics, ethics, and emotion.* Abingdon: Routledge.

Reid, H. L. (2012). *Introduction to the philosophy of sport.* Plymouth, UK: Rowman & Littlefield.

Simon, R. L, Torres, C. R., & Hager P. F. (2015). *Fair play: The ethics of sport* (4th ed.). Boulder, CO: Westview Press.

Suits, B. (1967). Is life a game we are playing? *Ethics 77*(3), 209–213.

Suits, B. (1978). *The grasshopper: Games, life, and utopia.* Toronto: University of Toronto.

Torres, C. R. (ed.). (2014). *The Bloomsbury companion to the philosophy of sport.* London: Bloomsbury.

CHAPTER 9

Sport Pedagogy and Physical Activity

BELINDA STILLWELL

LEARNING OBJECTIVES

1. Define *sport pedagogy*.
2. Outline the history of the physical education profession.
3. Describe the types of research conducted in the area of sport pedagogy.
4. Summarize the future direction of sport pedagogy.

KEY TERMS

academic learning time in physical education (ALT–PE)

action research

analytic research

Comprehensive School Physical Activity Program (CSPAP)

curriculum

descriptive research

domains of learning

formative assessment

games-based approach

instruction

instructional time

managerial time

moderate-to-vigorous physical activity (MVPA)

motor activity

National Physical Activity Plan (NPAP)

national standards

observational research

pedagogy

philosophical orientation

physical activity

physical education

pedagogy
The art, science, or profession of teaching.

qualitative research
quantitative research
sport pedagogy
summative assessment

teacher movement
teaching behaviors
wait time

sport pedagogy
Pedagogy that encompasses school programs of physical education as well as community-based club programs of sport and fitness.

What Is Sport Pedagogy?

Pedagogy is defined as the art, science, or profession of teaching. In addition to teaching, pedagogy includes the development of instructional programs, plans to implement those programs, and assessment of the programs' outcomes. Thus, the term **sport pedagogy** encompasses both school programs of physical education and community-based club programs of sport and fitness. The focus of this chapter will be on physical education, with references to sport and fitness, considering especially how this knowledge is applied within and beyond the school walls.

physical education
A planned, sequential program of curricula and instruction that helps students develop the knowledge, skills, and confidence needed to adopt and maintain a physically active lifestyle.

Oftentimes, the terms *physical education* and *physical activity* are used interchangeably, but they are not the same thing. **Physical education** "is a planned, sequential program of curricula and instruction that helps students develop the knowledge, skills, and confidence needed to adopt and maintain a physically active lifestyle" (American Alliance for Health, Physical Education, Recreation and Dance, 2011, p. 9). The Society of Health and Physical Educators (SHAPE America) has defined four essential components of a high-quality physical education program: (1) the opportunity to learn, (2) meaningful content, (3) appropriate instruction, and (4) student and program assessment (SHAPE America, n.d.a). In contrast, **physical activity** is defined as voluntary movement intentionally performed to achieve a goal in sport, exercise, dance, or any other movement experience (Hoffman, 2005).

physical activity
Any bodily movement that requires the use of energy by the individual.

domains of learning
The fundamental motor (psychomotor) skills, social (affective) skills, and thinking (cognitive) skills necessary to promote lifelong health and well-being.

Although increasing the level of physical activity in physical education classes is a high priority, it is not the only goal. Physical educators simultaneously seek to equip students with the motor, social, and critical thinking skills necessary to promote lifelong health and well-being. These skills are collectively referred to as the **domains of learning**. Although all of the domains are essential in teaching and learning, the psychomotor domain is emphasized in physical education, because this is the only class in which students learn how to move.

In order to provide students with a quality physical education, a set of **national standards** has been developed to complement other academic areas, such as art, social science, and math. The five standards define a physically literate person and are intended to guide teachers in planning the **curriculum** and **instruction** for their students (SHAPE America, n.d.b):

1. The physically literate individual demonstrates competency in a variety of motor skills and movement patterns.
2. The physically literate individual applies knowledge of concepts, principles, strategies, and tactics related to movement and performance.
3. The physically literate individual demonstrates the knowledge and skills to achieve and maintain a health-enhancing level of physical activity and fitness.
4. The physically literate individual exhibits responsible personal and social behavior that respects self and others.
5. The physically literate individual recognizes the value of physical activity for health, enjoyment, challenge, self-expression, and/or social interaction.

STOP AND THINK

How do physical education and physical activity differ?

national standards
Five standards developed by SHAPE America that define a physically literate person and are intended to guide teachers in planning the curriculum and instruction for their students.

curriculum
What will be taught (e.g., nontraditional games, dance, educational gymnastics).

instruction
How the curriculum is delivered (e.g., instructional formats, curriculum models, teaching strategies).

SHAPE America   SOCIETY OF HEALTH AND PHYSICAL EDUCATORS®

Grade-Level Outcomes for K-12 Physical Education

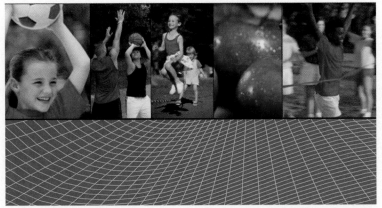

STOP AND THINK

Reflect on your elementary, middle, and high school physical education programs. Do you think you met the five national standards that define a physically literate person by the end of your high school career in physical education?

Ultimately, the physical educator decides what activities students will participate in, as well as which teaching strategies, instructional formats, and curriculum models will be used. For a detailed history on the development of physical education standards, see Siedentop and van der Mars (2012).

The History of Physical Education

Although various forms of sport, fitness, and physical education existed before 1885, it was not until 1886 that the first state legislation requiring physical education in schools was passed in California (Siedentop & van der Mars, 2012). Prior to this, several pioneering women and men built a strong foundation to support an expanding interest in the development of a full-fledged profession. One of the most influential of these pioneers was Dr. Delphine Hanna.

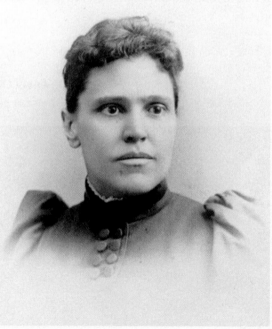

Dr. Delphine Hanna.   Courtesy of LOC

Dr. Delphine Hanna established the first women's professional physical education program at Oberlin College in Ohio in 1885. Dr. Hanna was the first woman in the United States, and possibly the world, to hold a professorship in physical education (Oberlin College Archives, 2014). Later, in 1903, she was appointed the first female full professor of physical education. Dr. Hanna also taught Luther Gulick (physical educator), Thomas Wood (new physical education developer), Jay Nash (creative leisure advocate), and Jesse Feiring Williams (physical educator, women's coach, author) (SHAPE America, n.d.c). Other female leaders who advocated for women in sport, fitness, and physical education included Ethel Perrin, Jessie Bancroft, Elizabeth Burchenal, and Blanche Trilling (**Box 9-1**).

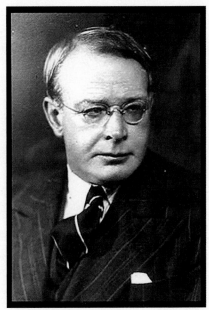

Thomas Wood.   Courtesy of LOC

Box 9-1   Historical Highlights of Pioneers in Physical Education

1825	Charles Beck becomes the first physical education teacher in the United States.
1831	Catherine Beecher publishes *A Course in Calisthenics for Young Ladies*. John Warren of Harvard writes the first theoretical treatise on physical education.
1837	Western Female Institute is founded by Catherine Beecher.
1861	Edward Hitchcock becomes the director of the Department of Hygiene and Physical Culture at Amherst College. Boston Normal Institute for Physical Education is founded by Dio Lewis.
1879	Dudley Sargent is appointed assistant professor of physical training at Harvard.
1883	Hartvig Nissen introduces Swedish gymnastics to the United States.

(continued)

1885	The professional physical education program at Oberlin College is established by Delphine Hanna.
1889	The Boston Normal School of Gymnastics, cofounded by Amy Morris Homans and Mary Hemenway, officially opens.
1890	Edward Hartwell becomes the director of physical training for Boston Public Schools.
1903	Luther Gulick is appointed director of physical education for New York schools. Delphine Hanna is appointed first female full professor of physical education.
1916	First state supervisor of physical education is named in New York.
1927	Rosiland Cassidy and Thomas Wood publish *The New Physical Education*.

D. Siedentop & H. van der Mars. (2012). *Introduction to physical education, fitness, and sport* (8th ed.). New York: McGraw-Hill.

Another important event took place around this time—the Boston conference of 1889. Organized by Amy Morris Homans (cofounder of the Boston Normal School of Gymnastics), this conference brought together prominent national and international leaders to discuss and evaluate the current activities and practices that were occurring in physical education, which were essentially different gymnastics systems (later called physical education). Known as the "battle of the systems," this forum fueled larger questions, such as "What should be the purpose of physical education?" and "How should that be purpose be achieved?" (Siedentop & van der Mars, 2012). Influenced by industrialization, urbanization, rising prosperity, and advances in transportation and communication, American society was fertile ground for sport to take root. As such, standardized sport quickly found its way into physical education curriculums, athletic programs in schools, and society as a whole.

Following the Great Depression and World War II, the explosion of sport for both women and men was championed by many well-known leaders. Continuing the work of earlier pioneers such as Theodore Roosevelt, who ushered in the Intercollegiate Athletic Association of the United States

(IAAUS) in 1906, and Blanche Trilling, who helped form the Athletic Conference of American College Women (ACACW) in 1917, several professional organizations that advanced the safe and humane participation of both men and women in competitive environments were established (**Box 9-2**).

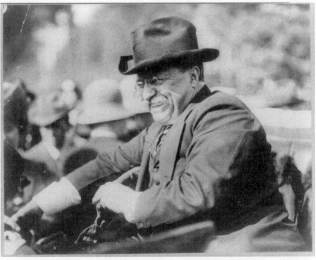

Theodore Roosevelt.

Courtesy of Library of Congress, LC-USZ62-12041

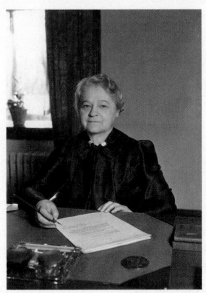

Blanche Trilling.

Courtesy of the University of Wisconsin-Madison (S05513)

Box 9-2 Historical Highlights of Organized Sport in the United States

1895   The Intercollegiate Conference of Faculty Representatives is formed (later known as the Western Conference or Big Ten).

1906   Theodore Roosevelt founds the Intercollegiate Athletic Association of the United States (IAAUS).

1917   Blanche Trilling helps form the Athletic Conference of American College Women (ACACW).

1941   Women's intercollegiate athletics is first organized on a national basis by the Division for Girls' and Women's Sports (DGWS).

1948   The Olympic Games begins again in the aftermath of World War II.

1950   The National Intramural Association is formed.

1956   The Tripartite Committee is formed by representatives of three organizations: the National Association for Physical Education for College Women (NAPECW), the National Association for Girls' and Women's Sport (NAGWS), and the American Federation of College Women.

1967   The Commission on Intercollegiate Athletics for Women (CIAW) is established.

1971   The Association for Intercollegiate Athletics for Women (AIAW) evolves out of the CIAW.

1972   Title IX of the Education Amendments is passed by the U.S. Congress.

1980   The NCAA offers women's Division I and II championships.

1983   The AIAW is phased out by the NCAA.

2002   Title IX is renamed the Patsy T. Mink Equal Opportunity Act after Patsy Mink, one of the principal authors of the amendment.

D. Siedentop & H. van der Mars. (2012). *Introduction to physical education, fitness, and sport* (8th ed.). New York: McGraw-Hill.

Although present in schools for many years, physical education consistently draws the most national attention in times of crisis, such as during the polio epidemic in the 1940s and 1950s; during World War II, when many draftees were excluded from service for poor fitness levels; the mid-1950s, when research showed that 60% of American children and adolescents failed a test of minimum muscular fitness compared to 9% of their European counterparts; and the recent obesity epidemic (Siedentop & van der Mars, 2012). While early views of physical education in the United States were heavily influenced by European gymnastic systems, a broader perspective was adopted at the beginning of the 20th century that included dance, sport, recreation, and fitness. This became known as the "new physical education." **TABLE 9-1** provides a brief overview of the **philosophical orientations** that

philosophical orientation
A particular perspective on how learning occurs.

TABLE 9-1   Philosophical Orientations that Have Influenced Physical Education

Period	Orientation	Emphasis	Result
Early 1900s	Progressive education	Every student is unique in terms of his or her physical, motor, social, and mental needs; therefore, a variety of activities should be offered to meet these needs.	Multiactivity model
1930s and 1940s	Human movement	The intellectual and emotional development of students.	Movement education
1960s and 1970s	Humanistic sport and physical education	Fully developing a student's potential through personal growth and self-development.	Personal and social responsibility model
	Lifelong wellness	Promotion of lifelong physical activity and healthy lifestyles that contribute to a student's lifelong fitness, wellness, and health through a combination of movement and classroom activities.	Concepts-based physical education model (now called the academic discipline model)
1980s	Experiential and adventure education	Helps students become responsible, caring, and contributing members of society.	Outdoor adventure model
	Play and sport education	Assists students in acquiring skills and developing an affection for the activities themselves.	Sport education model Teaching games for understanding (TGFU) model
1990s	Ecological approach	Increases students' moderate-to-vigorous levels of physical activity (MVPA) with the ultimate goal of contributing to a healthy lifestyle.	Health-optimizing physical education (HOPE) model

Modified from D. Siedentop & H. van der Mars. (2012). *Introduction to physical education, fitness, and sport* (8th ed.). New York: McGraw-Hill.

have shaped physical education over time as a result of social, cultural, and political influences.

Why Study Sport Pedagogy?

Sport, dance, fitness, nontraditional, and outdoor activity programs are accessible to the public through school programs like physical education and athletics as well as community-based centers and organizations. It is important that teachers and community leaders in these programs receive the best possible training in order for their students and participants to receive quality movement experiences that will last a lifetime. Sport pedagogy provides the essential training to effectively deliver these programs to children and adolescents from diverse backgrounds. Students who study sport pedagogy learn how to create a positive learning environment, plan curricula, deliver effective instruction, assess motor skills, and expand their own physical capabilities. Many become licensed physical educators in public schools, coaches, and before- and after-school physical activity specialists. Some credentialed physical educators also become Adapted Physical Educators (APE). These individuals are interested in working with students with physical and intellectual disabilities in the school setting. This additional authorization requires further coursework and field experiences typically available in comprehensive kinesiology departments. Your interest may also extend beyond the school day to include coaching athletes with disabilities in competitive community programs, the Special Olympics, or Paralympics. The ability to teach well holds value for all kinesiologists. Whether you are teaching eighth graders to play Ultimate frisbee, working one-on-one with an athlete recovering from an injury, or helping a toddler explore the swimming pool, knowing what to do, when to do it, and how to do it will help ensure a successful learning experience.

STOP AND THINK

Identify ways in which daily, quality physical education can address the current obesity epidemic.

Major Topics in Sport Pedagogy

In this section, we will examine the major topics that surround the four key components of a quality physical education program, as outlined by SHAPE America. These include the opportunity to learn, meaningful content,

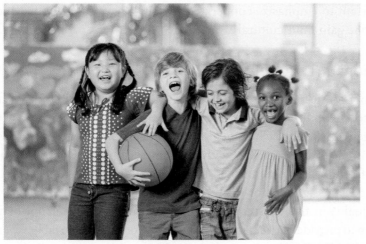

© Gagliardilmages/Shutterstock

appropriate instruction, and student and program assessment (SHAPE America, n.d.a).

OPPORTUNITY TO LEARN

According to SHAPE America, the opportunity to learn means that all students—kindergarten through high school—are required to take physical education. The total instructional time per week should total 150 minutes for elementary school students and 225 minutes per week for middle and high school students. Physical education class sizes must be consistent with those of other subject areas, such as science or math, in order to provide a safe environment with ample attention to all students. Lastly, all instructional periods need to be led by a qualified physical education specialist who provides a developmentally appropriate program with access to adequate equipment and facilities.

MEANINGFUL CONTENT

Meaningful content entails a written, sequential curriculum for prekindergarten through 12th grade that is based on national or state standards for physical education. Included in this curriculum is the instruction of a variety of motor skills and fitness education designed to enhance the psychomotor, cognitive, and affective development of every student. It is especially important to emphasize cooperation through physical activity, which can help one gain multicultural awareness.

APPROPRIATE INSTRUCTION

Appropriate instruction requires the full participation of all students, including those with little or no movement experience, as well as those with disabilities. Effective teachers achieve this inclusion through well-designed lessons that provide students with ample in-class practice opportunities and out-of-school assignments that support learning. Moreover, physical activity is never assigned as or withheld as punishment.

Quality instruction requires mastery of a number of teaching behaviors known to provide participants with an educational and enjoyable experience. Essential **teaching behaviors** include teacher movement; providing meaningful feedback; and minimizing instructional, managerial, and waiting time.

teaching behaviors
Verbal or nonverbal actions the teacher performs, such as instructional time or teacher movement.

teacher movement
Where the teacher goes within the activity area.

TEACHER MOVEMENT

Teacher movement patterns track where the teacher goes within the activity area. These patterns can be easily seen by dividing the activity area up into four quadrants, as shown below:

During the lesson or activity time, an observer would simply chart where the teacher moved by marking an "X" in that quadrant (a video camera can also be used). At the end of the observation period, the activity area might look like this:

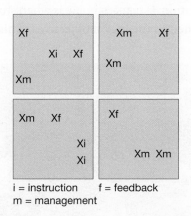

In addition, the observer could also chart what the teacher did after arriving at the new destination. For example, if the teacher moved from quadrant A to quadrant B to deliver feedback to a student, the observer might put a lowercase "f" next to the "X" to denote feedback. The observer may use an "i" for instruction or an "m" for management. The newly coded activity area would look like this:

i = instruction　　f = feedback
m = management

Movement allows the teacher to deliver meaningful feedback (f), provide additional instruction (i), or manage (m) any behavioral issues that might arise to help students stay engaged and on-task.

TABLE 9-2 Types of Feedback

Type of Feedback	Example
Positive	"Keep up the good work, Stephanie."
Corrective	"Remember to follow through."
General	"Excellent job today everybody."
Specific	"Great job squaring your shoulders up to the basket, Douglas."
Nonverbal	Thumbs up

instructional time
Time students spend watching or listening to the teacher.

managerial time
When students are involved in tasks that are not related to the lesson objectives, such as time spent taking roll, getting into groups, or putting away equipment.

MEANINGFUL FEEDBACK

Delivering meaningful feedback is a crucial part of effective teaching. Student performance can be greatly enhanced when teachers deliver the appropriate feedback at the right time. Different types of feedback include positive, corrective, general, specific, and nonverbal (**TABLE 9-2**).

MINIMIZING INSTRUCTIONAL, MANAGERIAL, AND WAIT TIME.

Instructional time is defined as the time students spend watching or listening to the teacher. This includes listening to explanations and directions or watching a demonstration. **Managerial time** is when students are involved in tasks that are not related to the lesson objectives. This could be time spent

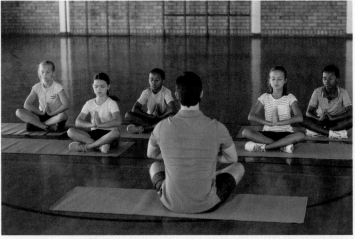

© wavebreakmedia/Shutterstock

taking roll, getting into groups, or putting away equipment. **Wait time** is when students do not have any task to do—they are simply "standing around" waiting for the next task to begin. Even though instructional time helps students understand key concepts, good teachers learn to decrease the amount of time students are passively listening and watching versus engaged in a movement task. Similarly, skilled teachers also minimize managerial and wait time for the same reason.

STUDENT AND PROGRAM ASSESSMENT

Student and program assessment is a fundamental part of a quality physical education program. Student assessment can be formative and/or summative in nature. **Formative assessment** is used as a checkpoint to evaluate student learning from day to day. An example might be a peer assessment that asks students to judge their classmate's passing skills during a small-sided basketball game. Peer feedback would help improve a classmate's passing effectiveness during future game play.

Conversely, **summative assessment** is used to find out what students have learned at the end of the instructional unit. For instance, after studying the rules of basketball, applying the rules in a game, and practicing refereeing skills, students would be assessed on their ability to officiate tournament play at the end of the unit. These assessments, whether formative or summative, are aligned with the physical education standards and written curriculum that has been established. Likewise, the entire physical education program must be assessed every 3 to 5 years. Such an assessment includes an evaluation of the four key components of a quality physical education program by key stakeholders.

These same behaviors are valuable to master when working in settings beyond the school walls, such as Boys & Girls Clubs, YMCAs, recreational centers, and fitness clubs. Participants led by qualified leaders that effectively supervise the activity area and reduce downtime will likely improve their motor skills, fitness levels, thinking abilities, and capacity for positive social interactions. Additionally, periodic reviews of the entire program (e.g., a YMCA afterschool program) would be conducted to reflect on meaningful change.

wait time
When students do not have any task to do; that is, they are simply standing around.

formative assessment
Assessment that is used as a checkpoint to evaluate student learning from day to day.

summative assessment
Assessment that is used to determine what students have learned at the end of a learning segment.

STOP AND THINK

Consider the four key components of a quality physical education program: (1) opportunity to learn, (2) meaningful content, (3) appropriate instruction, and (4) student and program assessment. What was your experience with these components during your elementary, middle, and/or high school years? How much physical activity did you encounter in your school physical education programs versus any movement-based programs you participated in outside of school?

What Can You Do with a Degree in Sport Pedagogy?

Most students who major in kinesiology with an emphasis in physical education intend to become teachers and coaches in the public schools, and some will go on to become athletic directors. In order to teach in the public school setting, students must complete an additional year enrolled in a full-time, university-level credential program. Some programs offer flexible scheduling that allow for more time to completion. Upon successful completion of a credential program, students earn a preliminary single-subject credential in physical education, which allows the holder to teach physical education at the K–12 level.

In terms of coaching, requirements vary by state, so be sure to check with your school administration or state association to confirm your state's requirements. Most states require certification courses, such as fundamentals of coaching; first aid, health, and safety for coaches; and concussion in sport. Like teaching, a set of national standards for sport coaches helps guide the profession and ensures the well-being of all athletes. Those who choose not to complete a credential or coaching certification program have a good foundation to work with school-aged participants in a variety of community-based activity programs.

Areas of Research in Sport Pedagogy

In this section, we discuss and provide examples of the most common methods used by researchers in sport pedagogy to ultimately improve teaching and learning in physical education as well as in other physical activity settings (Thomas, Nelson, & Silverman, 2011). Specific areas of study include the analysis of teacher and student behaviors, teacher effectiveness, classroom management, curriculum development and implementation, student achievement, and the degree to which students come to adopt and value a physically active lifestyle. **TABLE 9-3** presents examples of questions that may be studied within sport pedagogy.

The research approach a researcher uses depends on the type of data he or she is interested in collecting and analyzing. Like other disciplines, research in kinesiology can be broadly categorized as quantitative, qualitative, or a combination of both (mixed model). Researchers engaged in **quantitative research** use traditional scientific methods to generate numerical data and seek to establish causal relationships between two or more variables

quantitative research Research that generates numerical data and seeks to establish causal relationships between two or more variables by using statistical methods to test the strength and significance of the relationships.

TABLE 9-3   *Sport Pedagogy: Example Research Questions*

Area	Example Questions
Teacher behavior	What kind of feedback do teachers provide?
	How much time do teachers spend in various teaching activities?
Student behavior	What types of interaction occur between classmates?
	How do students spend their time in classes?
Teacher effectiveness	What characteristics make a teacher effective?
	What teaching strategies are most effective?
Classroom management	What types of routines and rules do teachers establish in their classrooms?
	How do teachers build a positive classroom climate?
Curriculum	Does a teacher's value orientation play a role in the curriculum they choose to teach?
	Is there an ideal physical education curriculum?
Student achievement	How are students assessed in physical education?
	In what ways are students involved in the assessment process?
Physically active lifestyle	Do students enjoy and value physical education beyond the school walls?
	Are there opportunities for students to be physically active throughout the school day?

Modified from D. Siedentop & H. van der Mars. (2012). *Introduction to physical education, fitness, and sport* (8th ed.). New York: McGraw-Hill.

(e.g., teacher and student behaviors) by using statistical methods to test the strength and significance of the relationships (Martin & McFerran, 2008). In contrast, researchers conducting **qualitative research** are interested in understanding the meaning individuals have constructed; that is, how people make sense of their world and the experience they have in the world (Merriam, 2009). With qualitative research, the data collected and analyzed are expressed in the form of words or images. These words can be acquired in several ways, such as through interviews, observations, or by examining existing documents, such as diaries and books. Images can come in the form of photographs or video clips.

DESCRIPTIVE RESEARCH

Descriptive research uses description, classification, measurement, and comparison to describe a population or phenomenon. Common descriptive research techniques include questionnaires, interviews, normative surveys,

qualitative research
Data collected and analyzed are expressed in the form of words or images to examine how people make sense of their world and the experience they have in the world.

descriptive research
Uses description, classification, measurement, and comparison to describe a population or phenomenon.

observational research
A technique used to observe and record behaviors that occur in a participant's natural setting.

motor activity
Activities that cause or produce motion.

STOP AND THINK

Review the types of questions studied by sport pedagogists in Table 9-3. Formulate two new questions that could be added to three of the areas presented in the table. For example, if you choose "teacher effectiveness," add two new questions to the existing questions that would be interesting to examine.

moderate-to-vigorous physical activity (MVPA)
Moderate-intensity physical activity is when a person is working hard enough to raise his or her heart rate and break into a sweat; vigorous physical activity is when a person is breathing hard and fast and his or her heart rate has increased significantly.

case studies, job analyses, developmental studies, correlational studies, epidemiologic research, and observational research (Thomas et al., 2011).

Observational research is a technique used to watch and record behaviors that occur in a participant's natural setting (Thomas et al., 2011). Observational research data have been gathered and analyzed since the early 1970s to find out what teachers and students have been doing during physical education classes. These types of studies most often yield numerical data (e.g., percentages, frequency, duration) to explain what is happening during class. The quantitative data can simply be reported or tested statistically to compare changes that occur over time or between classes.

Two key student variables that have been scrutinized over time are the quantity and quality of **motor activity** during physical education class. Results from this literature found that students were spending less than 30% of their time engaged in motor activity, while the remaining time was spent in managerial or instructional time (Siedentop & Tannehill, 2000). Based on these data, guidelines have been established by experts to help teachers increase their students' motor activity time by decreasing managerial, instructional, and wait time. These guidelines suggest that teachers and students spend less than 10% of the class period engaged in management time and less than 5% in waiting time. Moreover, each episode of instruction should last 1 minute or less. Occasionally, instructional time may exceed 1 minute if the teacher is introducing new information or if the topic is safety oriented.

EXPERIMENTAL RESEARCH

One way to think about quantitative research is to consider an experiment. For instance, we can create a scenario in which a researcher is interested in finding out if a games-based approach increases the amount of **moderate-to-vigorous physical activity (MVPA)** and **academic learning time in physical education (ALT-PE)** experienced by students during a series of soccer lessons (think of ALT-PE as the time students spend on task). To accomplish this, a researcher could set up an experiment comparing students using the

TABLE 9-4   Games-Based vs. Direct Teaching Approach

Games-Based Approach	Direct Teaching Approach
Students learn to solve problems within the context of small-sided games.	Skills and strategies are often isolated in drill-like activities before allowing students to "play the game."
Framework	**Framework**
Game 1: Students are given a game problem to solve (e.g., how to maintain possession) while participating in small-sided games.	*Explanation*: The teacher explains and demonstrates passing skills.
Questions and answers: Students engage in a question-and-answer session with the teacher following Game 1.	*Guided practice*: Students pass back and forth with a partner while the teacher provides feedback.
Practice task: Students practice a skill or strategy designed to solve the game problem in small, game-like groups.	*Independent practice*: Students continue to practice passing on their own.
Game 2: Students return to game play to apply the skill (passing) or strategy (give and go) previously practiced.	*Game*: Students play a game.
Closure: Students compare Game 1 and Game 2.	

games-based approach (Teacher A's class) with students taught using a direct teaching approach (Teacher B's class; **TABLE 9-4**). The amount of time students were engaged in MVPA and ALT-PE would be recorded in both classes, and the results would be compared using the appropriate statistical tests. The results might show that those students who were taught using the games-based approach were more active and successful when performing the tasks associated with each of the lesson goals than those taught using a direct teaching approach.

Continuing with our example, a researcher could convert this quantitative study into a qualitative study by exploring the personal experiences of students who participated in both classes. To achieve this, the researcher might conduct focus group interviews, forming small groups of students from each class and asking them questions about their movement experiences during the soccer unit. Sample questions might be: "Tell me about your experiences in class," "What did you like most about coming to class?" "What did you like least about coming to class?" and "Would you change anything about the way class was conducted?" The researcher might conclude that those who participated in the games-based approach felt more engaged and

academic learning time–physical education (ALT–PE) Time during class when students are successful and actively engaged in accomplishing the goals of a lesson.

games-based approach Approach to learning that allows students to discover what to do in a game and then how to do it.

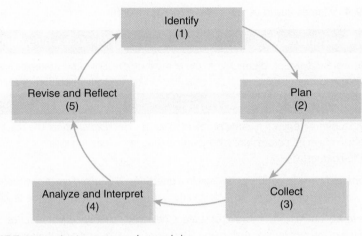

FIGURE 9-1   Action research model.

Data from Monet, Julie. (2014). Action Research Model. California State University, Chico.

successful than those who experienced the direct teaching approach. Lastly, the researcher could blend both of these studies and use a mixed-method approach to construct a deeper analysis of student experiences.

ACTION RESEARCH

action research
Type of research typically undertaken in a school setting by teachers who are looking for ways to improve instruction and increase student achievement. Also referred to as *action participatory research*.

Action research, also called *participatory action research*, has gained in popularity in recent years. **Action research** is typically undertaken in a school setting by teachers who are looking for ways to improve instruction and increase student achievement. The approach is similar to the experimental approach but it puts the teacher (as researcher) and her class (as participants) at the center of inquiry (**FIGURE 9-1**). Generally speaking, action research provides teachers the opportunity to work on areas they are curious about or challenged by in order to improve their effectiveness and, in turn, maximize student learning. It presents a systematic way to change both the teacher and the environment in which they work. In keeping with the games-based approach, see **Box 9-3** as an example of how this process might be applied to physical education.

Box 9-3 An Action Research Example

Step 1: Identify

To get started on an action research project, identify the following:

- A focus of interest or problem based on the needs of your students.
  Example: Students are not fully engaged in the lesson.

- A question to guide the project.
  Example: Will using the games-based approach improve students' physical engagement during a soccer unit?

- The current level of student performance in relation to the interest or problem stated.
  Example: At what level are students currently participating in sport units? To answer this, collect data from several sources to get a clear picture on where students are before the intervention occurs (e.g., observations, self-assessments).

- Resources to increase your knowledge and skills with regard to the interest or problem stated.
  Example: Broaden your own knowledge and experience in using the games-based approach.

Step 2: Plan

- Develop an intervention.
  Example: Create a unit plan on soccer using the games-based approach.

- Determine the assessments you will use to help answer the question.
  Example: Use several types of assessments to gather evidence (e.g., game-play peer assessments, video recordings of students in action).

- Determine when to assess students.
  Example: Collect pre-, mid-, and post-unit data.

Step 3: Collect

- Collect and organize the data.
  Example: Gather and organize game-play peer assessments and video recordings of students in action.

Step 4: Analyze and Interpret

- Look for patterns, trends, and insight among the data.
  Example (analyze): What themes emerge from the data? For example, did students' decision-making skills in game situations improve? Did this result in more movement?

Example (interpret): Compare your findings with other research studies on the games-based approach.

Step 5: Revise/Reflect

- Revise your question and/or intervention.
  Example (intervention): Extend the unit plan to include sports that are conceptually similar in nature to soccer, such as field hockey.
- Reflect on what you have learned. How will this research change your practice?
  Example: What have you learned from this project? How will this inform the next group of students you teach?

RESEARCH AND TECHNOLOGY

To help capture data during studies, researchers often use technologies that enable them to measure variables efficiently and accurately. Devices that have proven useful in research in this field include heart-rate monitors, activity monitors, pedometers, and video. The advantages and disadvantages of heart-rate monitors, activity monitors, and pedometers can be found in Welk and Meredith (2008). Continuing with our action research example, researchers might use heart-rate monitors and video recordings to gather data on the quantity (MVPA) and quality (ALT-PE) of student engagement to help them answer their question(s).

ANALYTIC RESEARCH

analytic research
Research conducted in the field of sport humanities, which includes sport history, sport philosophy, and sport literature.

The field of sport humanities also offers a rich avenue for research in sport pedagogy. This area includes sport history, sport philosophy, and sport literature. Through **analytic research**, sport historians critically analyze their findings in order to provide perspective on the past in relation to the present and future. Sport philosophers are interested in examining topics such as sport ethics, the value of physical activity, and mind–body relationships. As noted by Siedentop and van der Mars (2012), "Sport literature explores the use of prose (written or spoken language), film, and poetry that focuses specifically on sport or sport themes as vehicles through which to examine basic human dilemmas and situations."

The Future of Physical Education

The future direction of physical education is being shaped by two primary forces: the 2016 U.S. National Physical Activity Plan (NPAP) and the Comprehensive School Physical Activity Program (CSPAP). What do these two programs have in common? Both promote the behavior of physical activity. This is a major shift in thinking from the country's earlier focus on physical fitness. Although physical fitness is still one of the anticipated outcomes of physical education programs, a person's ability to improve his or her physical fitness is in many ways related to his or her genetics. For instance, a person's ability to enhance cardiorespiratory endurance or alter body composition often depends on biological factors such as muscle fiber composition and the presence or absence of chronic illness, disability, or a permanent medical condition. The potential to be physically active is ultimately a matter of adopting a healthy lifestyle. In this case, people can choose to eat better and increase their daily physical activity level.

> **STOP AND THINK**
>
> Use a library database such as the Physical Educators Index, SPORTDiscus, or PubMed to locate a research article focused on sport pedagogy. After reading the article, decide what research approach was used to answer the research question (e.g., descriptive, experimental, action research, analytical, or something else). Determine if the study was qualitative and/or quantitative.

NATIONAL PHYSICAL ACTIVITY PLAN

The 2016 **National Physical Activity Plan (NPAP)** created by The National Physical Activity Alliance (a nonprofit organization) outlines a vision for America: "One day, all Americans will be physically active and they will live, work, and play in environments that facilitate regular physical activity" (NPAP, 2016). The aim is to create a national culture that supports physically active lifestyles by improving health, preventing disease and disability, and enhancing quality of life. The plan is an inclusive set of policies, programs, and initiatives that are directed at increasing the levels of physical activity across the U.S. population, and it involves hundreds of private- and public-sector entities. It is organized into nine societal sectors: (1) business and industry; (2) community recreation, fitness and parks; (3) education; (4) faith-based settings; (5) healthcare; (6) mass media; (7) public health; (8) sport; and (9) transportation, land use and community design (NPAP, 2016).

National Physical Activity Plan (NPAP) A plan to create a national culture that supports physically active lifestyles by improving health, preventing disease and disability, and enhancing quality of life.

STOP AND THINK

In what ways does your community promote physically active lifestyles? Use the eight sectors outlined in the NPAP to help you formulate your answer.

Comprehensive School Physical Activity Program (CSPAP)
Goal that all schools provide a physical activity program with the following five components: (1) physical education, (2) physical activity during school, (3) physical activity before and after school, (4) staff involvement, and (5) family and community involvement.

Of special interest to the sport pedagogist is the education sector, and, in particular, Strategy 6, which reads: "Educational institutions should provide pre-service professional training and in-service professional development programs that prepare educators to deliver effective physical activity programs for students of all types" (NPAP, 2016). Additionally, each strategy is accompanied by suggested tactics to help achieve the overarching plan. For Strategy 6, a recommended tactic is to "Prepare physical education teachers to assume the role of school physical activity director, coordinating programs that are consistent with the Comprehensive School Physical Activity Program model" (NPAP, 2016).

COMPREHENSIVE SCHOOL PHYSICAL ACTIVITY PROGRAM

In an effort to gather baseline data related to progress toward the NPAP, the American Alliance for Health, Physical Education, Recreation, and Dance (AAHPERD) conducted a survey in 2011 titled the Comprehensive School Physical Activity Program (CSPAP) survey. This ongoing survey is also being used to inform AAHPERD's *Let's Move!* Active Schools (n.d.) initiative and is aimed at ensuring that every school provides a **Comprehensive School Physical Activity Program (CSPAP)** with quality physical education (AAHPERD, 2011). A CSPAP consists of five components: (1) physical education, (2) physical activity during school, (3) physical activity before and after school, (4) staff involvement, and (5) family and community involvement.

The AAHPERD survey found that less than 17% of schools are providing a CSPAP (see results from CSPAP survey for complete details, AAHPERD, 2011). In the conclusions, AAHPERD states that schools should be fully prepared to provide physical activity opportunities for their students, because school accounts for the majority of waking hours for most children and adolescents. Equally, schools should employ a director of physical activity (DPA) whose expertise and training would be helpful in coordinating the CSPAP, and that this individual would most likely be a physical educator. Other agencies and documents that support physical activity in schools

STOP AND THINK

In what ways did your elementary, middle, and/or high school promote physically active lifestyles? Use the five components of the CSPAP to aid in your evaluation.

include the Institute of Medicine, the Physical Activity Guidelines for Americans put forth by the U.S. Department of Health and Human Services, the White House Task Force on Childhood Obesity Report to the President, and *Healthy People 2020* (as reported by AAHPERD, 2011).

Despite the fact that physical education continues to face many challenges (e.g., large class sizes, marginalization, lack of resources), its importance cannot go unnoticed in helping to achieve a physically active population. Besides expanding physical activity opportunities in and beyond the school walls, it will be critical to create federal and state policies and secure funding to support movement programs. We must continue to strive to create equitable physical activity opportunities across the population. It will take collaboration at the local, state, national, and international levels to achieve this vision.

CHAPTER SUMMARY

In this chapter, you learned that sport pedagogy covers both school-based physical education programs and a variety of community-based movement programs. Even though physical education, sport, and fitness programs have been around for many years, 1886 marked the first state legislation requiring physical education in schools. Four key components that comprise a quality physical education program are the opportunity to learn, appropriate instruction, student evaluation, and program assessment. Most students who study sport pedagogy intend to become physical education teachers in the public schools, and a few become leaders in movement-based programs beyond the school walls.

Both qualitative and quantitative research methods are used to analyze teacher and student behaviors, teacher effectiveness, classroom management, curriculum development and implementation, student achievement, and the degree to which students come to adopt and value a physically active lifestyle. These variables also serve to inform instructors and coaches working in nonschool settings. Lastly, the CSPAP and the NPAP hold great promise in guiding Americans toward increased physical activity.

DISCUSSION QUESTIONS

1. With regard to your option area (e.g., physical education, exercise science, dance), what role do you feel you could play in achieving the vision of the NPAP?
2. Is your college campus designed to promote physically active lifestyles?
3. Respond to the following statement: Physical education is an academic subject.

4. How are physical educators and nonschool physical activity specialists similar? How are they different?

5. Why is research in sport pedagogy important?

REFERENCES

American Alliance for Health, Physical Education, Recreation and Dance. (2011). *2011 Comprehensive School Physical Activity Program (CSPAP) Survey Report.* Reston, VA: Author.

Hoffman, S. J. (2005). *Introduction to kinesiology* (3rd ed.). Champaign, IL: Human Kinetics.

Let's Move! Active Schools. (n.d.). Retrieved from http//www.LetsMoveInSchool.org

Martin, E., & McFerran, T. (2008). *A dictionary of nursing.* Oxford, UK: Oxford University Press.

Merriam, S. B. (2009). *Qualitative research: A guide to design and implementation.* San Francisco: Jossey-Bass.

Monet, J. (2014). Action research model. California State University, Chico. Retrieved from http://www.csuchico.edu/teacher-grants/actionresearch/ar_model.shtml

National Physical Activity Plan. (2016). About the Plan. Retrieved from http://www.physicalactivityplan.org/theplan/about.html

Oberlin College Archives. (2014). RG 30/324 Delphine Hanna (1854–1941). Retrieved from http://www.oberlin.edu/archive/holdings/finding/RG30/SG324/biography.html

SHAPE America. (n.d.a). What constitutes a quality physical education program? Retrieved from http://www.shapeamerica.org/advocacy/positionstatements/pe/loader.cfm?csModule=security/getfile&pageid=4704

SHAPE America. (n.d.b). National PE standards. Retrieved from http://www.shapeamerica.org/standards/pe/

SHAPE America. (n.d.c). A brief history of the Midwest district. Retrieved from http://www.aahperd.org/about/districts/midwest/history.cfm

Siedentop, D., & Tannehill, D. (2000). *Developing teaching skills in physical education* (4th ed.). Mountain View, CA: Mayfield.

Siedentop, D., & van der Mars, H. (2012). *Introduction to physical education, fitness, and sport* (8th ed.). New York: McGraw-Hill.

Thomas, J., Nelson, J., & Silverman, S. (2011). *Research methods in physical activity.* Champaign, IL: Human Kinetics.

Welk, G. J., & Meredith, M. D. (Eds.). (2008). *Fitnessgram/Activitygram reference guide* (3rd ed.). Dallas, TX: The Cooper Institute.

CHAPTER 10

Sociology of Sport, Exercise, and Physical Activity

MAUREEN SMITH AND KATHERINE M. JAMIESON

LEARNING OBJECTIVES

1. Describe the general scope of the field of sociology of sport, exercise, and physical activity.

2. Outline the general history and major events in the field of sociology of sport, exercise, and physical activity.

3. Define key terms used in the field of sociology of sport, exercise, and physical activity.

4. Describe key concepts and themes of sociology of sport, exercise, and physical activity.

5. Discuss the applications of sociology of sport, exercise, and physical activity to various careers in kinesiology and human movement.

6. Describe research areas within sociology of sport, exercise, and physical activity.

KEY TERMS

analytic knowledge techniques
cultural conditions
cultural theories
culture
emergent sport

experience knowledge techniques
historical context
landscape knowledge techniques
social currents
social facts

sociological imagination
sociology of sport, exercise, and
  physical activity

status quo
structural components
structural theories

What Is Sociology of Sport, Exercise, and Physical Activity?

Do you ever wonder why physical education is required in American schools? Have you ever thought about what physical education and sport were like for your parents, or your grandparents? Or for citizens in some European countries, where sport teams have their origins in city clubs and are not affiliated with the educational system? Have you noticed how much money and public resources flow into certain levels of sport and physical activity? If you have pondered these and related issues, you are on your way to developing a sociological imagination. Throughout this chapter, we will invite you to develop what C. Wright Mills (1959) called the **sociological imagination**, or a manner of seeing one's personal biography as deeply linked with broader societal conditions.

Sociology of sport, exercise, and physical activity is the study of sport as a social phenomenon. Studying sport from a sociological perspective is challenging work. Much of American culture is enamored with sport, with Super Bowl Sunday considered an unofficial national holiday, numerous television channels and radio stations devoted to sport, taxpayers voting to publicly fund arenas for sport teams, and millions of youth playing sport year-round. Yet, despite this love for sport, American sporting practices are also reflective of broader social inequalities and social problems, such as teenagers burning out from early sport specialization, coaches and parents yelling at referees, high schools cutting teams to solve budget issues, and the increasing incidence of health issues related to a lack of physical activity, including diabetes, cardiovascular disease, and obesity. This is what sport sociologist Stan Eitzen (2012) refers to as "paradoxes of sport," or the notion that sport is fair *and* foul. These contradictions make a critical examination important, but also tricky, because many people do not want to think about the seamier side of sport. A sport sociologist has much work to do!

What does it mean to study sport from a sociological perspective? Throughout this chapter, we will suggest that sport of course requires physical activity, but that it is never only physical, and that it is also deeply

sociological imagination
Framework used by C. Wright Mills to think about the world around us, taking into account how the individual is connected to the "bigger picture."

sociology of sport, exercise, and physical activity
Academic study of sport as a social phenomenon.

influenced by the broader cultural conditions in which it takes place. This simply means that even those things we take for granted as "natural" or "right" in our everyday lives, like sport, have evolved in response to broad societal conditions. These broad societal conditions typically are understood as issues of access, atmosphere, and historical context. Thus, learning to think about and see sport as *more than the physical*—as also cultural—is a requirement for anyone applying a sociological analysis to sport and physical activity. As a starting point, we have to think about what we mean by sport. Although much of the early work in the sociology of sport focused on traditional sport, more recently the field has taken a much more inclusive approach to studying sport, defining it more broadly to include exercise, physical activity, physical education, competition, recreation, dance, and physical culture. Currently, programs in kinesiology prepare students for professions and careers that go well beyond that of physical education teacher and coach to include wellness, fitness, personal training, strength and conditioning, athletic training, sport management, sport psychology, exercise physiology, and biomechanics. All of these areas of study are interested in physical activity. At the root of kinesiology is physical activity.

A next step in becoming attuned to the broad cultural contours of sport and physical activity is to define **culture**. All too often, the term *culture* is misunderstood as being synonymous with race or ethnicity. Although race and ethnicity are certainly relevant in a conceptual understanding of culture, they are not one and the same. Throughout this chapter, when we invite you to think about sport and physical activity as "cultural" practices, we are referring to the dominant and common language, ways of life, and role expectations that govern our everyday interactions in the social world. This governance of our interactions happens in formal and informal ways. For example, when a school-age boy expresses interest in trying out for the dance team rather than the football team, he may face informal governance in the form of social questions and accusations from peers about his gender identity, sexuality, physical competence, and so on. As well, he may face formal governance if the school is unaccustomed to having boys on the dance team and thus does not offer him equitable access and resources for his participation on this team. The shared knowledge that leads each of us to engage in these acts of governing social life is precisely what we refer to as culture.

Sociologists of sport and physical activity approach the study of human movement from a variety of social science perspectives. As mentioned earlier,

culture
Dominant and common language, ways of life, roles, and expectations that govern our everyday interactions in the social world.

STOP AND THINK

Identify and explain three different cultural norms that influence your own participation, or lack of, in physical activity, exercise, or sport.

sociologists of sport are not as interested in the actual physical aspects of the movement, but instead are more concerned with the cultural, political, economic, and historical conditions of human engagement in physical activity.

Sociology of sport and psychology of sport share some areas of study, such as sport fans, aggression, body image, and performance-enhancing drugs, among others. But the two approaches to studying these aspects of sport are quite different. A sport psychologist is working with individual athletes and movers, often in efforts to improve or enhance their performance, sometimes to help motivate them to show up to the gym. A sport sociologist is more interested in thinking about the conditions of individuals as connected to the broader group, whether athletes, coaches, fans, or sport parents, and how these individuals have been shaped by structures and cultures that create the conditions for them to participate in their activities. A sport sociologist is not quite as interested in figuring out how to make Usain Bolt run faster. Instead, the sport sociologist is more interested in the conditions that make one's elite or everyday involvement in physical activity a possibility. How did Bolt decide to participate in track and field instead of another sport, perhaps equally suited for a tall, lanky body, such as volleyball? Did his early days in track and field include the involvement of his parents? What conditions have helped foster the great success of sprinters in Jamaica?

Sport historians and sport sociologists also share some academic space; sport historians study the past, which at one point was the sport sociologist's present. The work each does can help inform the other. Think about it this way. Let's go back to Olympic Champion, Usain Bolt. A sport historian might examine the history of track and field in Jamaica, as well as the history of Jamaica in the Olympics. These histories help the sport sociologist think about the historical conditions Bolt and his fellow sprinters face in their quest for speed. In developing one's sociological imagination, historical conditions are relevant factors in thinking about the present.

Even if you decide that the sociology of sport and physical activity is not the career for you, a social-science understanding of sport can lend you helpful tools in your chosen field within kinesiology, as well as in your home communities. The tools of the field will assist you as a sport parent, organizer of youth/club sport, or professional working at a health club, community center, exercise studio, and so on. We would argue that a sociological imagination is an asset for anyone interested in creating a physically active society.

A Brief History of the Sociology of Sport, Exercise, and Physical Activity

Examples of the broad cultural value of sport have been around since the Olympics of ancient Greece, when only men could compete in the Olympic Games and only men could watch these sporting festivals. This was an early example of the "gendered nature" of sport, or the use of gender as a central organizing principle in major sport events. It was these highly organized and state-governed sporting contexts, as well as less formal forms of sport, that caught the interest and attention of social scientists. Even as far back as ancient Greek society, sport is observable as part of the significant rituals and human development issues of the time. Thus, sport was central to religious rituals and was part of the holistic development of the preferred citizen.

The sociological study of sport has emerged at the intersection of the discipline of physical education and various humanities and social science disciplines. As the field of physical education developed, the discipline evolved, moving from one that was rooted in anatomy and the study of the body, as well as the most effective ways of teaching and training, to include subdisciplines, or different ways of studying human movement that expanded beyond the physical. Some of the historical landmarks in the sociological study of sport follow.

In 1964, noted motor-learning specialist Franklin Henry of the University of California, Berkeley, wrote an article arguing that physical education was an academic discipline, not just a professional program to train physical education teachers, as it had been offered up until that point in time. Henry's call to arms might be considered the start of the field of kinesiology, at least in the United States, although this trend was also taking root in other parts of the world. Among the areas of study Henry listed as part of this academic discipline was sociology.

In 1965, Kenyon and Loy authored the article "Toward a Sociology of Sport" in the *Journal of Physical Education, Recreation, and Dance*, one of

STOP AND THINK

- How many different ways can you think of to describe the study of sociology of sport, exercise, and physical activity?

- How can this knowledge be useful for a variety of careers and community positions, such as coach, personal trainer, sport manager, recreational exerciser, or parent of a young athlete?

the leading physical education journals at the time. In that same year, a collection of scholars met in Europe to form the International Committee for the Sociology of Sport, which recently celebrated its 50th anniversary as the International Sociology of Sport Association in 2015 with a grand celebration in Paris, France.

At the end of the turbulent decade of the 1960s, Berkeley sociologist Harry Edwards, the founder of the Olympic Project for Human Rights, penned *Revolt of the Black Athlete* (1969), one of the first books that discussed sport as a political and cultural enterprise. Loy and Kenyon (1969) continued their work in the field and published one of the first textbooks in the sociology of sport, titled *Sport, Culture, and Society: A Reader on the Sociology of Sport.*

Soon thereafter, another book, *Meat on the Hoof: The Hidden World of Texas Football*, by Gary Shaw (1972), revealed the behind the scenes of college football, exposing the sport fan and nonfan alike to the seamy side of sport. At around the same time, New York Yankees pitcher Jim Bouton published his locker room tell-all, *Ball Four*. Many readers were shocked at the intimate details of professional athletes in the locker room, others were offended, and some were disappointed that Bouton shared the secrets of the fraternity. What these books from popular culture tell us is that readers of the time, as well as athletes of the time, were interested in thinking about sport in new and critical ways. They were willing to think about the machinations of the sport industry and move beyond the extolled virtues of sport. It is no accident that much of this comes in the years following various protests by college athletes for improved conditions on their campuses. In 1973, Harry Edwards authored *The Sociology of Sport*, one of the first comprehensive examinations of sport from a sociological perspective.

The North American Society for the Sociology of Sport (NASSS) was formed in 1978 by faculty attending a symposium focused on the sociology of sport. According to the NASSS, the organization was established by Andrew Yiannakis and Susan Greendorfer and included 19 additional founding members (NASSS, n.d.). The organization began publishing the *Sociology of Sport Journal*. The International Sociology of Sport Association (ISSA), established in 1965, also publishes a journal, *International Review for the Sociology of Sport*. Professional organizations and journals serve as gathering spaces and resources for scholars in the field and those interested in learning more about the field and its various applications.

Most courses offered in the sociology of sport are located in kinesiology departments, although many sociology departments are also offering courses and programs in this area. Initially, sport was viewed by academics with some suspicion, with faculty in physical education departments examining sport from a critical perspective, while others considered it trivial and not worthy of serious study. However, as sport has grown in popularity, so has the academic study of sport. This has resulted in sport being studied by scholars in a wide range of academic disciplines, from kinesiology and sociology to anthropology and American studies, among others (Nixon, 2010).

STOP AND THINK

- What is the importance of journals and conferences to the development of the field of sociology of sport, exercise, and physical activity?

- How do books written for popular culture audiences influence the field of sociology of sport, exercise, and physical activity?

Major Topics in Sociology of Sport, Exercise, and Physical Activity

Reading through the table of contents of most sociology of sport textbooks, you might be surprised at the range of topics covered in such a focused course. Major topics such as gender, race and ethnicity, and socioeconomic class are central to the discipline, as well as how these subjects interact with other topics, such as youth sport, socialization, and commercialization. Within each of these topics, one might focus on specific aspects, such as parent involvement in youth sport or the socialization of identified groups, such as rock climbers or cheerleaders. Many texts address the major spheres of sport, and sometimes will have entire chapters devoted to each of these spheres: economics, education, family, media, politics, and religion. More recently, the topic of sport for individuals with disabilities is being included in textbooks, as well as sport across the life span. One exciting element of the field is how it continues to grow and change, expanding its topics and subjects of study as society also grows and changes (Coakley, 2015; Eitzen & Sage, 2009; Sage, 2011).

PREPARING TO ASK AND ANSWER SOCIOLOGICAL QUESTIONS RELATED TO SPORT, EXERCISE, AND PHYSICAL ACTIVITY

As discussed earlier, C. Wright Mills developed a framework for how we can think about the world around us. He dubbed his approach as the *sociological imagination*. Developing a sociological imagination is critical to studying sport and physical activity from a sociological perspective. Mills described the sociological imagination as the individual's ability to connect his or her individual experiences to the broader society. He suggested that one employs a sociological imagination by considering how one's own issues are connected to the "bigger picture," and contended that historical conditions needed to be considered. One's individual troubles and challenges are connected to broader social ills, Mills contended. We are each a product of our times; thus, the decisions made and actions taken by individuals are guided by societal conditions, and are not merely the acts of a solitary individual. How can we apply this sociological imagination to thinking about sport and physical activity?

Everyone has the potential for a sociological imagination, sometimes we just need encouragement and permission to tap into this perspective. One must have the desire, willingness, and ability to shift the focus from one's own personal experiences to instead observe that experience as the result of broader social patterns. For social scientists, broad social patterns are typically observed as a constant linking of historical context, cultural conditions, and structural components of a society. **Historical context** means the current circumstances of a given time period. For example, what's happening politically and economically? In essence, what is the "historical setting" in which the event occurs? **Cultural conditions** refer to ideas behind human actions and societal norms that already inform our beliefs and practices before we are even aware of their existence. **Structural components** include the major spheres of social life that offer stability and transmit traditions. Thus, education, religion, family, politics, economy, and mass media are all structural components of daily life in the United States. Developing the skills and informed intellect to ask questions that place personal experiences into articulation with larger social patterns is crucial, and goes far beyond having an opinion about sport in one's community or society.

Let's think about how we might use the sociological imagination in thinking about an everyday activity like running. An exercise physiologist thinks about running in terms of performance outcomes and physiological variables, maybe even connecting a subject to machines to measure VO_2max or heart rate. The machines are used to calculate and determine the subject's output. Outside the laboratory setting, runners compete without the tethering of lab instruments, and the ways we might think about their

historical context
The circumstances of a given time period.

cultural conditions
Ideas behind human actions and societal norms that inform our beliefs and practices, often before we are even aware of their existence.

structural components
Major spheres of social life that offer stability and transmit traditions.

performance go beyond their VO$_2$max or cardiorespiratory system. A biomechanist is looking at gait patterns; for example, does the foot pronate or supinate? Sport sociologists, armed with their sociological imagination, think about and ask questions that are difficult to measure with any type of machine: What other factors contribute to a runner's success or failure that are not measured by instruments? Why did the individual choose running? What sorts of spaces do they choose to run in? For example, do they live in a neighborhood that allows them the safety and freedom to run at night and on sidewalks? What sorts of equipment is needed for running? What factors influence the decision to compete in an organized run? Some races are expensive, costing the participant in excess of a $100 entry fee. What sort of lifestyle is conducive to running? You might see Kenyan runners winning marathons and wonder how one country dominates this sport. What conditions in Kenya might contribute to success in running? And conversely, what conditions exist in the United States that do not foster long-distance running? Some might suggest that there are many competing alternatives from which youth can choose. Others would point out the common practice in the United States of parents driving children to and from school and other activities, not allowing them to run from location to location. Others would cite a general lack of support for running, from the minimal television coverage to lack of government financing to the celebration of other sports. What historical events have contributed to the increase in people running? Why are more people (especially women) running half marathons, marathons, and Tough Mudders? All of these ideas would be cultural conditions and provide the historical context for the sport sociologist in thinking about running. These factors are all part of the sociological imagination.

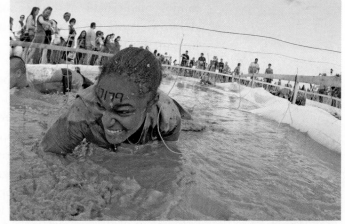

© Z2A1 / Alamy Stock Photo

STOP AND THINK

Think of a topic or issue related to sport, exercise, and/or physical activity, such as the Olympic Games, Zumba, steroid use in sport, optional physical education classes in high school curriculums, or any other of the almost unlimited questions that are possible. Come up with a list of questions a sport sociologist might ask about your topic.

WHY APPLY SOCIOLOGICAL KNOWLEDGE TO SPORT AND PHYSICAL ACTIVITY?

Why do kinesiologists invite students and community members to apply a sociological perspective to sport and physical activity? An overarching goal of sociological analyses of sport is to be able to create a more physically active society. Three subsequent goals that guide the application of social science to sport are:

1. The development and cultivation of cultural competencies
2. Identifying and understanding structural conditions (access points, components of society that one needs to learn how to navigate to get to engage in movement; that is, resources such as family, economy, education)
3. Acknowledging the historical moment/context (i.e., the sociological imagination)

Throughout this chapter, we propose a critical social science, or a perspective that suggests that the **status quo**—the typical way of being in the everyday—is inherently unequal and needs revision; we desire better outcomes in all levels of sport, including major profit-generating sport, high-organized sport, and low-organized sport (leisure). Thus, we are moved to ask critical questions of sport, such as the following: For whom is sport planned? How are public resources made available for sport? Who has access to sport? Who benefits from current social arrangements within sport settings? In what ways do contours of difference (race, class, gender, sexuality, ability) show up in sport?

This does make our field different. Here is where tapping into your sociological imagination can be crucial: When you develop the capacity for the sociological imagination, you then become excited about your own role in change; that is, in your own power to influence the historical moment.

Why ask sociological and cultural questions of sport? What does it offer? It offers a critique of power and provides frames for cultural analyses. It helps us to take the focus off individual- and identity-level politics and performance and moves the focus to societal structures and ideas that have influenced and reinforced the systems of power. This is a challenge for students and professionals in the broader field of kinesiology, where much of one's work might be with a singular person, an individual client; we need to think about all these individuals as part of patterns and trends—structures of dominant ideologies. Helpful in this regard is the work of Emile Durkheim (1982), who in his social analysis utilized what he called **social facts** and

status quo
The typical way of being in the everyday (i.e., the "way things are").

social facts
A fixed institution or civil governance structure that may influence how one performs their everyday roles as student, parent, worker, etc. This fixed governance takes the form of laws and public policy and even penalty for breaking such public contracts.

social currents, which he defined as two social influences that shape human social behavior. A social fact operates as a fixed institution or civil governance structure that may influence how one performs their everyday roles as student, parent, worker, etc. This fixed governance takes the form of laws and public policy and even penalty for breaking such public contracts. A social current is the more "in-the-moment" or short-term but deeply influencing "feelings" in a collective setting that shape the same everyday roles. Examples of these aspects are emotions and group experiences that go beyond the individual and that emerge when people are part of a larger group. Think about how a crowd at a sporting event is swept up in the emotions of the contest, whether it is the mob at the gladiator contests in ancient Rome or the loud and rowdy conditions of a Seattle Seahawks football game, and the fans who brag about breaking the decibel record with their crowd noise. These emotions, which sometimes lead to fans beating up other fans, booing a player, or storming the field, would be examples of Durkheim's social currents. Note that it does not need to be played out in front of thousands of fans; it could be hazing activities in a high school football locker room. For example, in Sayreville, Pennsylvania, a group of senior football athletes were accused of hazing their younger teammates in front of their other teammates. We might think about what those other teammates were feeling in response to the scene, and what led them to not stop the activity. Some would call this football culture, the culture of hazing, but it is also a social current. Thus, despite the somewhat fixed roles of parent, worker, and law-abiding citizen, in certain contexts of experiencing a "collective conscience," everyday citizens may act differently.

> **social currents**
> The short-term but deeply influencing "feelings" in a collective setting that shape the same everyday roles.

STOP AND THINK

Identify an example of how sociology of sport research can provide reasons for upsetting the status quo in a way that promotes opportunities for and access to physical activity.

STOP AND THINK

Consider the various responses to San Francisco 49er quarterback Colin Kaepernick when he decided to kneel during the national anthem as a means to bring attention to police brutality and racial and social injustice. How does the term collective conscience come alive for you in thinking about sport as a politicized space?

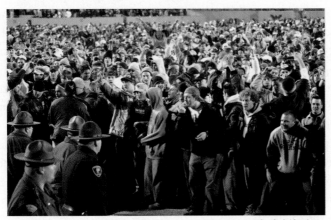

© Sean Brady / Getty Images

THEORY AND PRACTICE IN THE SOCIOLOGY OF SPORT, EXERCISE, AND PHYSICAL ACTIVITY

Sociologists of sport and physical activity use a variety of theories to explain and understand sport. Most of us begin with our own sense-making and assessment of the best approach to daily challenges. Our theorizing is based on ideas we have developed over time by making careful observations, talking to others, and looking for patterns. This practice of personal, everyday theorizing, however, has its limitations compared to more formalized, scientific ways of knowing. The point is that theorizing is a practice in which many of us engage each and every day of our lives. For example, when you decide to ride your bike to work, rather than drive your car, it is likely you will consider several factors, including the weather, distance, physical challenge, work requirements upon arrival, and perhaps safety issues. The ways that you integrate this knowledge toward informed assertions about your best time of departure, how to dress, and what you may need upon arrival is a practice that parallels scientific theorizing. Social scientists carefully gather and generate information (data) regarding various components of sport settings/activities, and then engage in a process of identifying relationships, meanings, and outcomes that may tell us something new about the role of sport in society.

Theoretical approaches to sport are often best understood when we can see their easy application to "real-life" settings and problems. For example, in San Francisco, with the influx of Google, Instagram, and other tech companies, many residents are being evicted from their homes in favor of higher rents and lucrative real estate deals. As a result of the new tech neighbors, many neighborhoods are changing in their demographics, which causes conflict with regard to certain issues. In a recent example, a public park in a San Francisco neighborhood that hosts many pickup soccer matches was a site of contested terrain. The city decided to begin issuing permits to allow groups to reserve the fields, and charging money to these groups, making it so that lower-income youth who habitually used the park space were no longer able to access the fields. In October 2014, three months after the incident, a video circulated of tech workers who had reserved a field verbally sparring with the youth, who challenged the workers to earn their way on to the field by playing a soccer match against them (Mission Local Staff, 2011). Many residents were upset that access to a public park was being restricted and were not supportive of the city's new policy that had not taken into account park users. As a result of protests, the city returned to its past practice of allowing anyone to access the fields at no fee. In rereading this short vignette of a neighborhood's contested use of public space, what structural forces do you see limiting or granting access to exercise? If you replied that one structural force is the city's decision to require permits for access to the park, at a cost, then you are correct. What sort of cultural forces are at play? Think about the shifting demographics of the neighborhood, with upper-income tech workers moving in and longtime residents being evicted to make room for premium residential space. One might wonder if the city's department of parks even thought about how its new, short-lived policy would impact the park's regular users.

Recall that a sociological perspective may be applied in everyday spaces and requires the willingness and ability to look beyond one's personal experiences and see these as reflective of larger patterns of social conditions in the social world. To be sure, well-honed sociological skills and knowledge around sport and physical activity may inform your work as a physical educator, leisure professional, athletic trainer, or coach. It is also quite likely that such a capacity for sociological analyses of sport may inform your own political activism and advocacy for meaningful physical activity in your home communities. Thus, as professionals who value lifelong physical activity, our best work is done when we are able to collectively imagine, investigate, and design communities with commitment and access to meaningful, daily physical activity.

Sociologists of sport use several scientific tools in order to imagine, investigate, and design physically active communities. The most prominent scientific tools for social scientists are theories, or tested explanations about the way society functions, and methodologies, or traditions of scientific investigation. In general, theories in sociology of sport may be categorized by their main focus or core explanation. Some theories focus on how entire social systems operate, including what counts as their major components (e.g., families, economy, education, religion, politics, etc.), and try to explain these systems and the role of sport within them as either harmonious or inherently unequal in structure. These **structural theories** explain broad societal systems and pose questions about how the system works to meet the needs of societal members, or not.

Alternatively, **cultural theories** attempt to explain the core values and collective meanings assigned to human interactions, including those that occur in sport and physical activity. Thus, a sport sociologist or other professional in kinesiology informed by cultural theories might study the dominant

structural theories
Theories that attempt to explain broad societal systems and pose questions about how the systems work to meet the needs of societal members, or not.

cultural theories
Theories that attempt to explain the core values and collective meanings assigned to human interactions.

landscape knowledge techniques
Research techniques that provide important information about different populations; includes surveys of large populations, community case studies, and census surveys.

experience knowledge techniques
Research techniques where the goal is to learn about the actual experiences of people involved in sport and physical activity settings; methods may include surveys, in-depth interviews, and focus groups.

analytic knowledge techniques
Research techniques that focus on the cultural meaning and values related to sport and physical activity; methods may include ethnography, including interviews.

ideas about the role of leisure-time activities or physical education classes in a particular community. The researcher might pose questions about the ways that ideas about gender or race or social class influence the thinking behind K–12 physical education curricula or the manner in which ideas about dis/ability influence the design of a public, leisure-time exercise program. If you think about your own high school experience, it is likely that sport held a prominent place in the broader school "culture." A cultural perspective will allow you to look more deeply at the culture groups that existed at your school, on what bases they were distinguishable, the sorts of social status that accrued to these different groups, and what role sport played in these social interactions and hierarchies.

In terms of methodologies or research techniques for sociological analyses, in general, sociologists engage in what we will call landscape, experience, and analytic knowledge techniques. When you read lengthy data tables that describe rates of participation in particular sports and physical activities, you are reading *social demography*, or data that helps to explain the sport and physical activity landscape. You may have participated in the U.S. Census, which is a study in social demography, or an attempt to count persons, living arrangements, income levels, leisure-time activities, and so on, in order to gain a large-scale glimpse of American life. **Landscape knowledge techniques** generate data that are quite informative about big patterns in a society, but they do not depict or explain other types of knowledge. Moving beyond landscape techniques, sport sociologists may apply a more in-depth and localized technique of research that underscores everyday lived experience. By employing **experience knowledge techniques**, sociologists of sport may actually talk with and observe real people in real sport and physical activity settings and then make some assertions about the role or importance of that particular physical activity setting in the lives of those particular people. A third technique privileges the application of theory to explain the meaning, impact, and use of sport or physical activity in both localized and collective (societal) contexts. This **analytic knowledge technique** would, for example, explain the use of bike riding en masse to disrupt the U.S. dependence on oil and to advocate for more public routes of transportation for nonmotorized vehicles. The analytic technique places sport and physical activity into a broader perspective on cultural context and human interactions—it is not so much about the sport activity, but about the human interactions that occur as part of the sporting space.

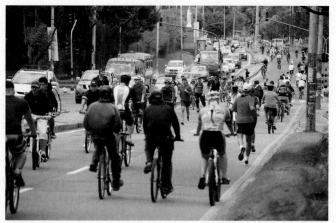

© Ivan_Sabo/Shutterstock

Each of these techniques—landscape, experience, and analytic—provide scholars (and future scholars, like you!) with the means to create new knowledge in the sociology of sport and physical activity. Let's take a closer look at each method of data collection and how each has been used to study sport and physical activity.

LANDSCAPE KNOWLEDGE TECHNIQUES

Landscape knowledge is important because it provides us with important information about different populations, such as parents of young athletes, consumers of sport, and organizers of sport and exercise, to name just a few. Certain methods work especially well in gathering the necessary data to produce landscape knowledge, including surveys of large sample populations, community case studies, and regular census surveys (e.g., the U.S. Census, which is conducted every 10 years). Surveys generally include focused questions around a particular topic, such as the one conducted annually by the Sports & Fitness Industry Association (SFIA; previously the Sporting Goods Manufacturers Association), which asks about physical activity involvement, equipment purchased, and expert services utilized in the past year. Do you recall completing a survey? Every day on ESPN's website, the viewers are asked to "vote" in the site's daily poll. Other sport websites ask viewers their opinions on topics, such as their feelings on the use of performance-enhancing drugs or concussions, two hotly debated topics. These types of surveys and casual polls are not the same as the scientific techniques employed by social scientists, who may also use online tools or even collect their data through telephone or in-person surveys. However, it is not the medium that determines the rigor; it is the application of the scientific method throughout the entire research process. This latter point is true for all of the methods described here.

The SFIA collects survey data annually to determine participation in over 100 sports, fitness, and recreation activities across the life span. Think about how this data might be used by different groups. Maybe a new high school is being built and the administration is trying to decide which sports to include in its athletic offerings. Or perhaps a city is designing a new park space and determining what sport and movement spaces to provide to its citizens. Such datasets are used to aid policy makers and program planners in thinking about resources for physical activity, such as indoor and outdoor space, types of equipment, and likely rates of use.

Within the landscape mode of knowledge production, a community case study may also employ survey techniques, but will likely do so in concert with other techniques, such as document analysis (e.g., public-policy or health-information brochures); community mapping of research-related sites and resources; and perhaps secondary data, such as health statistics by the Centers for Disease Control and Prevention (CDC) or other large databases that offer community-based information. In terms of examining healthy lifestyles in the United States, specifically cardiovascular disease, the Framingham Heart Study (a project of the National Heart, Lung, and Blood Institute and Boston University) has been conducting a community-based case study of health behaviors and longitudinal health outcomes for over 60 years. *Longitudinal* means that a study has been conducted over an extended period of time, such as over a lifetime or perhaps over generations. In fact, in the Framingham Heart Study, the researchers are conducting interviews and data collection with the third generation of participants, the grandchildren of the original cohort. The health data from this community in Massachusetts has become a key information resource for the general population.

EXPERIENCE KNOWLEDGE TECHNIQUES

Experience approaches to knowledge production may also use the techniques mentioned previously, but they do so with a distinguishing goal in mind—to learn about the actual experiences of people in sport and physical activity settings. One method in examining such experiences is through interviews with participants. In this way, the researcher will go well beyond survey questions that might ask for limited responses to more open-ended questions that seek to better understand the meaning of experiences in sport and physical activity. These interviews focus on the ways informants might describe their own interactions, access points, and social support systems related to their physical activity. For example, rather than simply asking how often one participates in a physical activity, a social scientist seeking to understand the experience of sport and physical activity might ask an informant to describe a key aspect of a particular event or to recall and describe a feeling related to a physical activity experience. For example, more individuals are participating in CrossFit. We might wonder why these people prefer CrossFit over aerobics or kickboxing or running on a treadmill. CrossFit has its own lingo and culture that many members find motivating and encouraging. They enjoy the support of "teammates," as well as the opportunity to measure themselves against their own daily performances; others might bristle at the yelling and cheering or the achievement-oriented measurements. But how would one obtain such information? Interviewing the participants would provide a social scientist with important data. These interviews could be conducted one on one, in pairs, or even in small groups, sometimes referred to as *focus groups*. Surveys and case studies could provide some of this data, but if the intent is to gain participant-centered understandings of experience, interview techniques may be the most appropriate method. Some researchers will develop a standard set of focused questions, whereas others will begin with a guiding question, allowing the participants to share their stories with little interruption or guidance. In fact, one might talk with the same participant about his or her interests and activities in physical activity and hear two different sets of responses based on the interview approach used. The interview could include a common set of questions posed to each informant, or it could simply proceed by asking informants to "tell me the story of CrossFit in this community today." As you imagine the different kinds of knowledge that will be gained regarding experience of sport and physical activity, also consider how such data may reflect a sociological imagination.

ANALYTIC KNOWLEDGE TECHNIQUES

When the research goal is one of deep, theoretical analyses, the techniques for knowledge production shift a bit to focus on symbolic meaning and cultural significance of sport and physical activity. In the previous two categories, one of the goals is to identify something "material" and "felt," such as rates of participation (landscape) or the actual experience of sport and physical activity. In the analytic mode of knowledge production, the focus is on cultural meaning and values related to sport and physical activity. Thus, rather than studying the actual experiences within one community's CrossFit gym, a social scientist working in analytic mode might study the cultural significance of CrossFit in an entire community, several communities, or in a national or global context. This type of research may also utilize those techniques described earlier, but it also typically requires integration of techniques, time in the field of inquiry, and a broad depth of sociocultural context. Thus, one might conduct an ethnographic study of a town to determine how much the residents value sport or physical activity, like that of *Friday Night Lights*, which was an ethnography of Texas high school football before it became a popular book, film, and television show. H. G. Bissinger spent 2 years in Odessa, Texas, studying high school football and describing its value and place in this community, both on and off the field. Bissinger (1990) described football in the context of economic conditions, educational policy, race, gender, local newspaper framings, and various social statuses within the town. This is an example of analytic knowledge production. In thinking about our CrossFit example and wanting to know more about the meaning of participants' experiences, you might find that interviewing the participants only tells you one part of the story. Perhaps you've watched a CrossFit session or even engaged in it yourself. Maybe you suspect that the stories being shared by the athletes are providing only part of the story. Using an ethnographic approach to studying the culture of CrossFit would provide a different, and perhaps more useful, technique to understanding the meaning of CrossFit and its culture to its participants.

Recall that the broad field of kinesiology and exercise and sport science has long been cross-disciplinary in nature, and yet it has relied largely on positivism (the privileging of scientific methods over other forms of inquiry) as its primary inquiry framework. As subdisciplinary areas, especially those connected to the social sciences, have advanced, so, too, have nonpositivist paradigmatic approaches to the study of human movement, physical activity, and the body. Little can be learned in attempts to "know" about the body without accounting for context, space, time, place, and so on. Thus, while landscape and experience types of knowledge remain useful in the sociological study of human physical activity, they are only two choices in a range of inquiry traditions and study designs that produce various types of knowledge. David Andrews (2008) argues that the study of the body cannot be reduced to the biological framing of bodily performance, but rather, he reminds us, "the active body is as much a social, cultural, philosophical, and historical entity as it is a genetic, physiological, and psychological vessel and needs to be engaged as such through rigorous ethnographic, autoethnographic, textual and discursive, sociohistoric treatment" (p. 49).

Through the application of various theoretical perspectives, the use of a variety of data generation techniques, and an intentional practice of communicating findings with at least three levels of audience (practitioners, including physical educators and coaches, scholarly peers, and public intellectualism), sociologists of sport and physical activity are able to study and explain the paradoxes of sport and much, much more. Clearly, producing meaningful, socially useful knowledge is hard work! Regardless of the overarching framework or specific methods utilized, it is incredibly demanding to identify a meaningful question, deploy the best set of research tools, and explain one's findings in an ethically informative and accessible manner. This may sound daunting, but it is also very interesting and some of the most fun a person can have! The sociology of sport, exercise, and physical activity presents unique challenges and opportunities for those willing to develop the proper skills for conducting research (Jamieson & Smith, 2016).

Case Study: Applying Your Sociological Imagination to Movement Settings

Reading through the table of contents of many sport sociology textbooks one can see the topics of inquiry. Typical chapter headings focus on social groups and categories of difference, such as race and ethnicity, gender, and socioeconomic class, to topics that engage with the intersections of these identities in specific settings, and also different spaces and forms; we might call these *traditional* and *emergent* forms. Other topics to be found are youth sport, deviance and violence, media, religion, politics, and socialization. An overarching assumption for sociologists of sport is that people practice physical activity and movement in a variety of forms. A second assumption goes beyond individual identities in understanding social groups and difference to understand sport as raced, gendered, and classed in its structure and relation to dominant culture. The fact that human beings experience social difference in an integrated or intersectional manner is a third assumption of sociologists of sport and physical activity. Intersectionality means that social organizing principles like race, gender, and social class are constantly intermingling to shape our daily experiences and interactions in our social world, including in sport. Thus, your teammate is not only white, but may be white, female, AND queer-identified, experiencing what some social scientists refer to as a *matrix of difference*. Finally, a fourth assumption for social scientists is that everyday people actively cocreate the physical activity spaces in their social worlds. We use these sociology of sport assumptions as a backdrop to the following application of the sociological imagination to a site for physical activity. We ask you to employ your sociological imagination in thinking about this social space for human movement.

EMERGENT SPORT: FROM CROSSFIT AND TOUGH MUDDERS TO THE BIGGEST LOSER

emergent sport
Activities that involve participants in new ways of exercise and sport, often including competition.

Before we dive into what we view as the area of **emergent sport**—that is, activities that involve participants in new ways of exercise and sport, often including competition—let's think about how we might first approach the area of fitness from a sociological perspective. One of the ways that sociologists might study exercise as a social and cultural phenomenon is to follow the development of the fitness movement in the United States. Certainly, individuals and communities engaged in physical activity before the fitness movement, but the fitness movement marks a societal-level change in our culture's view of exercise. Thanks to Dr. Kenneth Cooper, aerobic exercise and its health benefits became common knowledge for most people. Prior to Cooper's landmark 1968 publication on aerobic exercise, folks had the good sense to "move," but no one had articulated to the masses the best way to move and for what benefit. Dr. Cooper and the Cooper Institute closed this information gap and generated national interest in aerobic exercise. Scientific evidence continues to support that aerobic exercise produces great health benefits, such as the landmark 1989 *Journal of American Medicine* study (Blair et al., 1989) that declared 30 minutes of physical activity a day would reduce death rates by 58%. This was not the Industrial Revolution or the break-up of the Soviet Union, but let's be clear that the fitness movement was a significant social movement that changed how Americans thought about and engaged in human movement. It shaped physical education curricula, afterschool programs, and family interactions and made way for the development of a hugely successful fitness industry—an industry that has and will employ many of us.

To be fair, Jack LaLanne had been producing exercise shows and designing exercise spas since the 1930s, such that he is sometimes referred to as the "godfather of fitness." His work predated that of the Cooper Institute and the new fitness industry. One thing that was so unique about LaLanne was his ability to capture the interest of people who were not athletes or elite performers. He found ways to sell the fitness movement to "everyone." LaLanne's exercise show can be viewed through gendered, nationalist, and moral framings. Even for LaLanne back in the 1930s, exercise was deeply tied to social and cultural values.

Take LaLanne, add Cooper, some old Jane Fonda videos, and a little bit of Nike and Reebok, and you have a fitness movement, all of which has contributed to the fitness industry—a powerful force in American culture. Today, this fitness culture includes CrossFit, Tough Mudders, Color Runs, and Zombie Runs, as well as reality television programs about weight loss, such as *The Biggest Loser*.

CULTURAL CONDITIONS

What are the cultural conditions that support such a variety of ways to exercise, as well as to compete as we exercise? More Americans, in all age groups, and including more women than ever, are participating (competing) in half marathons, marathons, triathlons, and endurance-based obstacle course events. What sorts of cultural conditions are part of this current trend? Why do you think more and more people are competing in Tough Mudders and then posting their photos on social media? With many of these events, the term *competition* is being turned on its head. Winning isn't the most important thing, but rather getting active and "just doing it." Few people try to run their first marathon with the goal of winning; instead, finishing is the goal.

With Color Runs, no time is kept, it is simply the activity of running and moving with others in a fun and relaxed environment. What do you think has led to this shift of just getting people out there and moving? What sort of relationship exists between Tough Mudder competitions and the American military? Do people like doing Tough Mudders because it makes them feel like they are supporting the military by doing an obstacle course with the proceeds going to Wounded Warriors? People compete as teams, and leave no teammate behind. Does this emphasis on teamwork encourage people? We see some similar forms of encouragement in CrossFit. These are some of the newest forms of exercise, engaging in militaristic challenges, being yelled at as a motivation, and sticking together as a team.

STRUCTURAL CONDITIONS

The fitness industry is privatized; we make no illusions that schools or cities should provide opportunities for fitness. Cities do provide public park space in some neighborhoods, but rarely offer programming in those parks for the general masses to improve their fitness. Several employers offer reduced membership fees or an on-site gym facility as a means to motivate their employees to engage in physical activity. What other institutions influence the structure of how we approach fitness? American legislation on health care and health insurance may have impacts on one's fitness and overall health. Should individuals receive lower deductibles in exchange for efforts to improve their health? Some governments provide their citizens with expanded opportunities for physical activity, health, and wellness. Do you see any ways the federal government works to provide and encourage physical fitness for its citizens?

HISTORICAL CONTEXT

We live in a post-9/11 moment that is somewhat reminiscent of the 1950s and the role of physical education in national defense following World War I and World War II. Proponents of physical education used war preparation as a rationale to justify the inclusion of physical education as a mandatory school subject. In today's post-9/11 political and economic moment, the fitness movement is focused on endurance-based fitness and on individual participation versus team-focused sports. The goal of sport is to develop affective traits, character, and so on that fit with America's sense of security and capacity to lead the world. When we think about the increased participation of women in the fitness movement, we can look to the role of medical doctors and sport organizations in excluding women from long-distance sports, such as the marathon. For example, the first time the marathon was offered for women in the Olympic Games was 1984. How do you think the emergence of women in the marathon connects with our earlier discussion of the Cooper Institute, the rise of aerobics, and even legislation such as Title IX that mandates that girls and women be provided equal opportunities in school sports with federal funding?

STOP AND THINK

Create a case study of your own. Be sure to consider the cultural conditions, the structural conditions, and the historical context. Provide evidence and ask questions in each of the three areas (cultural, structural, and historical).

What Can You Do with a Degree in Sociology of Sport, Exercise, and Physical Activity?

Most students in kinesiology and exercise science are required to enroll in a sociology of sport, exercise, and physical activity course. At the undergraduate level, a degree in sport studies, which will include sociology of sport, is more likely to be offered than a focused degree in sociology of sport. Sociology of sport is sometimes offered at the master's and doctoral degree levels, with the goal of becoming a university faculty member. Throughout this chapter, we have tried to help you see the relevancy of the sociology of sport for *all* kinesiology and exercise science students; being able to ask and answer sociological questions and employing your sociological imagination are essential skills for an individual interested in working within the broad field of human movement.

CHAPTER SUMMARY

In this chapter, we have provided you with an overview of the sociology of sport, exercise, and physical activity. Sociologists of sport, exercise, and physical activity, in seeking to improve the access to and quality of physical activity for all, employ Mills's sociological imagination as a means to understand the culture of human movement. Specifically, we encourage you to think about the cultural contexts of your own individual experiences in movement and how you might explain your experience as it relates to broader social and cultural conditions. We also urge you to think about the historical moment, and consider what is it about the time period that creates the conditions for people to engage in various movement practices. Channels devoted to watching others play poker, stuff hot dogs in their mouth, play video games, and exercise as a means to compete to lose weight—these are new "sport" competitions in our culture. We have more and more kids playing sport, and more and more kids dropping out of sport. More women are running half marathons and challenging themselves in physical contests than ever before. Countries are deciding they no longer want to be considered to host the Olympic Games. And millions and millions of people on Saturday and Sunday afternoons join together to cheer on their teams, all while others lack access to safe spaces for exercise and physical activity. We hope you take up the challenge of using your sociological imagination in your kinesiology studies to think about the ways our various professions and careers can be agents of social change.

DISCUSSION QUESTIONS

1. What is the sociological imagination, and how is it applied to kinesiology?
2. What sorts of questions, evidence, materials, and methods are central to the sociology of sport?
3. How do the techniques of landscape knowledge, experience knowledge, and analytic knowledge differ? How do they complement one another?
4. How do cultural conditions, structural conditions, and historical context inform and impact our understanding of social issues in kinesiology?

REFERENCES

Andrews, D. L. (2008). Kinesiology's inconvenient truth and the physical cultural studies imperative. *Quest, 60,* 46–63.

Bissinger, H. G. (1990). *Friday night lights.* Reading, MA: Addison-Wesley.

Blair, S. N., Kohl, H. W., III, Paffenberger, R. S., Clark, D. G., Cooper, K. H., & Gibbons, L. W. (1989). Physical fitness and all-cause mortality. *Journal of the American Medical Association 262*(17), 2395–2401.

Bouton, J. (1970). *Ball four.* New York: World.

Coakley, J. J. (2015). *Sports in society: Issues and controversies* (11th ed.). Boston: McGraw-Hill.

Cooper, K. H. (1968). *Aerobics.* Philadelphia: Lippincott.

Durkheim, E. (1982). *The rules of the sociological method.* Edited by Steven Lukes. New York: Free Press. (Original work published 1895.)

Edwards, H. (1969). *Revolt of the black athlete.* New York: Free Press.

Edwards, H. (1973). *The sociology of sport.* Homewood, IL: Dorsey Press.

Eitzen, D. S. (2012). *Fair and foul: Beyond the myths and paradoxes of sport* (5th ed.). Lanham, MD: Rowman Littlefield.

Eitzen, D. S., & Sage, G. H. (2009). *Sociology of North American sport* (8th ed.). Boulder, CO: Paradigm Publishers.

Jamieson, K. M., & Smith, M. M. (2016). *Fundamentals of sociology of sport and physical activity*. Champaign, IL: Human Kinetics.

Kenyon, G. S. & Loy, J. W. (1965). Toward a sociology of sport. *Journal of Physical Education, Recreation, and Dance, 36*(5), 24–25, 68–69.

Loy, J. W., & Kenyon, G. S. (1969). *Sport, culture, and society: A reader on the sociology of sport*. Toronto: Macmillan.

Mills, C. W. (1959). *The sociological imagination*. New York: Oxford University Press.

Mission Local Staff. (2014, October 11). Mission Playground this morning. *MissionLocal*. Accessed at http://missionloca.org/2014/10/mission-playground-this-morning/

North American Society for the Sociology of Sport. (n.d.). About NASSS. Retrieved from http://www.nasss.org/about/about-nasss/

Nixon, H. L. (2010). Sport sociology, NASSS, and undergraduate education in the United States: A social network perspective for developing the field. *Sociology of Sport Journal, 27*, 76–88.

Sage, G. H. (2011). *Globalizing sport: How organizations, corporations, media, and politics are changing sport*. St. Paul, MN: Paradigm Publishers.

Shaw, G. (1972). *Meat on the hoof: The hidden world of Texas football*. New York: St. Martin's Press.

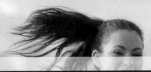

CHAPTER 11

Adapted Physical Activity

TAEYOU JUNG

LEARNING OBJECTIVES

1. Define *physical activity* and *adapted physical activity* (APA).
2. Identify the two main roots of APA.
3. Explain how APA can impact issues of growing importance in the United States, such as the obesity epidemic and the aging population.
4. List the common types of APA service programs.
5. Identify career options related to APA.
6. Describe common research approaches in APA.

KEY TERMS

adaptation
adapted aquatics
adapted physical activity (APA)
adapted physical education (APE)
corrective physical education

disability
inclusive fitness trainer
person-first attitudes and language
physical activity

What Is Physical Activity?

physical activity
Any bodily movement that requires the use of energy by the individual.

Physical activity is at the core of what we study in kinesiology. It is not easy to define a term so commonly used without much thought. You may find various technical definitions of physical activity in the field of kinesiology. Some definitions are quite narrow, whereas others are overly broad and inclusive. In the *2008 Physical Activity Guidelines for Americans* (**FIGURE 11-1**), physical activity is defined as "bodily movement that is produced by the contraction of skeletal muscle and that substantially increases energy expenditure" (U.S. Department of Health and Human Services, 2008, pg. 2). Another frequently

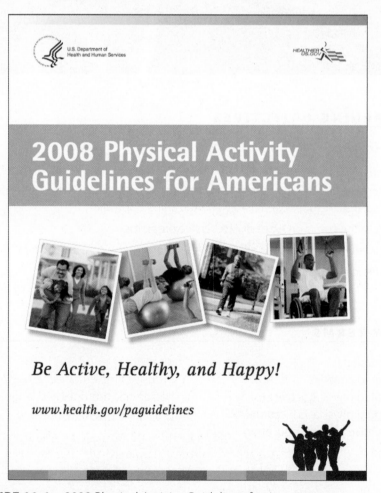

FIGURE 11-1   2008 Physical Activity Guidelines for Americans.
Reproduced from U.S. Department of Health and Human Services (2008). "2008 Physical Activity Guidelines for Americans." Page 1. http://health.gov/paguidelines/pdf/paguide.pdf

cited definition of physical activity is that it is "intentional, voluntary movement directed toward achieving an identifiable goal" (Newell, 1990, pg. 270). The common denominators in these definitions are that physical activity is a health-enhancing bodily movement that is purposeful and voluntary in its nature and also a vigorous form of movement that increases one's energy expenditure above a basic resting level. In this chapter, we will adopt our own definition of physical activity as health-enhancing bodily movement that elevates energy expenditure.

STOP AND THINK

Describe physical activity in your own words, and discuss how it is related to your career plan or area of academic interest.

WHAT IS ADAPTED PHYSICAL ACTIVITY?

When you have a disability or major health issue, you may be unable to carry out regular physical activity. For example, you would not recommend the same strength-training routine that you perform as a 20-year-old college student for an 85-year-old adult with Parkinson's disease. An older adult with aggravating pain in the knee due to arthritis can be better accommodated by exercising in water, where she can have her body weight supported by buoyancy, resulting in less pain. Similarly, you may need to modify the rules of a game when teaching basketball to a child with cerebral palsy in a wheelchair. These are practical situations in which you might consider modifying the physical activity.

When you modify a physical activity to accommodate the special needs of participants, you can simply refer to it as **adapted physical activity (APA)**. Of course, APA is defined in many different ways by scholars in the field and by its context (**FIGURE 11-2**). The International Federation of Adapted Physical Activity (IFAPA, n.d., 2004) defines APA as a:

adapted physical activity
A field of study of physical activity that is modified for people with special needs to promote healthy and active lifestyles.

> … cross-disciplinary body of knowledge directed toward the identification and solution of individual differences in physical activity. It is a service delivery profession and an academic field of study that supports an attitude of acceptance of individual differences, advocates access to active lifestyles and sport, and promotes innovation and cooperative service delivery programs and empowerment systems. APA includes, but is not limited to, physical education, sports, recreation, dance and creative arts, nutrition, medicine, and rehabilitation.

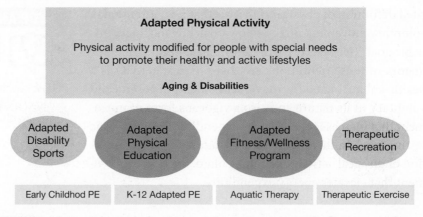

FIGURE 11-2 Adapted physical activity concept map: Definitions and programs.

One of the most prominent scholars in the field of APA, Claudine Sherrill (2004, pg. 5), defined it as "the umbrella term for services that promote an active, healthy lifestyle by remediating psychomotor problems that interfere with goal achievement and self-actualization." Greg Reid (2003, pg. 15) introduced his version of the definition as, "adaptations that could facilitate physical activity across a wide range of individual differences."

Depending on the context, APA can be defined as service delivery, an academic specialization or discipline, a profession, a set of beliefs that guide practice, an attitude of acceptance and empowerment, or a process or product that pertains to physical activity for people with special needs. For the purpose of this chapter, we choose to use a simplified definition of APA; it is a field of study of physical activity that is modified for people with special needs to promote healthy and active lifestyles. It is one of the academic specializations within kinesiology. In APA courses, you will learn various principles, theories, and applications in kinesiology that are related to populations with special needs, such as disabilities, chronic medical conditions, or aging-related health issues. APA service programs may encompass multiple forms of physical activity, such as adapted physical education, adapted sport (e.g., Paralympic sport, wheelchair sport), adapted fitness, therapeutic recreation, adapted aquatics, and therapeutic exercise.

In the United States, the APA field historically has put more emphasis on children with disabilities; thus the term **adapted physical education (APE)** has been frequently used in university programs and courses in place of APA. However, to be technically correct, APE is a part of APA, which is a widely accepted term in the international context. Also, with the growing population of older adults, we are seeing an increasing trend of APA courses and programs in the United States focusing on adults with disabilities and older adults with geriatric health conditions, in addition to children with disabilities. Therefore, life span physical activity for people with different abilities can be referred to as APA.

> **STOP AND THINK**
>
> Describe APA in your own words, and explain how it differs from physical education.

adapted physical education (APE) Physical education that has been adapted and/or modified so it is appropriate for children and youth with disabilities. This service is federally mandated for all students with disabilities. It includes physical fitness, fundamental motor skills and patterns, and individual and group games and sports, and may also cover aquatics and dance.

A Brief History of APA

Physical activity and exercise have been used for remedial and therapeutic purposes throughout history. Even the ancient Greeks, Romans, Indians, and Chinese used physical training and exercise to heal injuries and treat medical conditions. The present form of APA has evolved from various bases of knowledge. The cross-disciplinary nature of knowledge in APA can be summarized in the following five roots: (1) medical gymnastics, which later evolved into corrective physical training, physical therapy, sports medicine, and therapeutic exercise; (2) special education, which later became special physical education, behavior management, and APE; (3) life-span human development, which laid a basis for motor behavior science; (4) social science, which is related to topics in disability awareness, attitude toward individual differences, and inclusive physical education; and (5) sport, dance, aquatic, and leisure studies, which developed into disability sport, dance therapy, adapted aquatics and aquatic therapy, and therapeutic recreation (Sherrill, 2004).

Of these five roots, the two major ones that established the foundation of APA are medical gymnastics and special education. The medical roots of APA can be traced back to Swedish medical gymnastics, developed by Per Henrik Ling (1776–1839), which later evolved into corrective physical education, physical therapy, remedial and restorative exercise, adapted fitness, and therapeutic exercise. The Swedish exercise system was imported into the United States by Nils Posses in the late 19th century and introduced into schools in Boston and in a teacher preparation program developed by Amy

Morris Homans, a professor in physical education at Wellesley College. In the early 20th century, *Exercise in Education and Medicine* by R. Tait McKenzie (1867–1938), a professor at McGill University in Canada, and *Corrective Physical Education* by Josephine Rathbone (1899–1989), a professor at Columbia University (**FIGURE 11-3**), were published. The concept of **corrective physical education** was dominant until around 1950, when people in the field realized that the term *corrective* was not entirely relevant to World War II veterans with amputation or spinal cord injury. The shift from medically-oriented physical training to sport-oriented physical education also occurred around this time. In addition, the benefits of sport participation in rehabilitation and the start of wheelchair sports was gaining more attention, prompting the need for a more inclusive term.

corrective physical education
An early name of APA that came from the medical root of physical education designed mostly for World War II veterans with amputation or spinal cord injury.

The special education root was initially developed for children with deafness, blindness, or intellectual disabilities. The use of sensorimotor training, developed by the French physician Jean-Marc Itard (1775–1839), who is often referred to as the "father of special education," was brought to the United States in late 19th century by his student, Edouard Seguin, who later helped found the American Association on Mental Deficiency. This was the first professional organization on disability, and was followed by the U.S. Council for Exceptional Children, established in 1922, which carried on the development of special education in the United States.

Finally, the term *adapted physical education* emerged in 1952. The Committee on Adapted Physical Education defined APE as "a diversified program of developmental activities, games, sports, and rhythms suited to the interests, capacities, and limitations of students with disabilities who may not safely or successfully engage in unrestricted participation in the vigorous activities of the general physical education program" (AAHPERD, 1952, p. 15). Prior to this, one could find various versions of the name used in textbook titles, including those on special physical education, development physical education, and remedial physical education.

The International Sports Organization for the Disabled was founded in 1963, and the International Special Olympics was created in 1968 with great support from the Kennedy family (**FIGURE 11-4**). The human rights movement of the 1960s and worldwide efforts to protect the rights of people with disabilities in the 1970s and 1980s led to many countries passing legislation to prohibit inequity and segregation in society based on disability. The International Federation of Adapted Physical Activity (IFAPA) was founded

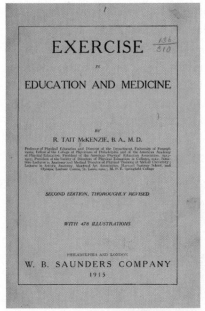

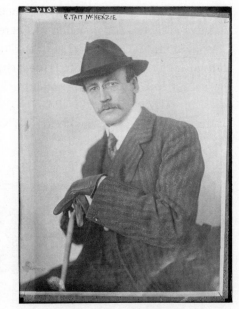

"Exercise in Education and Medicine" by
R. Tait McKenzie. W.B Saunders Company, 1915.

Library of Congress, LC-B2- 3014-2

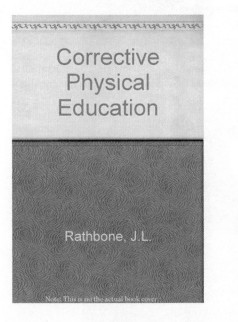

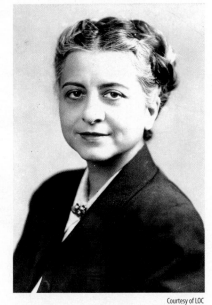

Courtesy of LOC

FIGURE 11-3 Early scholars and textbooks in APA: R. Tait McKenzie (top) and Josephine Rathbone (bottom).

in 1973 with the goal "to give global focus to professionals who use adapted physical activities for instruction, recreation, remediation, and research" (Eason, Smith, & Caron, 1983, p. xi). Other professional organizations were formed, including the National Consortium for Physical Education and Recreation for Individuals with Disabilities (NCPERID) in 1973, the Adapted Physical Activity Council (APAC) in 1984, and the North American Federation of Adapted Physical Activity (NAFAPA) in 1994) (Figure 11-4).

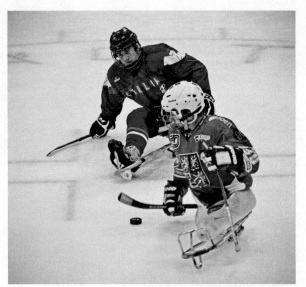

© ROBERTO ZILLI/Shutterstock

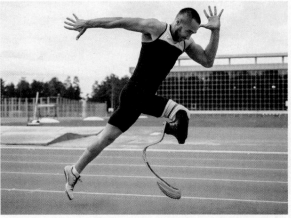

© sportpoint/Shutterstock

FIGURE 11-4   Paralympic winter and summer athletics.

Major Topics in APA

WHAT IS ADAPTATION?

The word *adapted* is derived from *adaptation*, which the dictionary defines as "the act or process of adapting" or "something that is changed or modified to suit new conditions or needs" (Collins English Dictionary, 2003). Thus, **adaptation** means an adjustment, change, modification, or accommodation made to meet the needs of an individual or the environment. It is a process that professionals use to accomplish goals and achieve positive outcomes through diverse service programs, including teaching, coaching, rehabilitation, fitness, sport medicine and recreation. The application of adaptation theory to APA, suggested by Ernst Kiphard (1983, pg. 26), emphasized the nature of motor adaptation as "individual and environmental interaction as a means of maintaining homeostasis" and "adaptation as a reciprocal process." Taken together, these definitions suggest that humans not only adapt to the environment, but also change the environment every time they respond to it.

WHAT IS APPROPRIATE LANGUAGE IN APA?

In the field of APA, special education, and rehabilitation service, we emphasize **person-first attitudes and language**. We refer to an individual who has a disability as a *person with a disability* instead of as a *disabled person*. Not only is this politically correct, but it is also more respectful, considering the fact that many individuals with disabilities have many abilities and often amazing talents. When referred to as disabled persons, much of which they are capable is completely ignored. It is more appropriate and empowering to focus on what they can do rather than solely on their disabilities.

The term **disability** is also an umbrella term, "covering impairments, activity limitations, and participation restrictions" (World Health Organization, 2001). According to the World Health Organization (WHO, 2001), "An impairment is a problem in body function or structure; an activity limitation is a difficulty encountered by an individual in executing a task or action; while a participation restriction is a problem experienced by an individual in involvement in life situations." Disability is not just a health problem, but rather a complex phenomenon reflecting the interaction between a person

STOP AND THINK

- Describe the two main roots of APA.
- Explain how APA differs from APE.
- List the major professional organizations in APA.

adaptation
Something that is changed or modified to suit new conditions or needs.

person-first attitudes and language
More appropriate and empowering way to refer to someone with a disability by focusing on what the person can do instead of solely on his or her disabilities.

disability
An umbrella term that encompasses impairments, activity limitations, and participation restrictions.

and society. The WHO officially states that overcoming the difficulties faced by people with disabilities requires interventions to remove environmental and social barriers and facilitate their inclusion in society.

Lastly, the term *handicap* is not commonly used due to its negative connotations. Some say that the term originated from the description of a person with amputation begging for money with his "hand in cap," and thus it is highly derogatory to use this term when referring to a person with a disability. However, this is in fact not the origin of the word. The term is actually derived from a 17th-century English game called "hand in cap," later shortened to *handicap* (Oxford Dictionary of English Etymology, 1966). It initially meant to "put someone at a disadvantage" in an attempt to equalize contests and games to make them fair. Later it was applied to other games, such as golf, polo, and billiards, as a means of giving a disadvantage to persons having a structural advantage in a game to make a fair competition. Soon after that, people started using handicap when referring to disabilities, noting that the person has a disadvantage. Due to its demeaning connotations, it is no longer used in the context of APA and rehabilitation.

HOW CAN APA IMPACT AGING AND DISABILITY?

According to the U.S. Census Bureau (2010), approximately one in five U.S. citizens (19.9%), or over 47 million Americans, reported having a disability as of 2010. If you add the prevalence of obesity (34.9% of adults with BMI greater than 30 kg/m^2) and extreme obesity (6.4% of adults with BMI over 40 kg/m^2) into that figure, the percentage of people with a disability is overwhelming. An increasing number of children are being diagnosed with developmental disabilities, including autism spectrum disorder, which affects 1 in 68 U.S. children (Centers for Disease Control and Prevention, 2014). Of children aged 3 to 17 years, 14% have developmental disabilities (Boyle et al., 2011). Also, childhood obesity has become a major epidemic, with over 30% of U.S. children determined to be overweight or obese (Ogden, Carroll, Kit, & Flegal, 2014).

In addition, it is estimated that by the year 2030 approximately 70 million people in the United States will be older than age 65, and this group is at a greater risk for developing aging-related health issues such as Alzheimer's, Parkinson's, stroke, senior fall risk, and other chronic diseases. According to the CDC (2009), 54% of people older than age 65 have at least one disability.

By studying APA, you can prepare yourself to meet this growing demand and make a meaningful impact on the quality of lives of this population.

Research has shown that people with disabilities are less active than those without disabilities and experience disparities in health (CDC, 2010). Engaging in regular physical activity is an important step for all people in leading healthy lives, including those with disabilities. Physiologically, people with disabilities have similar needs to promote their health and prevent unnecessary diseases. The U.S. Surgeon General recommends that everyone participate in moderate physical activity on a daily basis (CDC, 2014). Although physical activity and fitness have been widely promoted in the media and the fitness profession has grown in the past decade, the majority of facilities and programs are designed for healthy individuals. Unfortunately, people with disabilities often encounter barriers to physical activity, which has profound negative effects (Rimmer, Wang, & Smith, 2008). Sedentary lifestyles often lead to secondary conditions, such as obesity, diabetes, and cardiovascular disease, which negatively impact health and quality of life and result in higher costs to society. It is imperative to have highly trained professionals in APA tear down the barriers and facilitate the opportunities for physical activity to meet the needs of this growing population.

It is well documented that people with disabilities benefit—physically, psychosocially, and cognitively—from physical activity. Unfortunately, the resources and number of knowledgeable professionals are inadequate for servicing this population. More well-prepared professionals are needed in the field of APA. Although situations may differ, depending on your university program and curriculum, successful completion of an APA program will prepare you for work as an adapted fitness trainer, adapted physical education teacher, adapted aquatics instructor, senior exercise instructor, rehabilitation exercise specialist, or APA coordinator in the public or private sector. You will be trained to enter the workforce and have a positive impact on the quality of lives of individuals with disabilities.

STOP AND THINK

Why should the use of terms such as *handicapped person* and *disabled student* be avoided?

WHAT COURSES ARE AVAILABLE IN APA?

The courses available in APA will vary depending on your university's specific kinesiology program and curriculum. Some APA programs have courses specifically designed to prepare you to become an adapted physical education teacher, following state guidelines. In this case, most courses are related to APE and pedagogical (teaching-related) content. Examples of the courses in this category may include those with titles such as Introduction to APE, Program Development and Implementation in APE, Motor Assessment in Children with Disabilities, Inclusive Physical Education for Children with Disabilities, Collaborative Team Teaching, Behavior Management, and Practicum in APE.

Other APA programs may have course offerings that pertain to a life-span approach to APA, so that the courses can prepare you to become an APA service provider or specialist who can work with people of different abilities at all ages. It is common that these APA courses often require you to enroll in a concurrent laboratory class or practicum at an APA service delivery program, which may be located on or off campus. This category would include classes with titles such as Introduction to APA, Adapted Sports, Adapted Aquatics, Medical and Pathological Aspects in APA, Assessment and Development of Individualized Program in APA, Adapted Therapeutic Exercise, Aquatic Therapeutic Exercise, Movement Science in Disabilities, Exercise Management for Individuals with Disabilities and Chronic Medical Conditions, APA Programming for Individuals with Physical and Neurological Disabilities, Policies and Management of APA Program, Clinical Practicum in APA, and Research Seminar in APA. These courses can prepare you to become a health and fitness professional who can promote healthy and active lifestyles among people with special needs.

WHAT DO APA SERVICE PROGRAMS LOOK LIKE?

APA programs are found in several settings, such as public and private schools, children's hospitals, rehabilitation centers, residential settings for adults with disabilities, community centers, university-based APA programs, faith-based activity centers, senior day care centers, assisted living or nursing home settings, wellness programs in retirement communities, horseback riding ranches, adaptive ski programs, adapted watersports centers, park and recreation facilities, adapted golf programs, Veterans Affairs hospitals, specialized rehabilitation or recovery exercise clinics, and commercial fitness centers. Some settings are geared toward APA services for children with disabilities, whereas others are designed to provide APA services to adults with special needs or older adults. Some services are offered in educational settings or community-service environments, whereas others take place in clinical or medical settings. Depending on your interest and career path, you could apply your knowledge of APA to different age groups, disability populations, or working environments. You could also choose to work in the public or private sector, which may be a for-profit or non-profit setting. Whatever setting you choose, you can use your knowledge and training to influence the quality of life of people with special needs.

The Center of Achievement through Adapted Physical Activity at California State University, Northridge, is an example of a university-based APA program that provides quality APA services for individuals with disabilities while providing field training opportunities for kinesiology students and health professionals (**FIGURE 11-5**). Currently, the center offers both aquatic- and land-based therapeutic exercise programs for approximately 400 individuals with special needs. The program participants may range

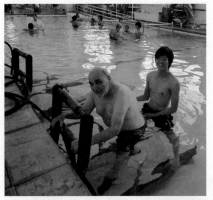
Courtesy of Taeyou Jung/ CSUN

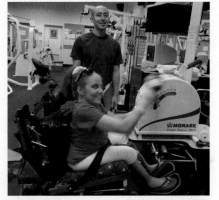
Courtesy of Taeyou Jung/ CSUN

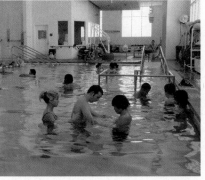
Courtesy of Taeyou Jung/ CSUN

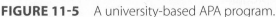
Courtesy of Taeyou Jung/ CSUN

FIGURE 11-5 A university-based APA program.

from a 3-year-old child with cerebral palsy to a 95-year-old client with Parkinson's disease. Independent clients with disabilities are often accommodated in a group class, whereas individuals with severe disabilities are assisted one-on-one by staff in individualized sessions either in water or on land. The center houses two main program areas: the Brown Aquatic Therapy Center, including four distinctively designed aquatic therapy pools with numerous aquatic exercise devices and underwater treadmills, and the Adapted Therapeutic Exercise Center, which has more than 100 pieces of accessible and adapted fitness equipment and a large expansion room for group classes, such as adapted yoga and dance classes. Undergraduate and graduate students in APA are actively involved in hands-on experience under clinical supervision and conducting clinical research to document scientific evidence of the various interventions offered.

Many ski resorts offer adaptive ski programs for individuals with special needs (**FIGURE 11-6**). At the Heavenly Mountain Resort in Lake Tahoe, California, the adaptive ski program's mission statement is "that everyone should have access to the thrill of skiing and riding." Their specially trained instructors provide a comprehensive adaptive ski program. The program focuses on personalized instruction for participants with disabilities to help build confidence and a love for snow sports in a safe environment.

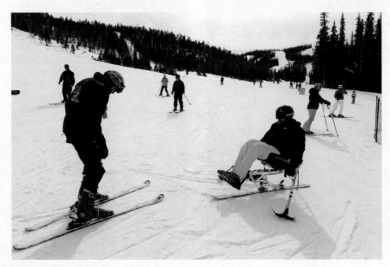

FIGURE 11-6   Adaptive ski program.
© Helen H. Richardson / Getty Images

The adaptive ski program offers individualized instruction for people with cognitive or developmental disabilities; bi ski for persons with disability of legs and arms; mono ski for persons with disability of legs but strong upper body; three track for persons with disability of one leg; four track for persons with disability of both legs, and one-on-one lessons for people with blindness or low vision.

STOP AND THINK

Identify three APA service programs that are available in or near the town in which you currently reside.

What Can You Do with Training in APA?

Options for careers in APA differ depending on your training and interests. If want to work with children with disabilities in an educational setting, you might want to go through an APE credential or certificate program. You can work as an APE teacher in a public or private school setting, teaching physical education for children with special needs. You may find APE teachers working in a special education school or working as a consultant or supervisor for a school district. APE specialists also work in children's hospitals or rehabilitation centers.

APA specialists may choose to work in clinical and medical settings for children or adults with special needs, such as medical hospitals, private clinics, rehabilitation centers, residential communities, university-based centers, adapted fitness or wellness centers, or commercial gyms. You can work as an APA specialist in a group home setting for adults with disabilities or for nonprofit disability organizations. Commercial gyms and fitness centers are hiring adapted fitness instructors or **inclusive fitness trainers** to accommodate members with disabilities or aging-related health issues. In addition, APA specialists who are trained in **adapted aquatics** or aquatic therapy can deliver services to children with disabilities in pediatric hospitals, community pools, or private physical therapy clinics. Specialized rehabilitation exercise centers and private fitness clinics are available for people with disabilities where adapted fitness trainers provide instruction in recovery exercises. Public offices in many counties and states also have APA specialists who deliver physical activity services for community members with special needs. Also, nonprofit disability organizations often place an APA specialist in the division of physical activity in each charter or regional office so that they can organize various physical activity and wellness programs for their members with disabilities.

inclusive fitness trainer
Fitness trainer who can assist people with special needs in an inclusive fitness setting.

adapted aquatics
Aquatic activities that have been modified for people with special needs.

If you have an interest in advancing your knowledge and training in APA, you may choose to pursue graduate study in APA or a related field. Upon completion of a graduate degree in APA, you might further your career in academic or research institutions, working as a university professor or researcher in APA or a related field, such as movement science in disabilities, rehabilitation science, neuromotor control, clinical biomechanics, public health, or gerontology (**FIGURE 11-7**). It is common for an APA professor at a university or community college to teach courses in APA while operating an APA service program on campus.

Lastly, if you are pursuing a career in allied health professions, taking courses in APA can be helpful. If you are interested in physical medicine and rehabilitation, physical therapy, occupational therapy, or rehabilitation nursing, courses in APA can provide great training background and hands-on experience before you advance into a professional graduate program.

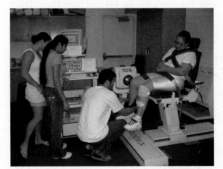
Courtesy of Taeyou Jung/ CSUN

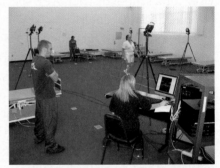
Courtesy of Taeyou Jung/ CSUN

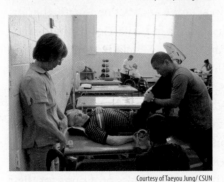
Courtesy of Taeyou Jung/ CSUN

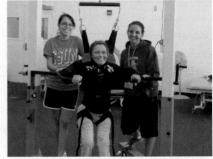
Courtesy of Taeyou Jung/ CSUN

FIGURE 11-7   Research activities in APA.

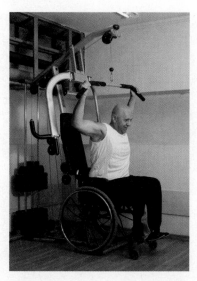

FIGURE 11-8   Accessible exercise equipment: Cybex Total Access weight machine.

© Yuriy Rachenkov/Shutterstock

In addition, if you are inclined to pursue an entrepreneurial path, the application of APA to the rehabilitation or retirement wellness industry can be promising, predominantly in assistive technology or adapted exercise equipment that integrate the concepts of universal design and accessibility for people with different abilities (**FIGURE 11-8**).

WHAT KIND OF WORK DO YOU ACTUALLY DO IN APA?

The following are the stories of real people who are currently working in the field of APA.

APE TEACHER

Andrea has been working as an APE teacher for a public school district in Virginia after completing her APE master's program and acquiring her certification (**FIGURE 11-9**). She is an itinerant APE teacher, assisting students with disabilities at four different schools in the district. She helps K–12 students with disabilities learn proper motor, fitness, and sport-specific skills in inclusive physical education and self-contained classes. She puts a great deal of effort in teaching her students lifelong physical activity and leisure skills

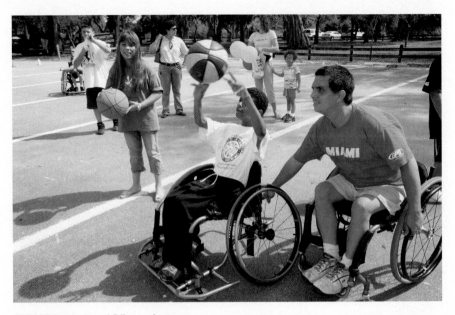

FIGURE 11-9   APE teacher.
© Jeff Greenberg / Alamy Stock Photo

through her APE curriculum. Andrea also attends her students' Individualized Education Program (IEP) meetings, where she develops the best possible service programs for her students in collaboration with other teachers and therapists. Andrea also works as an APE consultant for nearby school districts. She assists school administrators and regular physical education teachers with the development APE curriculum or lesson plans and often shares her tips for challenging cases at the schools.

ADAPTED AQUATICS INSTRUCTOR

Ella is a clinical coordinator of an adapted aquatics program at a university-based APA center (**FIGURE 11-10**). She is a certified aquatic therapy specialist and inclusive fitness trainer. Her aquatic program provides adapted aquatics services for children with disabilities as well as aquatic therapeutic exercise for adults with disabilities. Ella is particularly passionate about helping children with autism in water. She uses her creativity in her lesson plan and instruction to make each session fun and effective. As a clinical coordinator, she is responsible for evaluating and developing individualized

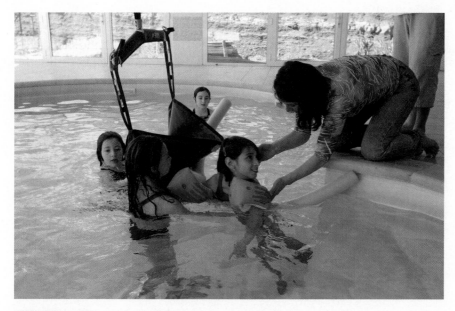

FIGURE 11-10   Adapted aquatics instructor.
© BSIP SA / Alamy Stock Photo

aquatic programs. She also teaches and supervises APA students in laboratory classes.

APA SPECIALIST AT A MEDICAL CENTER

For the past 7 years, Sylvia has been working as an APA specialist in a multiple sclerosis center that is affiliated with the neurology department at a major university hospital in California. While she was in an APA graduate program, she was inspired by her aunt who was diagnosed with multiple sclerosis (MS) and motivated to focus her research on exercise for individuals with MS. Through her master's program in APA, she gained vast knowledge and hands-on skills that she could apply to helping people with MS in clinical settings. In addition, Sylvia was able to network with many professionals in MS organizations while she conducted her graduate research. Her research endeavors helped her acquire a unique APA position at the medical center. She enjoys instructing group and individualized exercise sessions for patients with MS. She is also collaborating with medical researchers for federally funded clinical trials on MS and exercise.

APA COORDINATOR IN THE PUBLIC SECTOR

Marcus is an outdoor enthusiast. He is an avid hiker, kayaker, and skier. After completing his program in APA, he found his dream job as a physical activity coordinator in a county office in Colorado. He is in charge of arranging and managing all physical activity programs in the county. He is dedicated to making adapted outdoor recreation programs more accessible to community members with disabilities. Marcus has been involved in an adaptive ski program for several years. Recently, he added an adapted kayak/canoe program to his summer activity calendar. He also created a summer camping program for children with disabilities. Marcus recruits and manages instructors for adapted yoga and dance classes offered at the county's community centers. He claims that his versatility in both outdoor recreation and APA makes his work performance highly appreciated by his county office.

ADAPTED FITNESS BUSINESS OWNER

Wesley uses his training in APA in combination with his exceptional communication and business skills to operate a private adapted fitness center for people with physical disabilities. After finishing his degree in kinesiology with a specialization in APA, he began as an adapted personal trainer to help people with disabilities in commercial gym settings and later at clients' homes. He has also worked in a couple of specialized fitness centers that provide mobility rehabilitation and therapeutic exercise services for clients with neuromuscular disabilities. Over the years, he developed new ideas about how to operate and manage an adapted fitness program. Last year, he opened his own adapted fitness center after converting an old gym and equipping it with various accessible and adapted exercise equipment. He has been also serving as a clinical site supervisor for university internship students. Wesley enjoys helping his clients while training interns in APA.

APA SERVICE PROGRAM DIRECTOR AT A COMMUNITY COLLEGE

Many community colleges offer physical activity classes for community members. Most also have specific courses for students with disabilities or older adults. Christopher is a professor at a community college in Oregon. He teaches several classes in kinesiology, including Introduction to APA. He is also the director of the APA service program on his campus, where he and his students instruct adapted classes for community members with special needs. Every Monday and Wednesday afternoon, his program offers a group adapted exercise session for individuals with disabilities using a large expansion room at the student recreation center. The program also provides a group aquatic class for older adults on Tuesdays and Thursdays. Every Friday afternoon, he and his students have fun playing with children with disabilities in the adapted motor skill clinic session. In addition, Christopher assists his church community with creating adapted programs for members with disabilities. He reminds us of what "total commitment" truly means.

ADAPTED FITNESS TRAINER IN A RECOVERY EXERCISE PROGRAM

Kyle is an adapted fitness trainer at a spinal cord injury (SCI) recovery center. The SCI recovery center offers nonmedical and physical activity–based intervention programs. When he first started working at the center about 10 years ago, it was the only SCI recovery program in the United States. He has recently been promoted to supervising director at a new site in New England as his company has expanded its franchised business to multiple locations across the United States and to other countries. Although he has additional administrative responsibilities as a director now, Kyle still enjoys working one on one with clients with SCI while supervising and training staff members.

APA RESEARCHER IN A UNIVERSITY

Lisa has always had a passion for helping children with disabilities. After completing her doctoral training in APA, she began working as a researcher for an infant motor development laboratory at a university in New York. Her research interests lie in studying motor skill development among infants and toddlers with developmental disabilities and investigating the effects of various early intervention programs. Lisa is also interested in childhood obesity among children with developmental disabilities and is investigating the relationship between young children's play patterns and incidence of obesity.

ADAPTED WELLNESS PROGRAM DIRECTOR AT A RETIREMENT COMMUNITY

John is a wellness program director at a residential retirement community in Florida. The upscale retirement home community has its own wellness center next to a small medical clinic and a golf course. He is responsible for managing all health and wellness classes offered at the center. While he was in his APA program, he learned how to develop and implement adapted fitness and aquatic exercise for older adults with disabilities. He also gained multiple certifications, such as a certified aquatic instructor certification from the Arthritis Foundation. He has created new fitness and wellness classes for his community members. John and his staff have also developed a few group and individual classes uniquely designed to accommodate older adults with chronic medical conditions such as arthritis, stroke, and Parkinson's disease. John enjoys watching people smile as he teaches group aquatic classes for older adults with arthritis. His adapted wellness program recently started to offer a group wellness walk and senior fall prevention exercise class.

WHAT CREDENTIALS OR CERTIFICATIONS ARE AVAILABLE IN THE FIELD OF APA?

If you are interested in pursuing a career in APA, you might want to consider obtaining a credential or certification. You may need to take prerequisite courses and accumulate a certain number of hours of practicum or field experience to be eligible to take certain certification exams. Most require you to complete continuing education units (CEUs) periodically to maintain your certification. Some certifications are specific to a population (e.g., Certified Arthritis Foundation Aquatic Instructor) or an intervention technique (e.g., Certified Halliwick Instructor). The following is an overview of just some of the various APA certifications.

CERTIFIED ADAPTED PHYSICAL EDUCATOR (CAPE)

If you are interested in working as an APE teacher or specialist for children with disabilities, you can apply for certification as a Certified Adapted Physical Educator (CAPE). This national certification has minimum criteria of a bachelor's degree in kinesiology, 12 units of coursework in APA, 200 hours of field experience, and a current valid teaching certification in physical education to be eligible to sit for the certification exam. The National Consortium for Physical Education and Recreation for Individuals with Disabilities (NCPERID) and the Adapted Physical Activity Council (APAC) have worked together to create the Adapted Physical Education National Standards. The national certification exam is based on 15 standards: human development, motor behavior, exercise science, measurement and evaluation, history and philosophy, unique attributes of learners, curriculum theory and development, assessment, instructional design and planning, teaching, consultation and staff development, continuing education, ethics, and communication. More information is available at *www.apens.org*.

CERTIFIED INCLUSIVE FITNESS TRAINER (CIFT)

The Certified Inclusive Fitness Trainer (CIFT) certification has been developed for APA health and fitness professionals who want to empower people with disabilities through adapted exercise and fitness programs. It is endorsed by two major professional organizations: the American College of Sports Medicine (ACSM) and the National Center on Health, Physical Activity and Disability (NCHPAD). The certification requires you to fully understand the exercise guidelines and precautions for people with disabilities and know how to utilize safe and adapted exercise methods. Minimum requirements for eligibility include current health/fitness-related certifications, as well as adult cardiopulmonary resuscitation (CPR) and automated external defibrillator (AED) certifications. The certification exam requires that you demonstrate competency in the following areas: exercise physiology and other exercise science, fitness and clinical exercise testing, exercise prescription and programming, safety, injury prevention and emergency procedures, human behavior and counseling, clinical and medical considerations, the Americans with Disabilities Act (ADA) and design, and disability awareness. More information is available at *http://certification.acsm. org/acsm-inclusive-fitness-trainer*.

AQUATIC THERAPY AND REHABILITATION INSTITUTE CERTIFIED (ATRIC)

If you are interested in adapted aquatics or aquatic therapy, a few certification options are available, including Adapted Aquatics Instructor certification and Aquatic Fitness Professional certification. One of the most comprehensive certifications in aquatic therapeutic exercise is Aquatic Therapy and Rehabilitation Institute Certified (ATRIC). The ATRIC exam is based on standards developed by a multidisciplinary committee of aquatic therapy and

STOP AND THINK

Select a specific career in APA that you find interesting and at which you think you would be most successful. What challenges and rewards do you see from such a career?

rehabilitation professionals. When you sit for the ATRIC exam, you will be tested on your knowledge and competency on standards in six areas: movement mechanics and science (anatomy, physiology, kinesiology and biomechanics), aquatic principles, basic principles and methods used in aquatic therapy and rehabilitation, professional responsibility, safety and risk awareness, and legal considerations. More information on ATRIC is available at *www.atri.org /ATRICertification.htm.*

Areas of Research in APA

Because of the cross-disciplinary nature of APA, researchers conduct research using a variety of methods and approaches. Common research methods in APA include surveys, questionnaires, observation, interviews, biomechanical measurements (e.g., motion analysis systems, force plates), physiological instruments (e.g., body composition measurements, metabolic analysis systems), and clinical evaluation tools (e.g., Test of Gross Motor Development [TGMD], Berg Balance Scale). Research can be qualitative or quantitative.

Researchers in APA can also focus on a specific population. For example, an APA researcher might focus research on physical activity and children with autism. Researchers in APA may also conduct theory-driven research by applying concepts such as adaptation, self-determination, dynamical systems theory, social constructivism, or ecological system theory.

Researchers evaluate intervention programs using a number of different approaches. The research approaches in APA can be categorized as follows: administrative and epidemiological studies, biomechanical studies, motor behavioral studies, pedagogical studies, physiological studies, and psychological studies.

ADMINISTRATIVE AND EPIDEMIOLOGICAL APPROACH

Researchers using an administrative and epidemiological approach might examine professional development, participation patterns in physical activity, barriers and facilitators, policies and procedures, cost-effectiveness, awareness and perception, and incidence and prevalence with regard to APA.

An example of a research study in this category is Rimmer, Riley, Wang, Rauworth, and Jurkowski's (2004) "Physical activity participation among persons with disabilities: Barriers and facilitators." In this study, the authors applied content analysis to tape recordings to identify barriers and facilitators associated with participation in APA programs/facilities among individuals with disabilities. They then identified various themes that emerged, such as environmental barriers, economic issues, emotional barriers, equipment barriers, information-related barriers, perceptions and attitudes, policies and procedures, and availability of resources.

BIOMECHANICAL APPROACH

With the biomechanical approach, researchers typically utilize biomechanical instruments to analyze movement patterns or investigate outcome measures in gait, balance, and sport-specific or other functional motor skills. Commonly used biomechanical tools include a three-dimensional motion analysis system, a posturograph (a computerized balance-measuring device), a force plate, and an accelerometer. An example of a study using this approach is Jung, Lee, Charalambous, and Vrongistinos's (2010) "The influence of applying additional weight to the affected leg on gait patterns during aquatic treadmill walking in people post-stroke." The authors used a three-dimensional underwater motion analysis system to examine the effects of using cuff weight for people with stroke in aquatic therapy and concluded that it could help people with hemiparesis walk better during aquatic gait training.

MOTOR BEHAVIORAL APPROACH

Common topics examined using the motor behavioral approach are related to motor development, motor learning, and motor control. Research in this area examines topics such as multitasking, coordination, skill acquisition, information processing, visual feedback, and emerging motor patterns. An example of a study using this approach is Wu, Looper, Ulrich, Ulrich, and Angulo-Barroso's (2007) "Exploring effects of different treadmill interventions on walking onset and gait patterns in infants with Down syndrome." The researchers investigated the effects of different treadmill gait training for infants with Down syndrome and found that high-intensity treadmill training promoted earlier walking onset and elicited favorable gait patterns.

PEDAGOGICAL APPROACH

Researchers in this category often examine research topics such as instruction, teacher preparation, inclusion, peer-tutoring, teaching effectiveness, active learning time, behavior management, and feedback. Klavina and Block's (2008) study, "The effect of peer tutoring on interaction behaviors in inclusive physical education," is a good example of research in this category. The researchers examined the effects of peer tutoring on physical, instructional, and social interaction behaviors between elementary school students with severe disabilities (SD) and peers without SD. They found that peer-mediated and voluntary peer support increased the instructional and physical interaction behaviors between students with SD and their peers, as well as activity engagement time.

PHYSIOLOGICAL APPROACH

Researches taking a physiological approach will examine topics such as aerobic capacity, lactate threshold, pain, fatigue, cardiorespiratory response, muscular strength, and energy expenditure. Physiological research instruments include tools that measure pulmonary gas exchange (telemetry metabolic gas analyzer), body composition (densitometry), muscular strength (dynamometer), and electrical activity of muscle (electromyography). A study by Parlser, Madras, and Weiss (2006), "Outcomes of an aquatic exercise program including aerobic capacity, lactate threshold, and fatigue in individuals with multiple sclerosis," is a good example of research in this category. The researchers examined the effects of aquatic exercise on cardiovascular fitness in people with MS and found positive outcomes in peak oxygen consumption and fatigue level without any adverse symptoms.

PSYCHOLOGICAL APPROACH

Researchers who take this approach study key topics such as motivation, perceived competency, depression, quality of life, attitude, and self-efficacy. An investigation by Todd, Reid, and Butler-Kisber (2010) titled "Cycling for students with ASD: Self-regulation promotes sustained physical activity" is a good example of research in this category. The authors examined how a self-regulation instructional strategy on sustained cycling, which included self-monitoring, goal setting, and self-reinforcement, could influence adolescents with autism. The results suggested that self-regulation interventions could promote motivation and help sustain participation in physical activity for adolescents with severe autism.

STOP AND THINK

Identify the research approach in APA that most interests you. In your own words, explain why you find this particular research approach interesting. Identify at least four possible research topics related to that approach.

CHAPTER SUMMARY

In this chapter, you have learned a great deal about the field of APA: What it is, where it came from, how it impacts society, how APA service programs are delivered, what careers options are available, and how research is conducted. You learned that APA involves the use of physical activity that is modified for people with special needs to promote healthy and active lifestyles. You also learned about the various types of APA service programs, including APE, adapted sport, therapeutic recreation, inclusive fitness, adapted aquatics, aquatic therapy, and therapeutic exercise. Career options in APA vary, and depending on your interest and training, they can be a fulfilling pathway to making a significant difference in the quality of life of people with special needs. Lastly, it is important for us to continue asking questions about the effectiveness of APA service programs. As you learned in this chapter, outcomes of APA programs and study of movements in people with disabilities can be examined in a number of different ways and through several different approaches.

DISCUSSION QUESTIONS

1. How does APA impact our society's issues related to aging and disability?
2. What is the function of an APA service program? Why are APA service programs important?
3. What are common topics of research in the field of APA?

REFERENCES

American Association for Health, Physical Education, and Recreation. (1952). Guiding principles for adapted physical education. *Journal of Health, Physical Education and Recreation, 23*, 15.

Boyle, C. A., Boulet, S., Schieve, L. A., Cohen, R. A., Blumberg, S. J., Yeargin-Allsopp, M., ... Kogan, M. D. (2011). Trends in the prevalence of developmental disabilities in US children, 1997–2008. *Pediatrics, 127*(6), 1034–1042.

Centers for Disease Control and Prevention. (2014). Community Report on Autism. Retrieved from http://www.cdc.gov/ncbddd/autism/states/comm_report_autism_2014.pdf

Centers for Disease Control and Prevention. (2009). Exercise/physical activity. Retrieved from www.cdc.gov/nchs/fastats

Centers for Disease Control and Prevention. (2010). CDC Health Disparities and Inequalities Report U.S. 2010. Retrieved from http://www.cdc.gov/mmwr/pdf/other/su6203.pdf

Centers for Disease Control and Prevention. (2014). Autism spectrum disorder. Retrieved from http://www.cdc.gov/media/releases/2014/p0327-autism-spectrum-disorder.html

Collins English Dictionary. (2011). Adaptation. Retrieved from http://www.collinsdictionary.com/dictionary/english/adaptation

Eason, R. L., Smith, T. L., & Caron, F. (Eds.). (1983). *Adapted physical activity: From theory to application. Proceedings of the Third International Symposium on Adapted Physical Activity.* Champaign, IL: Human Kinetics.

International Federation of Adapted Physical Activity. (2004). By laws. Retrieved from http://www.ifapa.biz/imgs/uploads/PDF/IFAPA%20By-Laws.pdf

International Federation of Adapted Physical Activity. (n.d.) Definition of adapted physical activity. Retrieved from http://ifapa-international.net/definition/

Jung, T., Lee, D., Charalambous, C., & Vrongistinos, K. (2010). The influence of applying additional weight to the affected leg on gait patterns during aquatic treadmill walking in people post-stroke. *Archives of Physical Medicine and Rehabilitation, 91*(1), 129–136.

Kiphard, E. (1983). Adapted physical education in Germany. In R. Eason, T. L. Smith, & F. Caron (Eds.), *Adapted physical activity: From theory to application* (pp. 25–32). Champaign, IL: Human Kinetics.

Klavina, A., & Block, M. E. (2008). The effect of peer tutoring on interaction behaviors in inclusive physical education. *Adapted Physical Activity Quarterly, 25*(2), 132–158.

Newell, K. M. (1990). Physical activity, knowledge types, and degree programs. *Quest, 42*, 269-278.

Ogden, C. L., Carroll, M. D., Kit, B. K., & Flegal, K. M. (2014). Prevalence of childhood and adult obesity in the United States, 2011–2012. *Journal of the American Medical Association, 311*(8), 806–814.

Oxford Dictionary of English Etymology. (1966). Handicap. Retrieved from http://www.oxforddictionaries.com/us/definition/handicap

Parlser, G., Madras, D., & Weiss, E. (2006). Outcomes of an aquatic exercise program including aerobic capacity, lactate threshold, and fatigue in individuals with multiple sclerosis. *Journal of Neurological Physical Therapy, 30*(2), 82–90.

Reid, G. (2003). Defining adapted physical activity. In R. D. Steadward, G. D. Wheeler, & E. J. Watkinson (Eds.), *Adapted physical activity* (pp. 11–25). Edmonton: University of Alberta Press.

Rimmer, J. H., Riley, B., Wang, E., Rauworth, A., & Jurkowski, J. (2004). Physical activity participation among persons with disabilities: Barriers and facilitators. *American Journal of Preventative Medicine, 26*(5), 419–425.

Rimmer, J. H., Wang, E., & Smith D. (2008). Barriers associated with exercise and community access for individuals with stroke. *Journal of Rehabilitation Research Development, 45*(2), 315–322.

Sherrill, C. (2004). *Adapted physical activity, recreation, and sport: Crossdisciplinary and lifespan* (6th ed.). Boston, MA: McGraw-Hill Higher Education.

Todd, T., Reid, G., & Butler-Kisber, L. (2010). Cycling for students with ASD: Self-regulation promotes sustained physical activity. *Adapted Physical Activity Quarterly, 27*(3), 226–241.

U.S. Bureau of the Census. (2010). Participation in selected sport activities: 2004. *Statistical abstract of the United States*. Washington, D.C.: Government Printing Office.

U.S. Department of Health and Human Services. (2008). *2008 Physical Activity Guidelines for Americans*. Retrieved from http://www.health.gov/PAGuidelines

World Health Organization. (2001). International classification of functioning, disability and health. Retrieved from http://www.who.int/topics/disabilities/en/

Wu, J., Looper, J., Ulrich, B. D., Ulrich, D. A., & Angulo-Barroso, R. M. (2007). Exploring effects of different treadmill interventions on walking onset and gait patterns in infants with Down syndrome. *Developmental Medicine and Child Neurology, 49*(11), 839–845.

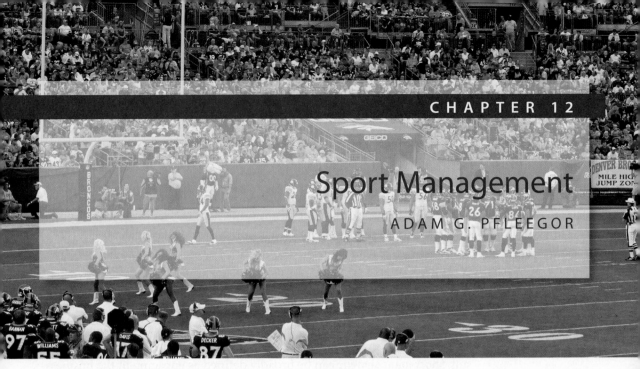

CHAPTER 12

Sport Management

ADAM G. PFLEEGOR

LEARNING OBJECTIVES

1. Define *sport management*.
2. Outline the academic history of sport management in the United States.
3. Describe the size and impact of the sport industry in the United States.
4. Define key terminology in sport management.
5. Describe the areas of industry and academic research in sport management.
6. Identify possible career choices with a sport management degree.

KEY TERMS

aesthetic sports
discretionary income
extreme sports
gross domestic sport product (GDSP)
mega events
National Collegiate Athletic Association (NCAA)

North American Society for Sport Management (NASSM)
popular sport media
power and performance sports
sabermetrics
sport management

sport management
The business-
related aspects
of producing,
managing, or
organizing spectator
events or sport-
specific products.

What Is Sport Management?

Sport is a concept that is often easier to describe than to define. For many of us, sport is, and has been, intertwined with our everyday lives in a variety of forms since our early youth. From virtually spectating (watching on television or Internet) the world's biggest mega events, such as the Summer and Winter Olympic Games, the FIFA World Cup, or the National Football League (NFL) Super Bowl, to participating in a competitive event or simply enjoying physical activity, sport permeates our daily existence and helps define and shape American society. Due to the immense popularity and international growth of sport, and specifically competitive spectator sport, the field of sport management has emerged from parent disciplines such as business management, business administration, and physical education as a standalone scholarly pursuit. **Sport management** can be broadly defined as engaging in the business-related aspects of producing, managing, or organizing spectator events or sport-specific products (**FIGURE 12-1**; Pitts & Stotlar, 2013). Essentially, every

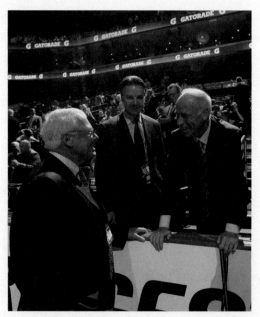

FIGURE 12-1   The field of sport management covers a wide spectrum of practices and career opportunities.
© Bruce Bennett / Getty Images

aspect of putting together a sport or recreational event or selling a sport product (organizing, promoting, marketing, advertising, etc.) can fall under the guise and direction of a sport management professional (Chelladurai, 2014).

Sport management encompasses a wide variety of sport types, settings, and industry segments (Parks, Quarterman, & Thibault, 2011). Types of sports include traditional head-to-head sports such as American football, soccer, and ice hockey; **aesthetic sports** such as figure skating, diving, and gymnastics; and **extreme sports** such as whitewater rafting, sky diving, and heli-skiing. Sport management can also be characterized by the broad number of settings in which it takes place, such as major professional sports, minor league sports, intercollegiate athletics, local recreation organizations, or municipal parks departments. It also encompasses a number of different industry segments, including marketing, sales, finance, and event management. Overall, sport management reaches throughout the sport industry, touching upon many activities, areas, careers, and segments.

Sport management has become one of the fastest-growing standalone degree programs in the United States. According to the **North American Society for Sport Management (NASSM)**, more than 475 sport management degree programs in the United States offer bachelor's, master's, or doctoral degrees. These degree programs, originating from Brooklyn Dodger's owner Walter O'Malley's suggestion that professional sport employees should gain industry-specific knowledge, provide a broad-based business or management degree with a focus on sport or recreation career opportunities at the undergraduate level and opportunities to focus in specific areas such as intercollegiate sport or sport marketing at the graduate level. Despite its prominent role on many academic campuses across the country, sport management as a degree program had a small-scale and humble start.

The History of Sport Management in the United States

Throughout the early to mid-1900s, several institutions across the United States offered individual courses focused on the administration (management) of sport and recreation. As early as 1911, a course at the University of Wisconsin taught students the intricacies of operating sporting events and running athletic teams (Seifried, 2015). Initially housed in physical education programs, the demand for courses focused on sport administration, especially in amateur settings such as youth or interscholastic sport, grew as the popularity of sport soared to new heights across the country. During this time period, several emerging

---

aesthetic sports
Sports that rely on agility, fluidity, beauty, and precision to showcase excellence. Aesthetic sports often include aspects of subjective judging where competitors compete in a parallel fashion, as seen in figure skating, diving, gymnastics, and synchronized swimming.

extreme sports
Countercultural, nature-based, or other sports that involve elements of personal danger. Examples include freestyle skiing, parasailing, cliff diving, and slacklining.

North American Society for Sport Management (NASSM)
The main sport management governing academic association in North America. Founded in 1985 by a group of sport scholars, NASSM hosts an annual conference and publishes the *Journal of Sport Management*.

STOP AND THINK

Sport management covers a broad spectrum of careers, tasks, and opportunities. In your own words, describe what sport management is and how it relates to your intended career choice.

scholars worked with students on dissertation research associated with sport administration tasks and concerns. Despite the increased focus on sport management courses and dissertation research, the first standalone academic program was not developed until 1966 at Ohio University. The master's degree in sport administration at Ohio University was started by Dr. James Mason after he was contacted by Brooklyn Dodger's president Walter O'Malley (**FIGURE 12-2**). O'Malley inquired of Mason where future professionals interested in working in sport, recreation, or leisure could go to secure a higher education focused on the industry. After considering the specific duties of sport administration and management professionals and how the set of knowledge differs from traditional physical education, business, and management programs, Ohio University accepted the first group of sport management

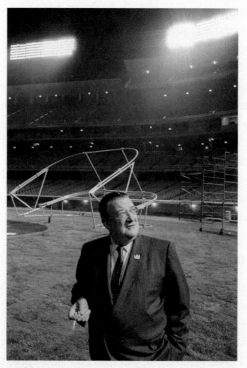

FIGURE 12-2   Brooklyn/Los Angeles Dodgers owner and executive Walter O'Malley ignited the discussion for the first sport management program.
© Phil Bath / Getty Images

students for the 1966 school year and ushered in a new academic field on college campuses (Parks et al., 2011).

From these early graduate programs, which focused on a broad-based sport management curriculum and field experience, the major has grown into a variety of general and specific curriculums worldwide. Although many undergraduate programs still offer a curriculum based on the model developed by Ohio University and supported by NASSM and the Commission on Sport Management Accreditation (COSMA), graduate programs provide future professionals the opportunity to specialize in industry-specific segments such as marketing, event management, facility management, parks and recreation, intercollegiate sports, sport management ethics, and other areas of expertise. However, several graduate programs continue to offer a general-knowledge curriculum aimed at providing students the opportunity to explore a plethora of career opportunities. In addition, academics in sport management have developed and published in a wide spectrum of journals dedicated to sport management research (**TABLE 12-1**) and share findings

TABLE 12-1   Academic Journals for Sport Management

European Sport Management Quarterly
International Journal of Sport Management
International Journal of Sport Management and Marketing
Journal of Amateur Sport
Journal of Contemporary Athletics
Journal of Issues in Intercollegiate Athletics
Journal of Legal Aspects of Sport
Journal of Sport History
Journal of Sport Management
Journal of the Philosophy of Sport
Journal of Sports Economics
Sport Management Education Journal
Sport Management Review
Sport Marketing Quarterly
Sport, Ethics, and Philosophy

TABLE 12-2   Academic Associations That Address Issues Related to Sport Management

| African Sport Management Association (ASMA) |
| Asian Association for Sport Management (AASM) |
| College Sport Research Institute (CSRI) |
| European Association for Sport Management (EASM) |
| International Association for the Philosophy of Sport (IAPS) |
| North American Society for Sport History (NASSH) |
| North American Society for Sport Management (NASSM) |
| Sport and Recreation Law Association (SRLA) |
| Sport Management Association of Australia and New Zealand (SMAANZ) |
| Sport Marketing Association (SMA) |
| World Association of Sport Management (WASM) |

STOP AND THINK

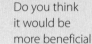

- Do you think it would be more beneficial for future professionals to specialize in a specific area of sport management or to study a broad-based curriculum?

- What are the pros and cons of each approach, and which would you personally find most appealing?

with other scholars and practitioners through a number of different professional associations (**TABLE 12-2**). Ultimately, the continued growth and success of all sport management programs is dependent on the growth of the sport industry and practical need for sport managers and administrators. Therefore, it is important to take a brief look at the size and growth of the sport industry in the United States (Fielding et al., 2011).

The Size of the Sport Industry in the United States

What is the current financial and economic impact of the sport industry? Examining the size and impact of the sport industry indicates consumer demand for sport event spectating, sport participation, and sport-related products, which can help predict future growth or decline of the sport industry and the role of sport in the overall economic climate. Although not specifically listed as its own industrial classification by the U.S. Census Bureau's North American Industry Classification System, several popular sport publications (e.g., *Sports Business Journal*) and various sport scholars have attempted to quantify the monetary size of the sport industry. With previous attempts showing a discrepancy of $200 to $300 billion a year in the **gross domestic sport product (GDSP)**, Millano and Chelladurai (2011) provided a comprehensive analysis of the size of the sport industry utilizing three measurement techniques to more accurately determine its financial impact. They determined that the size of the sport industry in the United States was conservatively $169 billion, moderately $189 billion, and liberally $208 billion. The differences between these three estimates can be attributed to the amount of leisure-time activity spending (e.g., country clubs, golf courses, social clubs) included in the estimate. The conservative estimate included none of this spending, the moderate estimate included some of this spending, and the liberal estimate included the entire amount.

No matter which estimate you deem most appropriate, the financial size of the industry is immense and comparable with even the largest industries in the United States, such as real estate, construction, agriculture, transportation, and education. The economic impact of the sport industry further indicates how important sport is to our society and bodes well for future sport management professionals seeking internships and entry-level positions. It is important to note that the sport industry has been relatively immune to the economic cycle when compared to other industries. During poor economic times, consumers still tend to spend discretionary funds on sport spectating and participation, similar to how consumers continue to spend money on movies, donuts, and coffee. This continued spending during poor economic conditions indicates that sport may act as a way for individuals to escape difficult day-to-day life situations and that many view sport as an essential part of American life.

Major Topics in Sport Management

As an industry and academic discipline, sport, and the management and administration of sport, is fast paced, dynamic, and demanding. Therefore, the major topics examined by scholars in peer-reviewed publications and **popular sport media** such as ESPN, NBC Sports, *Sports Illustrated*, and other outlets are consistently changing and evolving based

---

gross domestic sport product (GDSP)
The financial (monetary) measurement of all sport-related goods and services produced in a country over a year.

---

popular sport media
The host of media outlets that televise, broadcast, and report on sport issues. These outlets are widely available to the general public and are not peer-reviewed by sport scholars. Examples include ESPN, CNN, *Sports Illustrated,* the Bleacher Report, CBS Sports, NBC Sports, and countless other networks and individuals that cover sport topics.

STOP AND THINK

Considering that sport is not listed as its own industrial classification by the U.S. Census Bureau, where would the GDSP indicated by Millano and Chelladurai fall compared to the size of other major industries in the United States?

Any casual sport fan encounters countless breaking stories dealing with sport. In your opinion, what is the most memorable story in the past few years concerning the management of sport? Why do you think it was important?

on breaking stories, new technologies, novel strategies, new rules of play, and the latest trends in the industry. Considering contemporary issues and developments across the industry, several major topics stand out in the current sport management discourse. It is imperative to remember that the topics listed and briefly described here are not the only major topics in the field, as the range of issues in sport management and administration is vast and diverse, much like its parent disciplines.

INTERCOLLEGIATE, INTERSCHOLASTIC, AND AMATEUR ATHLETICS

National Collegiate Athletic Association (NCAA)
Organized into three separate divisions, the NCAA overseas intercollegiate sport contests and championships for American institutions of higher education. Currently, it has more than 1,200 member institutions from all 50 states.

The complete integration of education and sport is unique to the United States, especially at the competitive intercollegiate level. Starting with the first intercollegiate rowing contest in the late 1800s, intercollegiate sport in the United States has grown into a multi-million-dollar business entity. The primary governing body of American intercollegiate sport, the **National Collegiate Athletic Association (NCAA)**, currently supports three competitive divisions with more than 1,200 institutions, hosts nationally televised contests and tournaments, and has member institutions with athletic department budgets fast approaching $150 to $200 million per year (**FIGURE 12-3**). The top intercollegiate football programs draw crowds of more than 100,000 fans for a single game, eclipsing those of the most-well-attended contests in the NFL. The popularity and financial prowess of college sport can be seen in the most recent NCAA March Madness (Division I basketball postseason championship tournament) television contract. The current deal agreed on in 2016 between the NCAA, CBS, and Turner Broadcasting is worth approximately $11 billion and extends the multimedia rights through 2032. In accordance with this deal, CBS, Turner Broadcasting, and both companies' affiliate stations (TNT, TBS, TruTV, CBS Sports), will show every game between the tournament's 68-team field live to consumers across the globe.

In addition to the popularity of college sport, high school athletics and youth/amateur sport continue to be cornerstones of American society. Young athletes of diverse race, ethnicity, socioeconomic status, and gender participate together starting in amateur athletics soon after birth. Due to their popularity, strict governing structures, and large financial ramifications,

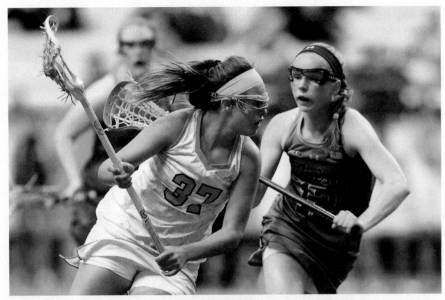

FIGURE 12-3   NCAA sport has grown into a multi-million-dollar business in the United States.
© Cal Sport Media / Alamy Stock Photo

amateur athletics—from youth contests to the intense competition of inter-collegiate sport—has developed into a major topic in sport management, for both scholars and practitioners. In fact, several academic journals, including the *Journal of Issues in Intercollegiate Athletics* and the *Journal of Amateur Sport*, focus solely on these issues, with researchers examining such things as the amateur status of athletes, the value of competition, pay-for-pay in high schools, and concerns and issues with the NCAA.

SPORT MARKETING AND REVENUE GENERATION

Because sport is an intangible, perishable entertainment product, the mar-keting of sport contests to a variety of individuals is crucial for consumer satisfaction; fan identification; repeat customers; and the financial viability and longevity of organizations, programs, and institutions. As intercollegiate and professional teams attempt to expand their fan base and create loyal cus-tomers, sport marketers utilize an array of information to appropriately price, promote, produce, and distribute the product to fans and nonfans alike. Sport marketing, personal and corporate selling, and revenue generation are similar in many ways to marketing aspects and concerns in general business and marketing environments; however, Mullin, Hardy, and Sutton (2007) note that sport marketing deserves unique attention because the product is intangible, perishable, and, most important, unpredictable. For example, marketing an upcoming blockbuster film is relatively straightforward because marketers know the exact product that will be provided to the customer, including the ending. In contrast, sport is unpredictable; the outcome is not predetermined, and thus marketers are required to focus on the potential of the contest and outside events such as halftime shows or giveaways (**FIGURE 12-4**).

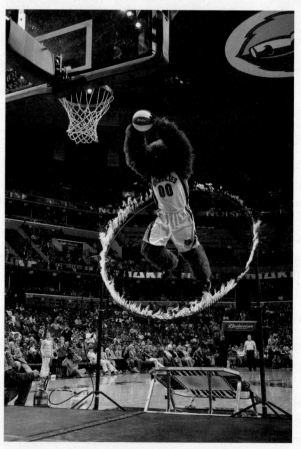

FIGURE 12-4   Due to the unpredictability of sporting events, sport marketers often promote halftime entertainment.

© Joe Murphy / Getty Images

In addition, fans attend games for countless reasons, and therefore will experience the game in different ways with different levels of attachment and attention. Thus, sport marketers need to consider all types of fans in their efforts to promote the organization or institution. Some primary subtopics examined in sport marketing are ticket sales, revenue generation, promotions, and pricing. These concerns are addressed in general sport management journals and more specifically in journals such as *Sport Marketing Quarterly* and *International Journal of Sport Management and Marketing*.

SPORT CONSUMER BEHAVIOR

Sport consumer behavior examines why and how consumers make purchasing decisions for sport products and experiences. Entwined with sport marketing and revenue generation, sport consumer behavior has emerged as a primary topic in its own right due to an organization's focus on attracting fans, retaining fans, and providing a quality consumer experience. An initial key component to sport consumer behavior is understanding spectator motivation. Much like its entertainment competitors, such as theater productions, movie showings, festivals, and concerts, attendees at a sport contest select to consume and spectate the contest for countless numbers of reasons. Some fans may be highly identified with the team and show their support through purchasing season tickets and attending every game in team-sponsored merchandise and painted faces, whereas the fan sitting next to them may be attending to impress a friend, love interest, or colleague and be more focused on interaction than with the game outcome (**FIGURE 12-5**). By better understanding why fans attend contests, sport managers and administrators can tailor the experience to increase consumer satisfaction and hopefully turn single-contest or sporadic attendees into repeat consumers of the team, event, or organization. These actions essentially turn nonfans and casual fans into diehards who follow the organization's every move. In recent years, Americans have seen a reduction in **discretionary income**, resulting in more intense competition between sport and other activities for people's entertainment dollars, making sport consumer behavior research more important than ever. Examining sport consumer behavior coupled with sport marketing and sales is critical to the long-term prosperity and viability of organizations and institutions. The many subtopics and dominant themes in sport consumer behavior

discretionary income The amount of money left over after an individual or family pays for necessities such as shelter, food, and clothing. Sport competes with other brands of entertainment, such as movie theaters, for this segment of money.

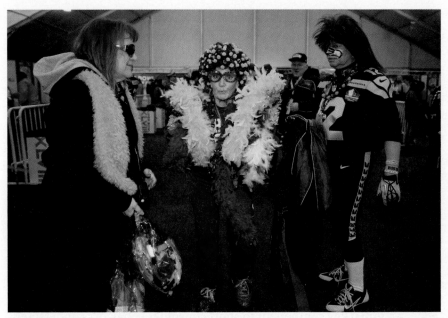

FIGURE 12-5   It is the goal of sport organizations to create highly identified or diehard fans.
© Jamie Squire / Getty Images

are showcased in general sport management, sport marketing, and sport economics journals such as *Journal of Sport Management, Sport Marketing Quarterly,* and *Journal of Sports Economics.*

SPORT FACILITY MANAGEMENT

The facilities that house professional and intercollegiate sport contests are regularly some of the largest structures and building projects in their respective towns and cities. In many cases, large-scale sport facilities have become signature architectural structures in communities that represent the community to outsiders and constituents alike. Because marketers, promoters, and managers cannot guarantee game scores, outcomes, or athletic excitement, they often rely on a facility filled with technology and amenities to satiate customer demands. As construction and architectural technology advances at a rapid pace, several stadiums have broken the $1 billion construction cost mark (e.g., AT&T Stadium in Arlington, Texas, and MetLife Stadium in East Rutherford, New Jersey) due to their location, size, and amenities. In fact, even renovations of existing facilities have approached or broken the $1 billion price tag (e.g., Madison Square Garden in New York City and Dodger Stadium in Los Angeles, California). The increased construction and development costs have stemmed from larger footprints, more luxury amenities, advanced technology, better concession options, and signature architectural features such as retractable roofs, viewing bridges, or massive high-definition television screens and jumbotrons (**FIGURE 12-6**).

Despite the need to keep up with competing organizations, the decision to tear down an old facility and construct a futuristic venue should not be taken lightly. This is due to the heritage and history accumulated in many venues as signature events, games, contests, or moments have become part of a structure's past. Overall, the construction of new facilities and the renovation of existing structures has become a key topic in sport management. Intercollegiate athletic departments are regularly competing with

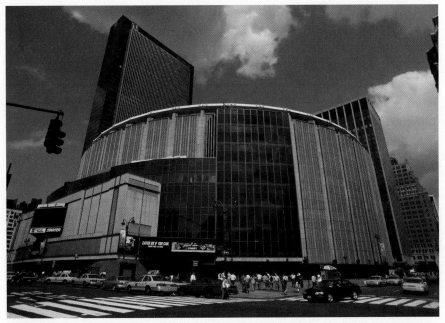

FIGURE 12-6   External view of the "world's most famous arena," Madison Square Garden in New York City.
© JTB MEDIA CREATION, Inc. / Alamy Stock Photo

one another through their venues to attract the best recruits and coaches, and professional organizations demand new facilities or threaten to relocate in order to increase the amount of generated revenue from their physical home (e.g., the NFL's St. Louis Rams relocating to Los Angeles for the 2016 season). Subtopics concerning sport facility management encompass construction and renovations; stadium locations; new technologies, such as smart seats and high-definition video screens; significance and maintenance of a facility's heritage and history; liability and risk; event management; fan experience; and franchise relocation decisions such as *European Sport Management Quarterly* and *Sport Management Review*.

SPORT MANAGEMENT ETHICS

As the financial, career, and public relations implications of competitive athletics increase, the propensity to bend or break the rules to gain an advantage also increases. Whereas other sport majors and fields such as sport philosophy, sport ethics, and sport sociology tend to focus on ethical actions of players and societal trends in athletics, sport management ethics focuses on decisions made by those in managerial and administrative roles. As highly structured activities, the many rules and regulations of sport can be manipulated, broken, or bent not only by players and coaches on the field, but also by administrators, managers, and other employees off the field to gain an advantage over other organizations, institutions, or companies. For example, in 2007, the NFL's New England Patriots were caught illegally videotaping the New York Jets's coaching signals. The event, which is commonly referred to as "spygate," involved managers and other organizational members breaking the league's rules to gain an advantage over their divisional rival.

In order to preserve the sanctity of competitive sport and the industry, a level or fair business playing field is sought by scholars and industry professionals alike. Therefore, research on ethical situations, ethical decision-making, and concepts of fairness permeate much of contemporary sport research. By quickly tuning in to ESPN, NBC Sports, or other popular sport programming, you will most likely see yet another story about an organization or institution breaking the rules. To help managers make better ethical decisions, research concerning sport management ethics has been featured in journals across the discipline, such as the *Sport Management Review*, but it is highlighted in the *Journal for the Philosophy of Sport* and *Sport, Ethics, and Philosophy*. Examples of current subtopics include the use of performance-enhancing drugs; concerns with leadership styles of managers; personnel decisions; and fair, competitive sport structures.

SPORT LAW

Legal and liability topics associated with the participation, management, and administration of sport are omnipresent at all levels of the industry. As sport participation and spectator attendance numbers continue to increase, the potential for catastrophic consequences also increases. The protection and safety of all involved at large-scale gatherings is paramount for the continued viability of local contests, intercollegiate sport events, professional athletics, and international **mega events**. From a participatory standpoint, sport and event managers must be cognizant of the safety of the athletes in order to maintain a safe environment and limit liability for their organization. These participatory safety concerns are magnified for physical **power and performance sports** such as American football, rugby, ice hockey, and other activities that physically match opponents directly against one another. However, safety and liability interests are present in all activities, regardless of the level of direct physical contact (e.g., cheerleading and figure skating). In addition to participant liability and safety, legal and liability topics are also important with regard to spectators. For example, the National Hockey League (NHL) decided to add nets behind the goals in 2002 to protect fans from flying sticks, pucks, and other objects. However, this decision was made retroactively after 13-year-old Brittanie Cecil died when she was struck by a puck while attending a Columbus Blue Jackets game for her birthday party. The NHL rightfully received harsh criticism for not proactively protecting fans. Specific subtopics for consideration for contemporary sport managers include Title IX laws and regulations, sport marketing and advertising issues, human resources problems and regulations, liability of attendees and fans, spectator and participant violence, and issues with sport facilities and event subcontractors. These, along with other subtopics in sport law, are addressed in general legal journals, sport management journals, and sport law journals such as the *Journal of Legal Aspects of Sport*.

mega events
Large-scale sporting events or festivals that occur infrequently or on a scheduled basis. Examples include the NFL Super Bowl, the FIFA World Cup, the Summer and Winter Olympic Games, and the Boston Marathon.

power and performance sports
Sport or athletic contests that involve direct physical contact between athletes or participants in order to secure the primary goals of the activities. These sports generally favor athletes who are bigger, faster, and stronger, rather than displaying the flexibility and artistry required in aesthetic sports.

Overall, the major topics in sport management are constantly evolving as new technologies, strategies, situations, and predicaments present themselves. What should be obvious from the descriptions in this section is that many of these topics are inherently intertwined with one another. Essentially, sport managers are attempting to market and sell their product to consumers and provide a quality product, all while maintaining ethical and legal principles in their organizations. At large organizations, such as those seen in the highest professional ranks or NCAA Division I athletics, individuals are often specialized and deal specifically with one particular topic or situation. However, in smaller organizations, such as minor league sport or NCAA Division III athletics, sport managers are regularly tasked with performing multiple duties and dealing with numerous types of situations. Noting this, let's take a look at some of the potential career opportunities available to future sport managers and administrators.

Career Opportunities with a Sport Management Degree

Career opportunities in sport management are diverse and constantly evolving. For students seeking a degree in sport management, future career prospects range from local recreational sport organizations, such as departments of parks and recreation, to international sport organizations, such as Fédération Internationale de Football Association (FIFA). For a small sample of potential career opportunities, see **TABLE 12-3**, which breaks down the opportunities into recreation- and sport-focused positions. Due to the breadth of the sport industry, the table only indicates a small number of selected opportunities, and therefore should not be considered a comprehensive assessment of potential careers.

Predominant Areas of Research in Sport Management

Much like the parent disciplines of sport management, such as physical education, business management, and business administration, the range of scholarship and research

TABLE 12-3   Selected Sport Management Career Areas

Area Served	Specific Opportunities
Recreation	Scheduling
	Programming
	Tournament director
	Public relations
	Media
	Budgeting and finance
	Event management
	Facility management
	Concessions management
	Marketing
	Sponsorship
	Officiating
	Coaching
Professional and intercollegiate sport	Public relations
	Media
	Budgeting and finance
	Event management
	Facility management
	Marketing
	Ticketing
	Sponsorship
	Sales
	Guest services
	Concessions management
	Video coordinator
	Video production
	Guest services
	Officiating
	Coaching
	Human resources
	Legal counsel
	Sport agent

sabermetrics
Term coined by Bill James to describe the quantitative study of baseball to predict player and team performance. Sabermetrics gained mainstream popularity with the release of the book, and subsequent movie, *Moneyball*.

in sport management is vast. **TABLE 12-4** indicates selected areas of research that are currently common in the field's academic journals. As you can see by the listed topics, researchers employ qualitative, quantitative, and mixed-methods approaches in their sport-specific research, ranging from structural equation modeling (SEM) and **sabermetrics** to ethical or sociological theory. Notably, many of the predominant areas of research coincide with the contemporary topics in sport management discussed previously in this chapter, as well as the potential career opportunities listed earlier in Table 12-3.

TABLE 12-4   Selected Areas of Research in Sport Management

Area of Interest	Topics Examined
Sport marketing	Consumer behavior
	Sponsorship
	Personal sales
	Corporate sales
Sport-for-development	Community development
	Economic development
	Sport-for-peace
Sociocultural	Diversity
	Politics
	Violence
	Gender
	Race
	Ethnicity
	LGBTQ athletes
Sport tourism	Globalization
	Place and sport
	Economic impact
Sport economics	Revenue generation
	Valuation
	Economic impact

TABLE 12-4   Selected Areas of Research in Sport Management (*continued*)

Area of Interest	Topics Examined
Sport finance	Budgeting Financial analysis Financial management Stadium financing
Sport leadership	Strategic leadership Crisis leadership Toxic leadership Organizational culture
Sport law	Human resources Strategic management Operations management Marketing management
Sport communication	Publication relations Sport media Social media
Sport ethics	Sport philosophy Management ethics Scholarship ethics Performance enhancement Decision-making Fair play

CHAPTER SUMMARY

In this chapter, you have learned about sport management as both an academic discipline and as a practical industry. Despite the vast array of major topics, research focuses, and career opportunities that characterize the field, we were able to begin to define sport management. From its humble beginnings as a single graduate program at Ohio University to the explosion of programs across the globe, future sport managers have a variety of choices concerning where and what to study in the field. As the popularity of sport at a variety of competitive levels (i.e., professional, intercollegiate, interscholastic, and youth) continues to blossom in the United States and across the globe, career opportunities in sport management are projected to continue to grow and diversify.

STOP AND THINK

- Taking a look at Table 12-4 and noting the wide variety of scholarship topics, which do you think will be the most important research areas in the future?

- Explain why you feel this way. What events have caused that topic to be of great importance to sport managers?

In the future, sport management practitioners will be required to rely on technology to accomplish daily tasks, such as marketing upcoming contests or events, selling tickets, organizing community rallies, designing sport stadiums or arenas, or hiring personnel. Overall, it is best to understand the field of sport management as a specialized discourse that emerged from its parent disciplines of physical education, business management, and business administration out of the necessity for a skilled and knowledgeable sport workforce.

DISCUSSION QUESTIONS

1. Several outspoken business leaders have criticized the sport management degree. For example, Mark Cuban, the oft-brash owner of the Dallas Mavericks, has bashed the degree and supported the idea that interested students pursue a general business or management degree instead. Considering the positives and negatives of both, what advantages (if any) does a sport management degree have over a general business or management degree for future sport industry professionals?

2. The rapid and continued expansion of the sport industry in the United States and across the globe was mentioned multiple times in this chapter. Due to this expansion, there have been a plethora of entry-level positions for sport management graduates. Do you foresee this expansion "bubble" bursting? In other words, at what point might we see a marked slowing in the growth and popularity of sport?

3. The academic and practical field of sport management overlaps with a variety of other sport and non-sport-related fields (e.g., sport psychology). What other fields do you think show the greatest overlap and congruency with sport management?

4. If you were a hiring manager for a professional sports franchise, what qualities would be most important to you when looking for new sport management employees? Explain your answer with an example and reasoning.

REFERENCES

Chelladurai, P. (2014). *Managing organizations for sport and physical activity: A systems perspective* (4th ed.). Scottsdale, AZ: Holcomb Hathaway.

Fielding, L. W., & Pedersen, P. M. (2011). Historical aspects of the sport business industry. In P. M. Pedersen, J. B. Parks, J. Quarterman, & L. Thibault (Eds.), *Contemporary sport management* (4th ed.) (pp. 50–69). Champaign, IL: Human Kinetics.

Millano, M., & Chelladurai, P. (2011). Gross domestic sport product: The size of the sport industry in the United States. *Journal of Sport Management*, 25, 24–35.

Mullin, B., Hardy, S., & Sutton, W. (2007). *Sport Marketing* (4th ed.). Champaign, IL: Human Kinetics.

Parks, J. B., Quarterman, J., & Thibault, L. (2011). Managing sport in the 21st century. In P. M. Pedersen, J. B. Parks, J. Quarterman, & L. Thibault (Eds.), *Contemporary sport management* (4th ed.) (pp. 4–27). Champaign, IL: Human Kinetics.

Pitts, B. G., & Stotlar, D. K. (2013). *Fundamentals of sport marketing* (4th ed.). Morgantown, WV: FIT.

Seifried, C. (2015). Tracing the history of sport management as a professional field and academic discipline. In M. T. Bowers & M. A. Dixon (eds.), *Sport management: An exploration of the field and its values* (pp. 17–38). Urbana, IL: Sagamore Publishing.

PART III

Integration of the Pillars

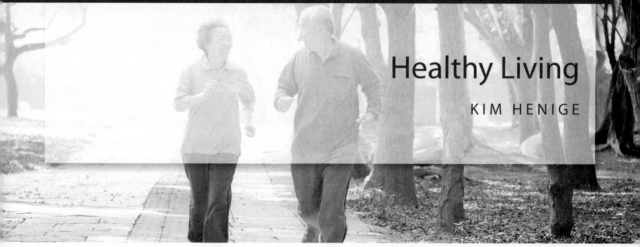

CHAPTER 13

Healthy Living

KIM HENIGE

LEARNING OBJECTIVES

1. Describe the importance of obtaining experience and applying course material to real-world scenarios.
2. List and describe the SMART components of good exercise goals.
3. List and explain the steps involved in beginning an exercise program.
4. Explain the transtheoretical model of behavior change and describe how it is used to motivate individuals participating in an exercise program.

KEY TERMS

aerobic capacity

blood pressure

body composition

bone density

cardiovascular disease

chronic health problems/
  chronic disease

diabetes

diastolic blood pressure

evidence-based principles

exercise prescription

flexibility

functional capacity

health-related components of
  physical fitness

hypertension

impact exercise

muscular endurance

muscular strength
obesity-related disease
osteoporosis
sedentary

stroke
systolic blood pressure
waist circumference
weight-bearing exercise

Case Study: Health and Wellness

sedentary
Participation in very little physical activity.

Lou and Sue are in their late 50s and, like most middle-aged Americans, are relatively **sedentary**. Other than performing household chores and yardwork and running the usual errands, the couple has made no special effort to be physically active in many years. Sue used to belong to a health club where she took step aerobics classes, but that was over 10 years ago. Lou played sports in high school and did some recreational running in his 20s and 30s, but has not done anything regularly since that time. As the years went by, both Lou and Sue made several failed attempts to become regularly active again. Each year when they saw their family physician for their physical exams, the doctor asked what they were doing for physical activity, and each year they told her they were getting ready to start a new workout program. That new workout program never began.

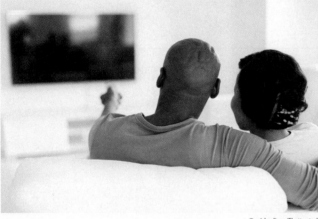

© michaeljung/Shutterstock

Sue works as an administrative assistant at a university, a job that requires her to sit most of the day. She occasionally walks across campus to deliver paperwork or attend meetings, but mostly stays within her building. Lou is a contractor who owns his own construction company. Like Sue, he spends a lot of time sitting at a desk or in meetings, but occasionally goes out in the field to walk job sites. Lou and Sue represent the typical American couple with sedentary jobs who have become increasingly sedentary in their free time as they got older. As a consequence of their inactivity, they are both about 30 pounds overweight, having each gained 1 to 2 pounds each year over the last 15 years. They have both begun to realize that they do not have the energy they used to have, and everyday activities such as climbing stairs and putting on their pants without leaning against a wall have become more difficult. They have three young grandchildren, and several times a year they like to take them to sporting events, amusement parks, and other places that require a significant amount of walking. Over the summer they took the kids to the local fair, and Sue felt herself getting winded trying to keep up.

In the last few years, Lou and Sue have had friends close to their age suffer heart attacks and strokes and

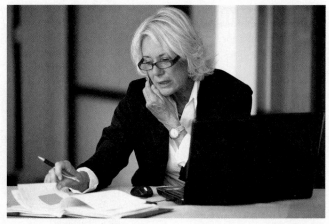

© Phovoir/Shutterstock

fall and break their hips. Lately when their friends get together, the conversation seems to go to their **chronic health problems**, stories of doctor visits, and complaints about the side effects of their medications. Realization that they are aging, which will likely cause a decline in their health and **functional capacity**, has increased their motivation to make healthy lifestyle changes, but they also worry about their ability to exercise safely. After so many years without exercising and images in the media of young, lean people sweating heavily in boot camp–style workouts, they wonder if they are now too old and unfit for exercise. In addition, Lou's father had a heart attack and died when he was 60 years old, and Sue's mother was diagnosed with **osteoporosis** in her early 60s. Mortality is becoming a reality, and they fear that one of them will be the next within their group to experience a major health event.

Sue's university has a kinesiology department where undergraduate students take a variety of courses related to fitness programming. Many of the courses include case study discussions and/or hands-on opportunities within teaching labs where they practice fitness assessment, **exercise prescription**, and exercise technique coaching on each other. Practicing skills on other students is helpful, but it does not expose them to the challenges often encountered when working with individuals in the real world. Some of the biggest challenges in fitness programming emerge when training people who have functional limitations or chronic health conditions and who are unfit, sedentary, overweight, unmotivated, inexperienced, and/or older. The typical kinesiology student is healthy, fit, active, experienced, and motivated to exercise. There is a large gap between the fitness level of the

chronic health problems/chronic disease
Health problems or diseases that begin gradually and last for an extended period of time.

functional capacity
A person's ability to participate in physical activity, including basic daily tasks.

osteoporosis
A disease in which bone density is reduced, increasing the risk of bone fracture.

exercise prescription
The details of an exercise program, including frequency, intensity, duration, and exercise mode.

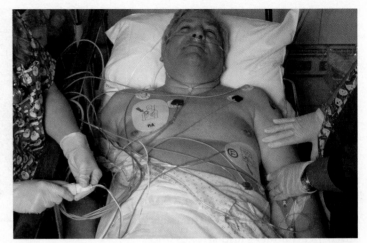

© Jones & Bartlett Learning

typical kinesiology student and the majority of people in society who need the most help. Unless students at this university have taken the initiative to find fitness-related jobs on their own, they graduate without ever gaining challenging, real-world experiences.

TWO COMMON PROBLEMS

Our case study presents two very common problems in American society. The first problem is that there is an aging couple who needs to lose weight, improve their functional capacity, and reduce their risk for chronic diseases such as cardiovascular disease and osteoporosis. On their own they have not been able to get motivated. They also have some fears about exercise, and they lack the knowledge needed to exercise safely and effectively on their own. The second problem is that at the university there are kinesiology students who need real-life, hands-on application and experience with exercise programming and administration.

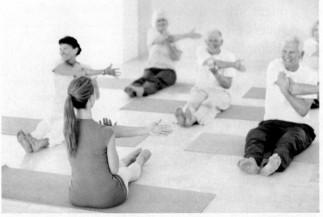

© kupicoo/Getty Images

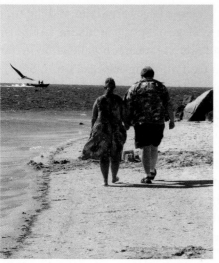

© Lisa F. Young/Shutterstock

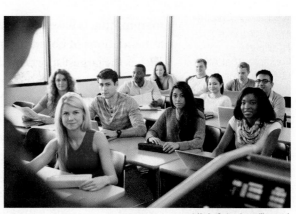

© Monkey Business Images/Shutterstock

A SOLUTION?

Over the summer, Sue received an email about a new staff and faculty fitness program on campus. The fitness program is led by students from the kinesiology department who work under the supervision of a kinesiology faculty member. Sue had heard of kinesiology, but was not quite sure what the students studied. After reading through the course catalog, Sue was surprised to learn that kinesiology students at the university study in a variety of areas, including dance, applied fitness, adapted physical activity, exercise science, athletic training, sport studies, and physical education. Sue contacted the kinesiology faculty member, Dr. Adams, who is in charge of the staff/faculty fitness program, and learned that it is led mostly by students within the applied fitness area. She was also told that the students are mostly seniors who have taken coursework in anatomy, physiology, biomechanics, exercise physiology, motor learning and control, motor development, exercise prescription, resistance training, group exercise training, injury prevention and treatment, exercise psychology, and more. Sue was especially pleased to find out that the exercise

STOP AND THINK

- What are the two common problems discussed in this section?

- How can departments of kinesiology help in solving these problems?

- Consider your parents, extended family, or older friends. Can you think of any individuals who might have similar issues or concerns as Lou and Sue? Can you think of any other issues or concerns that may be common with the middle-aged and/or older population?

- What types of real-life, hands-on experiences have you had with regard to applying your knowledge of kinesiology?

- What are some things you can do to find opportunities to gain these types of experiences?

evidence-based principles
Principles that have been developed based on sound and objective scientific research.

programming is based on integrated, **evidence-based principles** and the recommendations of both the American College of Sports Medicine (ACSM), which is the largest sports medicine and exercise science organization in the world, and the National Strength and Conditioning Association (NSCA), which is considered the worldwide authority on strength and conditioning. In her conversation with Dr. Adams, Sue also found out that each university employee is allowed to bring a guest. That evening Sue went home and told Lou about the program; they agreed that it was a good opportunity for them to receive the professional guidance and motivation they needed to begin exercising again. Although they were still a little apprehensive about whether they would fit into the program, they decided to give it a try.

STOP AND THINK

Take a few minutes and visit the ACSM website at *www.acsm.org*. Go to the "Student Corner" and access the many useful tools and resources available. Browse through the "Public Information" section to view the free educational resources. How do you think ACSM can benefit you as a student? As a fitness professional?

HEALTH EVALUATION

The first step when beginning a new exercise program is a *health evaluation* of the individual to make sure it is safe for him or her exercise and to determine whether there is a need for *physician clearance* before beginning the exercise program. A health questionnaire and **blood pressure** evaluation can determine whether the individual should see a physician for clearance before beginning a new exercise program. A simple and commonly used health questionnaire is the Physical Activity Readiness Questionnaire (PAR-Q; **FIGURE 13-1**).

blood pressure
The force of blood on the blood vessel walls.

systolic blood pressure
Pressure in the blood vessels while the heart is contracting and ejecting blood.

diastolic blood pressure
Pressure in the blood vessels when the heart is relaxed and refilling with blood.

Lou and Sue showed up on the first day of the program and are given paperwork to complete, including a liability waiver, the PAR-Q, and a general questionnaire. The general questionnaire addresses their past experience with physical activity, exercise preferences, goals, previous/current injuries, and limitations. Both Lou and Sue answered "no" to all of the questions on the PAR-Q form. If any question had been answered with a "yes," they would have been referred to their physician for clearance prior to beginning the exercise program. After completing the forms, a student obtained their blood pressure measurements. Sue's blood pressure was 110/80 mm Hg, a normal reading, but Lou's was high, 160/90 mm Hg. The top number is called the **systolic blood pressure**, and 140 mm Hg or above is considered high. The bottom number is called the **diastolic blood pressure**, and 90 mm Hg or above is considered high. It was an

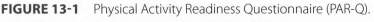

FIGURE 13-1   Physical Activity Readiness Questionnaire (PAR-Q).

Reproduced from Canadian Society for Exercise Physiology, PAR-Q & You: A Questionnaire for People Aged 15 to 69, CSEP, 2002.

exceptionally hot August day, and Lou had just walked across campus, which can temporarily increase blood pressure, so he was asked to sit and relax for 15 minutes and have his blood pressure rechecked. At the recheck his blood pressure was 150/90 mm Hg, lower than the first reading, but still elevated. Dr. Adams explained to Lou that his blood pressure was elevated and asked him if he had ever been told he had high blood pressure. Lou did not ever recall having a high reading and was troubled to hear he may have high blood pressure. Dr. Adams explained that blood pressure varies from day to day, and that it could just be an unusual and temporary occurrence for him. Lou was asked to come back the next day for a recheck. That night Lou and Sue went home and discussed the high reading. Although they knew they were not doing everything thing they could to live a healthy lifestyle, this was the first time either of them had been told they may have a major health condition. High blood pressure is referred to as **hypertension**, and it is a disease that affects over 80 million

> **STOP AND THINK**
>
> What is the PAR-Q? What is its purpose?

hypertension
High blood pressure; a chronic disease.

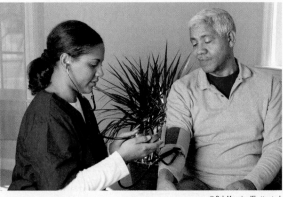
© Rob Marmion/Shutterstock

health-related components of physical fitness
The components of physical fitness that are associated with good physical health, including body composition, muscular strength, muscular endurance, aerobic capacity, and flexibility.

body composition
The proportion of total body weight made up of fat mass and fat-free mass.

muscular strength
The ability of skeletal muscles to generate force.

muscular endurance
The ability of skeletal muscles to generate force, repeatedly.

aerobic capacity
The ability to perform prolonged, large-muscle, dynamic exercise at moderate to high levels of intensity.

flexibility
The ability of the joints to move freely through their normal range of motion.

adults in the United States (American Heart Association, 2016). Hypertension does not have any symptoms, but it is associated with an increased risk for heart disease and stroke. Due to the fact that Lou's father died of heart disease, they were especially concerned.

PHYSICIAN CLEARANCE

The next day Lou went back for a recheck, and his blood pressure was, again, high. Due to the high reading, Lou was told he would need clearance from his physician before he could begin the exercise program. Lou called his physician the next day and made an appointment to talk to her about his blood pressure and the fitness program.

Before Lou saw his physician, he assumed that if his blood pressure was high, she would tell him that it was not safe for him to exercise. His blood pressure was indeed high, and the doctor started Lou on blood pressure medication. But to his surprise she cleared him for exercise and told him that if he exercised regularly and lost weight, he may be able to reduce his dosage or even come off of the medication someday.

FITNESS ASSESSMENT

Before beginning a fitness program, it is important to assess the individual's current body parameters and fitness level. Once the individual's current status is known, it can be used to identify weaknesses, create an individualized exercise prescription, and set measurable and attainable goals. Common *fitness assessments* include body weight, circumferences, and the **health-related components of physical fitness** (**body composition**, **muscular strength**, **muscular endurance**, **aerobic capacity**, and **flexibility**).

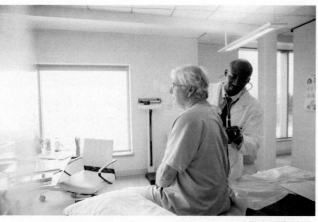

© Hero Images/Getty Images

The students measured Lou's and Sue's body weight, **waist circumference**, flexibility, muscular endurance, muscular strength, and aerobic capacity. These parameters were chosen because they are related to the physical concerns expressed by Lou and Sue, including cardiovascular disease and osteoporosis risk, and the ability to climb stairs, walk distances, and put on pants without leaning against a wall. As they were having their waist measurements taken, the student explained that waist circumference is a reliable predictor of **obesity-related disease**. Women with waists greater than 35 inches and men with waists greater than 40 inches are at a substantially increased risk for chronic diseases such as hypertension, **diabetes**, **cardiovascular disease**, and **stroke**. The sit-and-reach test was used to measure flexibility, the plank hold test was used to measure core muscular strength and endurance, the push-up test was used to measure upper body muscular strength and endurance, the 30-second chair stand test was used to measure lower body muscular strength and endurance, and the 1-mile walk test was used to measure aerobic capacity. After completing all of the testing, Lou and Sue each sat down for a consultation with one of the kinesiology students. During the consult, the student was able to help Lou and Sue create SMART goals for their exercise program (**TABLE 13-1**).

GOAL SETTING AND EXERCISE PRESCRIPTION

On the general questionnaire, both Lou and Sue expressed that they want to lose weight and be more physically fit. These are very common goals, but also very broad ones. Students in kinesiology learn about *goal setting* and

waist circumference
Measurement of waist size, usually in inches.

obesity-related disease
A disease for which obesity is a possible contributing risk factor.

diabetes
A disease in which blood sugar is high; a chronic disease.

cardiovascular disease
A disease of the heart and blood vessels, sometimes referred to as heart disease; a chronic disease.

stroke
Reduced blood flow to the brain that causes cell death; a chronic disease.

TABLE 13-1   SMART Goals for the Fall Semester (3 months)

Fitness Component	Lou	Sue
Body composition	Reduce waist circumference from 45 to 42 inches.	Reduce waist circumference from 38 to 35 inches.
Flexibility	Increase sit-and-reach distance from 7 to 9 inches.	Increase sit-and-reach distance from 13 to 15 inches.
Core muscular strength and endurance	Increase plank hold time from 30 seconds to 1 minute.	Increase plank hold time from 20 seconds to 1 minute.
Upper body muscular strength and endurance	Increase push-ups from 9 to 18 repetitions.	Increase push-ups from 4 to 12 repetitions.
Lower body muscular strength and endurance	Increase 30-second chair stand from 11 to 16 repetitions.	Increase 30-second chair stand from 10 to 15 repetitions.
Aerobic capacity	Increase 1-mile walk time from 15 to 12 minutes.	Increase 1-mile walk time from 20 to 15 minutes.

STOP AND THINK

• What is a physician clearance, and when is it necessary?

• Do you know anyone who has hypertension? If so, ask them if they know the benefits of exercise. Be sure to recommend that they see their physician for clearance before beginning a new exercise program.

• Search the Internet for free educational resources about hypertension and exercise. Once you find a resource, do you know how to judge its value? Not all online resources are reliable. Talk to your instructors or the librarians at your school for help in identifying reliable online resources.

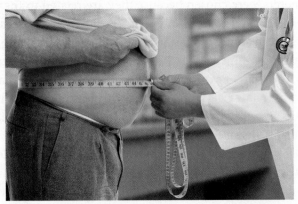
© kurhan/Shutterstock

how to help individuals write effective goals. A common guideline recommended for writing goals is to make them "SMART." SMART stands for specific, measurable, attainable, relevant, and time framed:

• *Specific*: The goal should not be general. For example, a general goal would be "to lose weight"; a more specific goal would be "to reduce waist circumference by

3 inches." Another general goal would be to "become more fit"; a specific goal would be to be able to "walk 1 mile within 15 minutes."

- *Measurable*: Measurable goals are clearly defined and usually quantifiable. There must be a clear way to determine whether the goal was attained, and this is one purpose of fitness assessment. If waist circumference is measured before beginning a program, then clear, specific, and easily measurable goals can be set. Waist circumference can be accurately measured with a measuring tape. If the goal is not specific, it is also not measurable. How would you measure whether someone had "become more fit"? Being "more fit" can mean many different things. Fitness has several components, including aerobic capacity, flexibility, muscular strength, muscular endurance, and body composition. It may take some questioning of the individual to determine how he or she interprets "more fit." It is useful to ask people if there is anything they cannot do now that they would like to be able to do, or if there is anything they struggle with that they would like to be able to do more easily. For example, Sue complained that she got winded when walking around the fair. The fitness professional should recognize that this is likely due to poor cardiorespiratory fitness, which can be easily measured with a timed distance test (e.g., 1-mile walk test). For each fitness component, multiple tests can be used to define one's current level and measure improvement.

- *Attainable*: Goals should be challenging, but also within the individual's physiological range (i.e., physical limits). Whether a goal is attainable is sometimes difficult to judge, and therefore some trial and error may be needed before an individual's attainable range is known. Not all goals are attainable. For example, depending on a person's body type, a 25-inch waist may be impossible; similarly, depending on one's genetic potential, a 5-minute mile may not be an attainable goal. Goals also need to be attainable within the time frame set for achievement of the goal.

- *Relevant*: The goal should be important and meaningful to the individual. For example, if a woman is told that a waist circumference

STOP AND THINK

- What is the purpose of assessing body parameters and fitness components?

- What are the common types of fitness assessment?

- What are the health-related components of physical fitness?

greater than 35 inches is associated with an increased risk for many chronic diseases, waist circumference becomes relevant to the individual (assuming she wants to prevent chronic disease). Another example of relevance relates to what an individual enjoys. If someone wants to improve aerobic capacity but does not like to run, setting a 5K race goal would not be relevant, and therefore not advised. Aerobic capacity can be improved in a number of different ways. It takes just a few questions to learn what an individual likes and does not like. If a man enjoys hiking, this "relevant" activity should be worked into his goal. Remember, the purpose of a SMART goal is to increase the chances that it will be achieved.

- *Time framed*: A specific goal date needs to be set on which the individual will be tested or checked to determine if the goal has been achieved. A good time frame is between 6 weeks and 3 months, because this provides enough time for physiological improvements to be made, but is not so long that the individual loses motivation. Regular feedback about progress is important when trying to maintain the motivation to continue. If large improvements are desired, a long-term goal can be set that can then be divided into short-term goals to measure progress toward the larger goal.

Successful goal attainment is partly due to the construction of the original goal. SMART goals provide a means for the fitness professional to design an exercise program that will best target the individual's desired results. Goals also promote motivation and provide the means for measuring success.

In summary, before they began the exercise program, Lou and Sue were taken through the standard phases of implementing a new exercise program: (1) they were screened for their health status to determine the safety of exercise and the need for physician clearance; (2) they were assessed to determine their current level of physical fitness, and (3) they set SMART goals. Kinesiology students learn about these steps in their coursework, but do not always have the opportunity to implement them in a real-world setting.

The next step in this process is to create a detailed *exercise prescription*. After talking to Lou and Sue about their goals and time availability, and also considering ACSM's exercise prescription guidelines, the plan for the semester was created. ACSM's exercise prescription guidelines have been developed over many years and are based on evidence-based principles.

THE FITNESS PROGRAM

Once the health evaluation, fitness assessment, goal setting, and exercise prescription have been completed, it is time to implement the program. Lou and Sue attended the *fitness program* regularly and learned a lot along the way. One day, the cardio portion seemed to include a lot of jumping, and Sue chose the modifications offered that eliminated all jumping. When a group exercise program is implemented, students need to present various options and modifications so that all participants are challenged equally. In a large group, there will be people with a variety of fitness levels and also a variety of limitations. One of the students, Carlos, noticed that Sue did not do any jumping. Carlos consulted with Sue's health and general questionnaires and saw that she did not list any previous injuries or limitations. During the cool down, Carlos stood next to Sue so he could talk to her before she left. When the cooldown ended, he asked her why she did not do any of the jumping, and she said she does not like to jump and also told him that she is a little afraid of the impact of jumping due to her mother's history with osteoporosis and a broken hip. Carlos remembered learning about the benefits of **weight-bearing** and **impact exercise** on **bone density** and was excited that he was going to be able to apply this knowledge for the first time. Carlos explained to Sue that bone density declines with age, but that some impact helps to slow the rate of loss because the body responds to stress by becoming stronger. He encouraged her to do a little bit of the lower-intensity jumping, but to pay careful attention to her body during and after the jumping to make sure she does not overdo it. She agreed to give it a try. When Sue left, Carlos told Dr. Adams what had happened and was pleased to report that he had applied information he had learned in class

STOP AND THINK

- What is the purpose of setting goals when beginning an exercise program?

- List and describe each component of a SMART goal.

- Write a goal you have for something you would like to enhance or improve about your personal fitness, and then evaluate how well it fits the SMART goal framework. If it does not completely fit the SMART goal framework, revise your goal so that it does.

- What is an exercise prescription?

- What does it mean to be an evidence-based principle?

---

weight-bearing exercise
Physical activity that requires an individual to support their body weight.

---

impact exercise
Physical activity that places stress on the bones.

---

bone density
The amount of bone tissue within the bones.

TABLE 13-2   Transtheoretical Model of Behavior Change Applied to Physical Activity

Stage	Description	Example Strategies
Precontemplation	• No intention to increase physical activity. • Unaware or ignorant of what inactivity is or the problems associated with inactivity.	• Raise awareness about the problems associated with inactivity by explaining the consequences and encouraging them to learn more on their own. • Raise awareness about the benefits of physical activity.
Contemplation	• Recognizes the need to become more physically active. • Thinking about increasing activity level, but not yet ready.	• Identify the barriers to becoming more physically active and strategies to overcome them.
Preparation	• Ready to increase physical activity soon (within the month). • May have already become more physically active.	• Develop a formal plan to increase physical activity. • Create an activity log to keep track of physical activity. • Create rewards for meeting goals.
Action	• Has become regularly physically active.	• Monitor progress toward short-term goals. • Identify potential obstacles that may interfere with the physical activity program and plan for them (e.g., plan for physical activity while on vacation). • Set a goal for an upcoming event, such as a 5K walk/run.
Maintenance	• Has been physically active regularly for at least 6 months.	• Be a role model and mentor to someone who would like to become more physically active.

Modified from J. O. Prochaska, C. C. DiClemente, & J. C. Norcross. (1992). In search of how people change: Applications to addictive behaviors. *American Psychologist, 47*(9), 1102–1114.

about exercise, bone density, and aging. Carlos also told Dr. Adams that he implemented the transtheoretical model that he had learned about in his exercise/sport psychology course. Dr. Adams was thrilled and asked Carlos to explain.

The transtheoretical model is a model of behavior change that states that individuals have different levels of motivational readiness when it comes to behavior change (**TABLE 13-2**). The model has five stages of change, and knowledge of an individual's current stage with regard to fitness can help fitness professionals identify the best strategies for promoting physical activity participation (Fahey, Insel, & Roth, 2014; Pekmezi, Barbera, & Marcus, 2010). The first stage of the model is precontemplation. People in the precontemplation stage do not recognize the need for a change, and therefore have no plan to change. These individuals feel that their current behavior is fine and does not need to be modified. Carlos realized that Sue was not aware of the value of jumping, especially as it relates to her, personally. As a result, Sue skipped the jumping portions of the exercise program, and probably would have continued to do so forever. Carlos remembered from his class that one way to move someone out of precontemplation and closer to behavior change is to raise his or her awareness. By telling Sue of the benefits of some impact and linking it to her fear of osteoporosis, and thus making it more relevant to her, he increased the chances that

STOP AND THINK

- Briefly explain the transtheoretical model of behavior change.

- How can fitness professionals use the transtheoretical model of behavior change?

- Search the Internet for free educational resources about exercise and bone health. Again, be careful to assess the reliability of each resource.

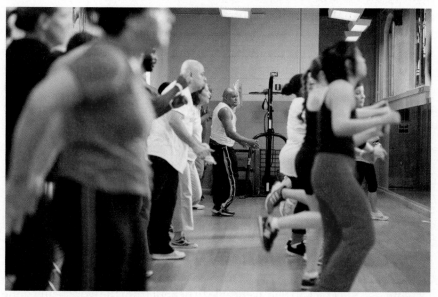

© Richard Levine / Alamy Stock Photo

Sue will add in some jumping, and therefore gain additional benefits from the exercise program. The next week, Carlos noticed Sue trying out some of the jumping exercises and watched her carefully to make sure she did not do too much. He talked to her after class and she said that it felt good and that she actually enjoyed it.

POST-ASSESSMENT, REEVALUATION, AND REVISION

At the end of the semester, Lou and Sue participated in a *post-assessment* during which all of their measurements were retaken. Post-assessment is essential because it provides information about the participant's progress toward the predetermined goals. If goals are not met, *reevaluation* of the fitness program and goals are necessary to try to determine why the goals were not met and then to *revise* the program and goals, as necessary, to promote future success. Once again, Lou and Sue each sat with one of the kinesiology students to discuss their progress and possibly reevaluate their goals. Both of them had reached most of their goals, but fell short on others. In the one-on-one meetings, the students reviewed their attendance records, exercise logs, goals, and test results to try to identify the reasons some of the goals were not met. They realized that some of the goals were not attainable, given the time frame. Together, Lou and Sue wrote a new set of goals, and the students developed a revised exercise plan for the next 3-month period. This timely feedback and reevaluation of goals is important to keep participants motivated and to prevent them from getting discouraged. Lou and Sue were able to experience some successes, reach some goals, but also learn that some of their initial expectations were too high.

Through the process described in this case study, kinesiology students were able to apply the principles of goal setting, motivation, and exercise prescription they had read in books and discussed in class. In doing so, they were able to experience the initiation of a new exercise program in the real world (**TABLE 13-3**) and gain even more knowledge from the process. At the same time, an older couple, Lou and Sue, were able to benefit from the work being done by the students.

STOP AND THINK

- What is a post-assessment, and why is it important?
- What conditions during post-assessment indicate a need to reevaluate the fitness program?
- What conditions during post-assessment indicate a need to revise goals?

TABLE 13-3   Steps to Beginning an Exercise Program

Step*	Description
Health evaluation	The participant completes a health questionnaire, such as the PAR-Q, and his or her blood pressure is taken. The health evaluation is used to determine whether exercise is safe for the individual and whether there is a need for physician clearance prior to beginning an exercise program.
Physician clearance	If health risks are identified during the health evaluation, the individual must visit his or her physician to determine whether he or she has any exercise limitations. The physician documents any limitations and provides the documentation to the fitness professional. This must be completed before any physical activity is performed, including testing.
Fitness assessment	Measurement of body parameters and fitness levels, including the health-related physical fitness components. Information gathered in the assessment is used to create an appropriate exercise prescription and to set measureable goals.
Goal setting and exercise prescription	The creation of SMART goals prior to beginning an exercise program helps guide the fitness professional in writing an effective exercise prescription to promote motivation and success.
Fitness program	Created by the fitness professional through exercise prescription and followed by the participant. The program is designed specifically to work toward achieving the predetermined goals.
Post-assessment	Retest the same body parameters and fitness levels measured prior to beginning the exercise program.
Reevaluation and revision	Information gathered from the post-assessment is used to evaluate whether the predetermined goals were met. Based on the evaluation, the fitness professional revises the goals and/or exercise program, as necessary, to promote future success.

*These steps are noted in *italics* throughout the chapter.

CHAPTER SUMMARY

Through the use of a realistic case study, you have learned about the positive implications of experience and application of your kinesiology course material. You have learned about the steps involved when an individual begins an exercise program. In the process of designing a safe and effective program, health screening, fitness assessment, and goal setting are essential. The SMART goal guidelines can be used to systematically create goals with the greatest chance for successful achievement and continued motivation. You learned the importance of periodic post-assessment, reevaluation, and revision of fitness goals and programming to ensure optimal participant success. You also learned about the transtheoretical model of behavior change, which can be used to help motivate individuals participating in an exercise program.

DISCUSSION QUESTIONS

1. Describe specific instances in your academic career (including high school) in which you had the opportunity to apply course material in real-world settings. What do you think were some of the benefits of those experiences?
2. Explain specific instances in your academic career (including high school) in which you did not have the opportunity to apply course material in real-world settings, but would like to have. What do you think were some of the disadvantages of not having those experiences?
3. What are the essential steps, in order, that should be followed when beginning an exercise program? Explain the elements and purpose of each step. For each step, what are some of the possible negative consequences if it is not completed?
4. How do the SMART components of good exercise goals promote positive experiences with physical activity?
5. If experience and application are not provided to you within your courses, what can you do on your own to get them?

REFERENCES

American Heart Association. (2016). About high blood pressure. Retrieved from http://www.heart.org/HEARTORG/Conditions/HighBloodPressure/AboutHighBloodPressure/About-High-Blood-Pressure_UCM_002050_Article.jsp#.V3pniKKfWCg

Fahey, T. D., Insel, P. M., & Roth, W. T. (2014). *Fit and well, brief edition: Core concepts and labs in physical fitness and wellness* (11th ed.). New York: McGraw Hill.

Pekmezi, D., Barbera, B., & Marcus, B. H. (2010). Using the transtheoretical model to promote physical activity. *ACSM's Health and Fitness Journal, 14*(4), 8–13.

Prochaska, J. O., DiClemente, C. C., & Norcross, J. C. (1992). In search of how people change: Applications to addictive behaviors. *American Psychologist, 47*(9), 1102–1114.

CHAPTER 14

Restoring Function

BELINDA STILLWELL

LEARNING OBJECTIVES

1. Describe the school and community services that are available to assist individuals with disabilities.

2. Identify the legislation associated with services to assist individuals with disabilities.

3. Explain the differences between adapted physical activity (APA) and adapted physical education (APE).

4. Identify career possibilities that involve working with individuals with disabilities.

KEY TERMS

adapted physical activity (APA)
adapted physical education (APE)
added authorization
allied health professional
American Physical Therapy Association (APTA)
Americans with Disabilities Act (ADA)
Article 30
case study evaluation (CSE)

Commission on Teacher Credentialing (CTC)
due process
free, appropriate public education (FAPE)
Individualized Education Program (IEP)
Individuals with Disabilities Education Act (IDEA)
Institute of Medicine (IOM)

International Federation of Adapted
   Physical Activity (IFAPA)
least restrictive environment (LRE)
major life activities
multidisciplinary conference (MDC)
Public Law 94-142

reasonable accommodation
Section 504 of the Rehabilitation Act
   of 1973
teaching credential
traumatic brain injury (TBI)

traumatic brain injury (TBI)
Brain dysfunction caused by an external mechanical force; usually results from a violent blow or jolt to the head or body.

case study evaluation (CSE)
An evaluation to assess an individual's current abilities to determine if he or she qualifies for special education services.

multidisciplinary conference (MDC)
The follow-up meeting after a school district has completed a case study evaluation of a child. The purpose of the meeting is to inform the parents of the results of the school's evaluation and the multidisciplinary team's recommendations.

Case Study: Care for Restoring Healthy Balance

It was June, and Mia had just finished sixth grade. She was looking forward to attending the new middle school in her neighborhood in the fall, but over summer break, she was excited about spending time with her friends at the pool. On a hot mid-July day, as Mia was practicing her forward dive, she slipped and hit her head on the diving board. Lifeguards rescued Mia, and she was transported to the hospital for care. After she was treated and stabilized, doctors told her parents that the **traumatic brain injury (TBI)** Mia sustained had affected her memory and balance. Mia received the appropriate medical follow-up over the remainder of the summer and was able to return to school in the fall. The case study in this chapter will demonstrate how kinesiologists and other allied health professionals can play a vital role in helping restore Mia's memory and balance over a lifetime of care and physical activity.

Upon arrival at her new school in the fall, Mia's parents gave the school written consent to assess Mia's current abilities via a **case study evaluation (CSE)** to see if she qualified for special education services. The school district had 60 days from the day of the request to complete the CSE and conduct a **multidisciplinary conference (MDC)**. Before this evaluation could take place or any services could be provided, Mia was required to complete a hearing and vision test to rule out any hearing or vision problems. The CSE included a series of steps: (1) a meeting with Mia; (2) a meeting with Mia's parents (guardians or surrogate parents); (3) a social development study; (4) a review of Mia's medical history; (5) a report on Mia's vision and hearing screenings; (6) an evaluation of school performance, including observations of Mia in her learning environment; (7) achievement testing; (8) cognitive testing (e.g., IQ tests, memory assessments); and (9) other specialized tests as needed, such as psychological evaluations, speech/language assessments, learning disability assessments, or a social work report (The Council for Disability Rights, n.d.).

The MDC was attended by anyone who had a vested interest in Mia's health and well-being. This included Mia (if appropriate), Mia's parents, Mia's teacher, a school district representative, the director of special education, anyone involved in testing Mia, service providers (e.g., doctor, physical therapist, social worker), school personnel familiar with Mia, others who had information to share about Mia, attorney or nonattorney advocates, or any other person providing support or making observations. At the conference, Mia's test results were presented, her problems and needs were described, and recommendations were made as to whether Mia was in need of special education services. The school then wrote a multidisciplinary summary report listing Mia's test results and special education services for which she was eligible. Any disagreements about the report's recommendations were documented, and a copy of the report was provided to Mia's parents (The Council on Disability Rights, n.d.). If Mia's parents disagreed with the conclusions of the MDC regarding her needs, they would submit a written request to the school district superintendent for an independent educational review.

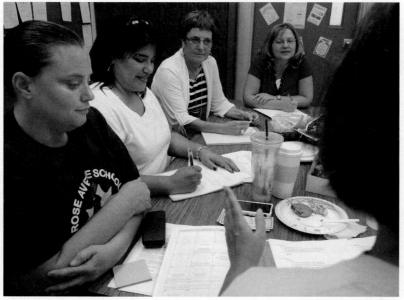

© ZUMA Press Inc / Alamy Stock Photo

Section 504 of the Rehabilitation Act of 1973
Civil rights law that prohibits discrimination against individuals with disabilities and ensures that children with disabilities have equal access to an education.

free, appropriate public education (FAPE)
Right of children with disabilities to have access to education, as guaranteed by the Rehabilitation Act of 1973 and the Individuals with Disabilities Education Act (IDEA).

reasonable accommodation
A school is required to take reasonable steps to accommodate a student with a disability unless it would cause the school undue hardship.

major life activities
Functions such as caring for one's self, performing manual tasks, walking, seeing, hearing, speaking, breathing, learning, and working.

KEY LEGISLATION

Regardless of whether a child with a disability is eligible for special education services, **Section 504 of the Rehabilitation Act of 1973** prohibits public schools from discriminating against students with disabilities and imposes an affirmative duty on schools to provide protections and reasonable accommodations to ensure access to a **free, appropriate public education (FAPE)** (The Council on Disability Rights, n.d.). For example, if the basketball coach cut Mia from the team simply because he did not want to be bothered by having a player on the team who had a disability, Section 504 would offer Mia protection against such unjust treatment. Similarly, a **reasonable accommodation** might be to provide a headset to muffle classroom noise Mia may experience during a math test. Section 504 defines a *disability* as "physical or mental impairments which substantially limit one or more major life activities. **Major life activities** include such functions as caring for one's self, performing manual tasks, walking, seeing, hearing, speaking, breathing, learning, and working" (The Council on Disability Rights, n.d.). Even though Section 504 does not provide funding to school districts for special education or related services beyond protections and accommodations, the

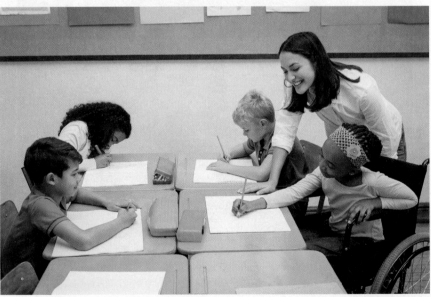

© wavebreakmedia/Shutterstock

Individuals with Disabilities Education Act (IDEA) provides financial support for specific disabilities, as defined by this law.

According to IDEA, a school district can receive federal and state funding for services provided for a child if that child is determined to have one or more of the following disabilities: autism; chronic or acute health condition; cognitive impairment; emotional/behavioral disorder; hearing/visual impairment; learning disability; orthopedic/health impairment; speech/language impairment; TBI; or visual impairment. IDEA has four distinct sections that are labeled A, B, C, and D. Part B of IDEA establishes the educational guidelines for schoolchildren 3 to 21 years of age. IDEA funds school districts that comply with the following six principles (American Psychological Association, 2013):

1. Every child is entitled to a FAPE.
2. When a school professional believes that a student between the ages of 3 and 21 years of age may have a disability that has a substantial impact on the student's learning or behavior, the student is entitled to an evaluation in all areas related to the suspected disability.
3. Each child identified as having a disability is entitled to an **Individualized Education Program (IEP)**. The purpose of the IEP is to lay out a series of specific actions and steps through which educators, parents, and the student may reach the child's stated goals.
4. A quality education and services for children with disabilities must be provided in the **least restrictive environment**, and those children should be placed in a "traditional" educational setting with students without disabilities.
5. The input of the child and the parents must be taken into account in the education process.
6. When parents feel that an IEP is inappropriate for their child or that their child is not receiving needed services, they have the right under IDEA to challenge their child's treatment through **due process**.

After Mia's evaluation was completed, it was determined that she qualified for special education and related services (**TABLE 14-1**). Her parents agreed with the results of the evaluation, and an IEP was created for Mia by a team of school personnel and Mia's parents. The IEP has two general purposes: (1) to establish annual goals for the child and (2) to state the special

Individuals with Disabilities Education Act (IDEA)
Federal law that outlines the rights and regulations for students with disabilities in the United States who require special education.

Individualized Education Program (IEP)
A legal document that defines a child's special education plan.

least restrictive environment (LRE)
A student who has a disability should have the opportunity to be educated with peers without disabilities, to the greatest extent appropriate.

due process
The legal requirement that the state must respect all legal rights that are owed to a person.

TABLE 14-1 Examples of Related Services

Service Area	Examples
Audiology	Provision of audiometric testing; recommendations for amplification systems; hearing aid orientations; habilitative activities (e.g., language habilitation, auditory training, speech reading, hearing conservation); and counseling and guidance of children, teachers, and staff regarding hearing loss.
Braillist/reader	Aides for students with visual disabilities who augment the educational program (e.g., reading/taping materials, brailling, or thermoforming material.
Counseling services	School guidance counselors, social workers, or psychologists who provide guidance directly in small groups or individual sessions through consultation with teachers or through crisis intervention.
Adapted driver education	Specially designed course to teach students with a disability to operate a car.
Adaptive technology	Specially designed devices or processes that enable a student with a disability to perform tasks more independently.
Interpreter	Specially trained individual who either interprets or translates.
Occupational therapy	Services designed to improve, develop, or restore functions impaired or lost through illness, injury, or deprivation; improving ability to perform tasks for independent functioning; or to prevent, through early intervention, initial or further impairment or loss of function.
Orientation and mobility	Services provided to a child with a visual disability designed to increase perception and mobility within his or her environments, with the goal of independent movement and living.
Parent counseling and training	Provision of assistance to parents in understanding and managing the special needs of their child and providing parents with information about child development.
Physical therapy	Services recommended and prescribed by a licensed medical examiner as necessary for students to benefit from an education.
Recreation	Activities that are therapeutic to accomplish behavioral or cognitive goals and objectives or that develop the constructive use of leisure time.
Rehabilitative counseling	Services focused specifically on career development, employment preparation, achieving independence, and integration in the workplace and community.
School health services	Administration of medication necessary to maintain the student during school hours.
Social work	Addressing problems in a student's living situation that affect his or her adjustment in school and mobilizing school and community resources to enable him or her to receive maximum benefit from his or her educational program.
Speech and language	Habilitation or prevention of communicative disorders.
Transportation	Services different from those normally provided that are required due to a student's disability.

Modified from The Council for Disability Rights (n.d.). A parent's guide to special ed/special needs. Retrieved from http://www.disabilityrights.org/appendix.htm

education and related services, as well as supplementary aids and services, that the public agency will provide to, or on behalf of, the child (Center for Parent Information and Resources, 2010). When the team wrote the IEP, they considered three main areas of school life: the general education curriculum (e.g., math, science), extracurricular activities, and nonacademic activities (e.g., school newspaper, school sports) (**TABLE 14-2**). One of the educational services that Mia received was **adapted physical education (APE)** until she was able to safely and/or successfully participate in general physical education without supplementary aids and services.

Extra IEP Content for Youth with Disabilities

For students approaching the end of their secondary school education, the IEP must also include statements about what are called *transition services*, which are designed to help youth with disabilities prepare for life after high school.

adapted physical education (APE) Physical education that has been adapted and/or modified so it is appropriate for children and youth with disabilities. This service is federally mandated for all students with disabilities. It includes physical fitness, fundamental motor skills and patterns, and individual and group games and sports, and may also cover aquatics and dance.

THIS IEP INCLUDES:			
Transition	☐		
Interm Service Plan	☒		

JAKE COUNTY
DEPARTMENT OF EDUCATION
INDIVIDUALIZED EDUCATION PROGRAM

CONFERENCE INFORMATION
Case #: __10-111111__
District: __10__
SID #: __1234567__
Date: __03/11/2013__
Type: __Annual Review__
Page: __1__

PERSONAL INFORMATION

STUDENT INFORMATION
Name: __John M. Smith__   ID #: __1234567__   DOB: __06/13/2004__   Gender: __M__
Address: __1234 Street Lane__   Age: __9__
Phone: __(123) 456-7890__   Languages/Mode of Communication: __English__   Grade: __2__
Primary Agency: __Jake County Schools__   School: __Gold Elementary School__

PARENT/GUARDIAN INFORMATION
Name: __Joan Smith__   Relationshipt to student: __Mother__
Address: __Same as above__
Phone (Home): __Same as above__   Phone (Work): __(123) 876-5432__
Languages/Mode of Communication: __English__   Interpreter Required? __No__

SPECIAL MEDICAL/PHYSICAL ALERTS
Mark all that apply: The student has: ☒ medical conditions and/or ☐ physical limitations which affect his/her
☐ learning ☒ behavior and/or ☐ participation in school activities
Mark all that apply: The student requires: ☒ medication and/or ☐ health care treatment(s) or procedure(s)
Other alerts? __Seasonal allergies - asthma__

TABLE 14-2   Contents of an IEP

A statement of the child's *present levels of academic achievement and functional performance*, including how the child's disability affects his or her involvement and progress in the general education curriculum;
A statement of measurable *annual goals*, including academic and functional goals;
A description of how the *child's progress* toward meeting the annual goals will be measured and when periodic progress reports will be provided;
A statement of the *special education and related services* and *supplementary aids and services* to be provided to the child or on behalf of the child;
A statement of the *program modifications or supports for school personnel* that will enable the child to advance appropriately toward attaining the annual goals, to make progress in the general education curriculum, to participate in extracurricular and other nonacademic activities, and to participate with other children with disabilities and children without disabilities;
An explanation of the *extent, if any, to which the child will not participate with children without disabilities* in the regular class and in extracurricular and nonacademic activities;
A statement of any *individual accommodations* that are necessary to measure the academic achievement and functional performance of the child on state and district-wide assessments;
The *projected date* for the beginning of the services and modifications and the anticipated *frequency, location, and duration* of those services and modifications.

Modified from Center for Parent Information and Resources. (2010). Contents of the IEP. Retrieved from http://www.parentcenterhub.org/repository/iepcontents/

IDEA requires that the first IEP be in effect when the child turns 16—or younger if determined by the IEP team—and it must include:

- Measurable *postsecondary goals* based upon age-appropriate transition assessments related to training, education, employment, and, where appropriate, independent living skills; and
- The transition services (including courses of study) needed to assist the child in reaching those goals.

Also, beginning no later than 1 year before the child reaches the age of majority under state law, the IEP must include:

- A statement that the child has been informed of the child's rights under Part B of IDEA (if any) that will transfer to the child on reaching the *age of majority*.

STOP AND THINK

What do you think school life would be like for children with disabilities if Section 504 of the Rehabilitation Act and the Individuals with Disabilities Education Act (IDEA) did not exist?

TABLE 14-3   Important Federal Laws Supporting Individuals with Disabilities

Year	Act	Importance
1968	Elimination of Architectural Barriers Act (Public Law 90-170)	Initial effort to ensure that particular federally funded buildings are accessible to persons with disabilities.
1973	Rehabilitation Act (Public Law 93-112)	Prohibited discrimination on the basis of disability.
1975	Education of All Handicapped Children Act (Public Law 94-142)	Mandated a free, appropriate education for all children and youths with disabilities, specifically including physical education.
1978	Amateur Sports Act (Public Law 95-606)	Recognized athletes with disabilities as part of the U.S. Olympic movement.
1990	Individuals with Disabilities Education Act (IDEA; Public Law 101-476)	Extended provisions of previous laws to young children.
1990	Americans with Disabilities Act (ADA)	Extended the broad protections of the Civil Rights Act of 1964 to people with disabilities.

Modified from DePauw (1996), as reported in D. Siedentop & H. van der Mars. (2012). *Introduction to physical education, fitness, and sport* (8th ed.). New York: McGraw-Hill.

ADAPTED PHYSICAL EDUCATION

APE is physical education for students with disabilities. It began as corrective physical education in the 1920s to meet the needs of children who had been paralyzed in the 1915–1917 polio epidemic and were now ready to attend school (Sherrill, 2004, as reported in Siedentop & van der Mars, 2012). As a result of legislative efforts from 1968 to 2004, APE flourished (DePauw, 1996, as reported in Siedentop and van der Mars, 2012). A summary of these laws is provided in **TABLE 14-3**. A key piece of legislation was the Education for All Handicapped Children Act of 1975, or **Public Law 94-142**. This act recognized physical education as a direct service and made specifically designed physical education programs available to all children with disabilities receiving a FAPE. IDEA is the reauthorization of Public Law 94-142, and it continues to emphasize FAPE, IEPs, LRE, and physical education as direct educational services.

Public Law 94-142
The Education for All Handicapped Children Act of 1975, which guarantees a free, appropriate public education to children with disabilities.

STOP AND THINK

Discuss how the traditional game of basketball could be modified for students in an APE class who are blind. Consider how the equipment, number of players, and rules could be adapted for student success.

BECOMING AN ADAPTED PHYSICAL EDUCATOR

teaching credential
A state-issued license to teach in public schools.

Students who are interested in becoming an adapted physical educator complete an undergraduate degree in kinesiology with an emphasis in sport pedagogy. This emphasis area might also be called a physical education teacher education (PETE) program. After successfully finishing the 4-year degree, students may qualify to enter a credential program to complete the necessary requirements for earning a teaching credential (license). A **teaching credential** in this area allows an individual to teach general physical education classes in kindergarten through 12th grade (K–12) public schools. (A credential is not ordinarily required to work in a private school setting.) Some institutions offer blended programs in which students can obtain both their undergraduate degree and teaching credential at the same time. This curriculum typically involves an additional semester of work. Blended programs also exist at the master's level at certain colleges and universities. Like the undergraduate blended program, a student at the graduate level can obtain both a master's degree and teaching credential simultaneously.

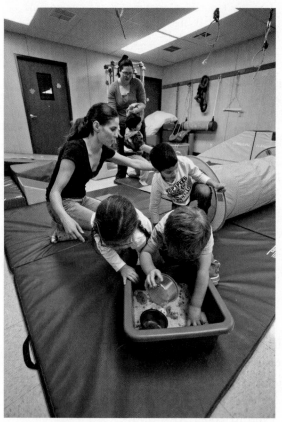

© Marmaduke St. John / Alamy Stock Photo

After receiving a credential, students can add other authorizations (subjects) to their existing credential to expand their teaching capabilities. Examples of these **added authorizations** are APE, music, math, and health science. To learn about coursework or other requirements in your state, contact your state's **Commission on Teacher Credentialing (CTC)** as well as the college or university you attend (Commission on Teacher Credentialing, 2010). One of the most common authorizations physical educators add to their existing credential is APE.

added authorization
Additional subjects that can be added to an existing teaching credential.

Commission on Teacher Credentialing (CTC)
State agency that regulates the issuance of teaching credentials to those who qualify.

Adding APE to an existing physical education credential is generally a smooth process because a physical educator's background is strongly supported by the subdisciplines in kinesiology (**TABLE 14-4**). Credential

TABLE 14-4   Sample Undergraduate Program in Kinesiology/Sport Pedagogy

Lower-Division Prerequisite Science and Math Courses

General Biology and Lab

Human Anatomy and Lab

Human Physiology and Lab

Introductory Statistics

Lower-Division Kinesiology Core Courses

Foundations of Kinesiology

Movement Forms: Dance, Sport, and Exercise and Lab

Upper-Division Kinesiology Core Courses

Foundations and Analysis of Human Movement

Historical and Philosophical Bases of Kinesiology

Sociopsychological Aspects of Physical Activity

Motor Behavior and Lab

Biomechanics and Lab

Physiology of Exercise and Lab

Physical Education Teacher Education (PETE) Option

Lower-Division Required Courses

Martial Arts

Basic Dance

Swimming

Fundamental Movement, Gymnastics, and Rhythms and Lab

Nontraditional Games and Activities and Lab

Analysis and Application of Games/Sports and Lab

Upper-Division Required Courses

Advanced Analysis of Dance Forms

Motor Development and Lab

Health-Related Fitness for K–12 and Lab

Introduction to Adapted Physical Education and Lab

Physical Education Content Development for Children and Lab

Physical Education Content Development for Adolescents and Lab

Learner Assessment and Technology in K–12 Physical Education and Lab

Note: Check with your university for additional requirements for becoming an adapted physical educator.

holders from other disciplines (e.g., music, English) often need to enroll in additional kinesiology coursework if they lack experience and knowledge in the movement sciences and sport humanities or pass a subject matter exam(s). Once you become an adapted physical educator, you will work with many other professionals in allied health fields to assist students with disabilities.

STOP AND THINK

Investigate institutions that offer APE programs. Find out what coursework, well as any necessary fieldwork experiences, you would need to complete in order to become an adapted physical educator.

In Mia's case, you would be part of the team that implements and reviews her IEP on an annual basis. As the adapted physical educator, you would work closely with other professionals identified within her circle of care. These individuals could be her occupational therapist, school counselor, physical therapist, or classroom teacher; they all share a common foundation of knowledge but bring a particular area of specialty to the IEP. For example, each of these professionals would have a basic understanding of psychological concepts and principles, but the school counselor would be one of the specialists in this area. Similarly, everyone would be aware of the importance of physical activity, but you, as the adapted physical educator, would be considered the expert in this area. Collectively, the whole team is instrumental in assisting Mia and her family in the restoration process.

As a result of the extensive planning, implementation, and assessment process Mia received throughout her secondary school years (grades 7–12), her memory and balance improved greatly. She was able to return to general physical education by the time she reached high school but still needed assistance in the classroom with her memory capabilities. In addition to her progress with the general education curriculum, Mia successfully participated on the yearbook staff, became a member of the art club, and volunteered at a community animal shelter during the summer months. She also learned how to operate a car in the adapted driver education course she took as a junior in high school. With the continued help of her occupational therapist, school counselor, and classroom teachers, Mia was able to graduate from high school with her peers. She was now ready to pursue the transition plan that was created for her just before she turned 16 years old. Embedded in this plan was her desire to attend art school full time while working part time in an art gallery and participating in leisure activities.

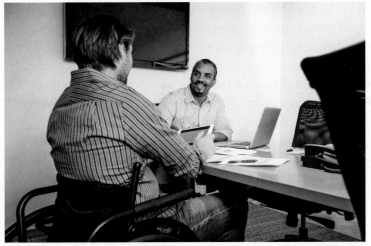

These new goals brought together a revised team of professionals that included a rehabilitative counselor, a social worker, and a recreational therapist, as well as the occupational therapist Mia had worked with throughout her secondary school career. Mia's rehabilitative counselor focused on preparing a career development plan with her to ensure progress toward an entry-level job in the art world upon graduation. Her social worker made certain she took advantage of the university resources available to her throughout her art degree program. The occupational therapist continued working with her to improve her memory skills by using assistive technology, and the recreational therapist introduced Mia to a cycling club in her community.

ADAPTED PHYSICAL ACTIVITY

After Mia completed her art degree, she looked forward to an upcoming job interview for a position as a curator at the local historical society. She was also thinking about getting back into the pool, realizing that she had not gone swimming since her accident in sixth grade. Although she was somewhat fearful, she decided to explore the local opportunities available to her. While searching the Internet, she discovered an adapted water-exercise class offered at a nearby recreational pool and went to observe the class and talk with the instructor. While chatting with the instructor after class, Mia found out that he was a kinesiology graduate and knew a lot about possibilities for **adapted physical activity (APA)** at the local, national, and international levels.

adapted physical activity (APA)
A field of study of physical activity that is modified for people with special needs to promote healthy and active lifestyles.

APA is a broader field of study that includes not only APE but also the delivery of services to individuals with disabilities to help promote a healthy and physically active lifestyle. Specifically, APA "is a professional branch of kinesiology/physical education/sport and human movement sciences, which is directed toward persons who require adaptation for participation in the context of physical activity" (International Federation of Adapted Physical Activity, n.d.). From a sport science perspective,

Adapted physical activity science is research, theory and practice directed toward persons of all ages underserved by the general sport sciences, disadvantaged in resources, or lacking power to access equal physical activity opportunities and rights. APA services and supports are provided in all kinds of settings. Thus, research, theory and practice relate to the needs and rights in inclusive as well as separate APA programs. (Sherrill & Hutzler, 2008, as reported by the International Federation of Adapted Physical Activity, n.d.)

Similar to APE, APA is addressed by federal legislation such as IDEA and the **Americans with Disabilities Act (ADA)**, but it acquires most of its support from **Article 30** of the United Nations Convention on the Rights of Persons with Disabilities (United Nations Enable, n.d.). See **TABLE 14-5** for the text of Article 30.

One of the most noted organizations in the field of APA is the **International Federation of Adapted Physical Activity (IFAPA)**. Founded in 1973 in Quebec, Canada, IFAPA is an "international, cross-disciplinary professional organization of individuals, institutions, and agencies concerned with promotion and dissemination of knowledge and information about adapted physical activity, disability sport, and all other aspects of sport, movement, and exercise science for the benefit persons who require adaptations to enable their participation" (IFAPA, 2014).

Even though APA most often involves individuals with disabilities, it may also apply to those who are obese, aged, or young or who have any other individual differences that may restrict participation in regular (non-adapted) physical activity.

TABLE 14-5   Article 30 of the United Nations Convention on the Rights of Persons with Disabilities: Participation in Cultural Life, Recreation, Leisure, and Sport

1.	States Parties recognize the right of persons with disabilities to take part on an equal basis with others in cultural life, and shall take all appropriate measures to ensure that persons with disabilities:
	(a) Enjoy access to cultural materials in accessible formats;
	(b) Enjoy access to television programmes, films, theatre and other cultural activities, in accessible formats;
	(c) Enjoy access to places for cultural performances or services, such as theatres, museums, cinemas, libraries and tourism services, and, as far as possible, enjoy access to monuments and sites of national cultural importance.
2.	States Parties shall take appropriate measures to enable persons with disabilities to have the opportunity to develop and utilize their creative, artistic and intellectual potential, not only for their own benefit, but also for the enrichment of society.
3.	States Parties shall take all appropriate steps, in accordance with international law, to ensure that laws protecting intellectual property rights do not constitute an unreasonable or discriminatory barrier to access by persons with disabilities to cultural materials.
4.	Persons with disabilities shall be entitled, on an equal basis with others, to recognition and support of their specific cultural and linguistic identity, including sign languages and deaf culture.
5.	With a view to enabling persons with disabilities to participate on an equal basis with others in recreational, leisure and sporting activities, States Parties shall take appropriate measures:
	(a) To encourage and promote the participation, to the fullest extent possible, of persons with disabilities in mainstream sporting activities at all levels;
	(b) To ensure that persons with disabilities have an opportunity to organize, develop and participate in disability-specific sporting and recreational activities and, to this end, encourage the provision, on an equal basis with others, of appropriate instruction, training and resources;
	(c) To ensure that persons with disabilities have access to sporting, recreational and tourism venues;
	(d) To ensure that children with disabilities have equal access with other children to participation in play, recreation and leisure and sporting activities, including those activities in the school system;
	(e) To ensure that persons with disabilities have access to services from those involved in the organization of recreational, tourism, leisure and sporting activities.

Article 30 of the United Nations Convention on the Rights of People with Disabilities. Retrieved from www.un.org/disabilities /documents/convention/convoptprot-e.pdf

According to IFAPA (2014), a variety of approaches can be taken to modifying physical activities to accommodate the unique needs of a particular individual. Examples include adapting the equipment, the task criteria, the instructions, the physical and social environments, or the rules.

In Mia's case, the following adjustments might have been made during her adapted water-exercise class:

	Mia's Need	Example Modification
Equipment	Improving and maintaining balance capabilities	Wears ankle weights in the water to help stabilize and strengthen the lower extremities.
Task criteria	Improving and maintaining balance capabilities	Performs a two-legged squat versus a one-legged squat.
Instructions	Improving memory capabilities	Instructor uses verbal cues and poster boards to reinforce critical elements of a movement (e.g., the squat: "keep knees aligned with ankles").
Physical environment	Improving and maintaining balance capabilities	Small amounts of turbulence are created by classmates to increase the amount of water resistance during squatting movements.
Social environment	Positive and successful movement experience	Encourage collaboration by working with a partner during the flexibility portion of class.
Rules	Positive and successful movement experience	Eliminate scorekeeping during a water game played at the end of class.

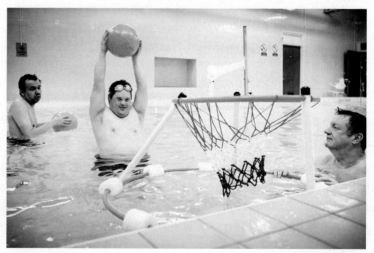

© Dean Mitchell/Getty Images

Mia was happy with the physical and emotional progress she made while attending her adapted water-exercise class. She not only felt stronger and more at ease around the pool again, but she made some new friends, whom she looked forward to seeing each week. Mia was also pleased to be given the head curator job she interviewed for at the local historical society. Reflecting on her past, she was apprecia-tive of the services she had received throughout her school

STOP AND THINK

Identify physical activity programs available in your community for individuals with disabilities.

career and the people who encouraged her along the way. Not only did these individuals rebuild her memory and balance skills, but they taught her the importance of advocating for others in similar situations. As a result of these interactions, Mia carried this compassion and knowledge with her as she began her working career.

When she arrived at the historical society, Mia soon discovered that more time and energy needed to be devoted to integrating individuals with disabilities into the fabric of the organization. Even though the museum met all ADA requirements regarding employment, public accommoda-tions, transportation, and telecommunications, she wanted to design a more focused campaign to increase public awareness. She began by setting up a

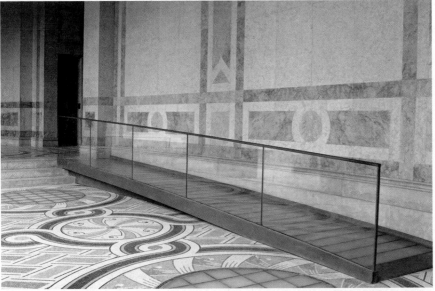

© Louise Heusinkveld / Alamy Stock Photo

yearly event calendar that included several novel programming and educational ideas that featured artists with disabilities. The following is a sample from her calendar for the summer months of June, July, and August:

June	July	August
New artist of the month	New artist of the month	New artist of the month
Speaker series	Speaker series	Speaker series
Internship opportunities	Internship opportunities	Internship opportunities
Community project with local school district	Sculpture workshop fundraiser	Sponsored sporting event fundraiser

STOP AND THINK

Think about your previous or current workplace. How did your place of employment meet the demands of the American with Disabilities Act?

To accelerate her efforts, Mia took advantage of updating the museum's webpage and Facebook page, and she established a Twitter account and blog to advertise upcoming events. Over time, her efforts paid off, and she was able to provide assistance to other historical societies that were interested in the same programming and educational ideas for and about individuals with disabilities.

CAREER POSSIBILITIES

You have already read about the many professions that impacted Mia's case throughout her life. During her secondary school years, she worked with an occupational therapist, a school counselor, a physical therapist, a classroom teacher, and an adapted physical educator. While attending college, she saw a rehabilitative counselor, a social worker, a recreational therapist, and an occupational therapist. Except for the adapted physical educator, these professions require specific degree programs and/or certifications that differ from that of kinesiology; however, these professions often include coursework common to kinesiology, such as biology, anatomy, physiology, psychology, or statistics.

Besides becoming an adapted physical educator, students interested in the broader field of APA can find college and university programs dedicated to providing coursework and field experiences in this area. These programs are most often offered at the master's level. One outstanding international program is Erasmus Mundus Master in Adapted Physical Activity.

The goal of this program is to educate students to become experts in movement and sport for persons with disabilities. Some graduates of this program have gone on to work with the Paralympic National Committees, international sports organizations, rehabilitation hospitals and clinics, and schools with children with special needs, and others have continued on to pursue a Ph.D. Other career opportunities in APA that use academic and nonacademic degrees include coaches for athletes with disabilities, recreation program developers, certified inclusive fitness trainers, psychomotor (movement) therapists, inclusive community program administrators, and disability sport administrators. Related careers in kinesiology that focus on the therapeutic and rehabilitative sciences are aquatics director, athletic trainer, biomechanist, cardiac rehabilitation specialist, epidemiologist (physical activity), exercise physiologist, sport psychologist, kinesiotherapist, and strength and conditioning coach.

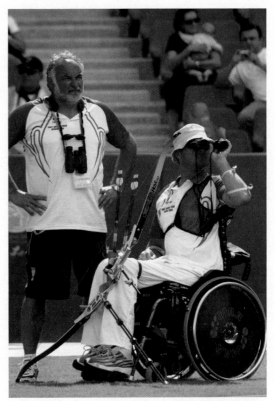

© Lucy Calder / Alamy Stock Photo

ALLIED HEALTH PROFESSIONS

According to the Association of Schools of Allied Health Professions (ASAHP, n.d.), **allied health professionals** are "involved with the delivery of health or related services pertaining to the identification, evaluation and prevention of diseases and disorders; dietary and nutrition services; and rehabilitation and health systems management, among others." The U.S. Code of Federal Regulations (CFR) defines allied health by exclusion. In other words, an allied health professional is any health professional who is not a physician, registered nurse, physician assistant, or doctor of osteopathy, dentistry, veterinary medicine, optometry, podiatric medicine, chiropractic, clinical psychology, or pharmacy. The CFR also specifies that individuals who possess a graduate degree in public health, health administration, social work, or counseling are important to health care, but are

allied health professional
A professional involved with the delivery of health or related services pertaining to the identification, evaluation, and prevention of diseases and disorders; dietary and nutrition services; and rehabilitation and health systems management; among others.

not considered allied health professionals. See **TABLE 14-6** for examples of allied health professionals.

TABLE 14-6   Examples of Allied Health Professionals

A

Anesthesiology assistant

Anesthesia technologist/technician

Athletic trainer

Audiologist

B

Behavioral disorder counselor

C

Cardiovascular technologist and technician

Clinical laboratory worker

Cytotechnologist

D

Dental hygienist

Dental assistant

Dental laboratory technician

Diagnostic medical sonographer

Dietitian

Dietetic assistant

E

Electroneurodiagnostic technologist

Emergency medical technician

Exercise science professional (personal fitness trainer, exercise physiologist)

G

Genetic assistant

H

Health information administrator and technologist

Health educator

Histotechnologist

Home health aide

K

Kinesiotherapist

L

Lactation consultant

M

Marriage and family therapist

Magnetic resonance technologist

Medical assistant

Medical dosimetrist

Medical illustrator

Medical librarian

Medical laboratory technologist

Medical transcriptionist

Mental health counselor

Music therapist

N

Nerve conduction studies technologist

Nuclear medicine technologist

Nutritionist

O

Occupational therapist

Occupational therapy assistant

Occupational therapy aide

Operating room technician

Ophthalmic medical assistant

Optometric assistant and technician

Orthotist

Orthotic and prosthetic technician

P

Perfusionist

Pharmacy assistant, aide, or technician

Physician assistant

Physical therapist

Physical therapy assistant

Physical therapy aide

Podiatric assistant

Poetry therapist

Polysomnographic technologist

Psychiatric aide or technician

R

Radiation therapist

Radiology assistant, technician, or administrator

Recreational therapist

Rehabilitation counselor

Respiratory therapist

S

Specialist in blood bank technology/transfusion medicine

Speech-language pathologist

Substance abuse counselor

Surgical neurophysiologist

Surgical assistant or technologist

V

Vocational rehabilitation counselor

Adapted from R. Arena, L. Goldberg, C. Ingersoll, D. Larsen, & D. Shelledy. (2011). Research in allied health profession: Why fund it? *Journal of Allied Health*, *40*(3), 161–166.

BROADER ISSUES IN THERAPEUTIC EXERCISE AND ALLIED HEALTH

Institute of Medicine (IOM)
Federal institute tasked with helping those in government and the private sector make informed health decisions by providing science-based evidence.

Just like those in the medical professions, experts in the therapeutic exercise and allied health professions are ethically bound to address common components advocated by the **Institute of Medicine (IOM)** in that the services delivered must be safe, person centered, timely, equitable, efficient, and effective (IOM, 2001, as reported by Arena, Goldberg, Ingersoll, Larsen, & Shelledy, 2011). Furthermore, the services provided must be theoretically sound, based on peer-reviewed results in published literature, and incorporate the perceptions and individual needs of patients. Together, these elements form what is called *evidence-based practice*. In the past, allied health professionals have blended theory (e.g., science, education, and medicine) and experience into practice without always testing their methods through rigorous research. According to Arena and colleagues (2011), this clinical approach arose for various reasons: (1) these professions were not yet mature, (2) there were more clinicians than researchers, and (3) these clinicians were not prepared to engage in research. But within the last 20 years, educational preparation has become more demanding, moving many certificate programs to 4-year baccalaureate degrees (e.g., athletic training, nursing) or even to advanced degrees (e.g., master's in occupational therapy and physician assistant), and finally on to doctoral degrees (e.g., audiology, physical therapy). This elevation in educational preparation has increased the number of faculty conducting research as well as preparing graduates to be better consumers of scientific literature and contributors to research in clinical practice.

In Mia's case, working with an interdisciplinary team of highly trained professionals whose practices were driven by evidence-based research has served her well. Because of these scholarly efforts, her treatments were safe; targeted to her needs; provided at the right time; and fair, efficient, and effective. Without well-researched interventions, Mia might have struggled unnecessarily when it came to living an independent and productive life. Although there is much work to be done in the area of research in the allied health professions, the **American Physical Therapy Association (APTA)** was one of the first organizations to publish a broad research agenda, which included the following items (Goldstein et al., 2011, as reported by Arena et al., 2011):

1. Basic research to evaluate genetic, anatomical, physiological, and environmental factors that impact disease, treatment, and recovery, as well as the ability of treatment to modify these factors.
2. Clinical research to develop and evaluate effective treatment methods, including timing, frequency, intensity, and dosage of optimal treatments and methods for predicting injury and recovery.

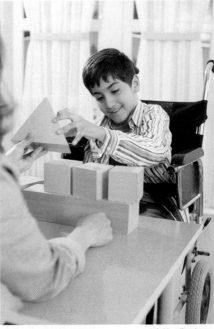
© fatihhoca/Getty Images

American Physical Therapy Association (APTA)
First professional organization to publish a broad research agenda for the allied health professions.

3. Educational research to determine the best methods of training clinicians and specialists for entry-level and advanced practice, life-long learning, and evidence-based practice.

4. Epidemiological research to determine the incidence of health conditions treated by physical therapists.

5. Health services research to evaluate the impact of treatment on healthcare costs and to determine the cost-effectiveness of interventions.

6. Workforce research to identify issues, best practices, and need for changes in scope-of-practice.

7. Measurement development and validation research to determine best measures for treatment effectiveness.

Allied health professionals must continue to work in teams with medical professionals and those in related fields to seek funding for high-quality research. This collaboration will enable providers to become creators of their own scientific base of knowledge rather than solely consumers of the literature of other fields.

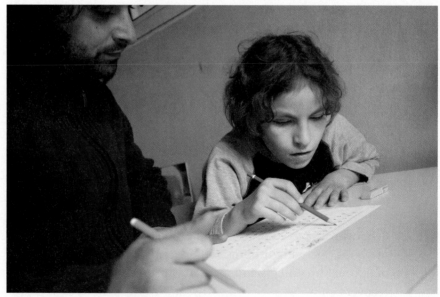

CHAPTER SUMMARY

In this chapter, you learned through a case study how educators and allied health professionals provided care and services to Mia throughout her secondary school and adult life to address a traumatic brain injury. You learned that these processes are supported by key legislative documents, such as Public Law 94-142, Section 504 of the Rehabilitation Act of 1973, the Individuals with Disabilities Education Act (IDEA), and the Americans with Disabilities Act (ADA). The differences between adapted physical education and the broader field of adapted physical activity were discussed, and the steps to become a credentialed adapted physical educator were identified. Possible career options in the allied health professions were introduced, along with a discussion of how professionals in these fields interact as members of multidisciplinary teams to assist individuals who require adaptation for participation in the context of physical activity.

DISCUSSION QUESTIONS

1. Why is the process to qualify for special education services necessary?
2. Where in society do you see the impact of the Amateur Sports Act?
3. How does Article 30 relate to your kinesiology option area?
4. Discuss the importance of evidence-based practice in kinesiology.
5. Is kinesiology an appropriate preparatory degree to move into an allied health profession?

REFERENCES

American Psychological Association. (2013). Individuals with Disabilities Education Act (IDEA). Retrieved from http://www.apa.org/about/gr/issues/disability/idea.aspx

Arena, R., Goldberg, L., Ingersoll, C., Larsen, D., & Shelledy, D. (2011). Research in the allied health professions: Why fund it? *Journal of Allied Health*, 40(3), 161–166.

Association of Schools of Allied Health Professions. (n.d.). Allied health professionals. Retrieved from http://www.asahp.org/definition.htm

Center for Parent Information and Resources. (2010). Contents of the IEP. Retrieved from http://www.parentcenterhub.org/repository/iepcontents/

Commission on Teacher Credentialing. (2010). Credential requirements. Retrieved from http://www.ctc.ca.gov/credentials/CREDS/add-cred-auth.html

International Federation of Adapted Physical Activity. (2014). Retrieved from http://ifapa-international.net/

Siedentop, D., & van der Mars, H. (2012). *Introduction to physical education, fitness, and sport* (8th ed.). New York: McGraw-Hill.

The Council for Disability Rights (n.d.). A parent's guide to special ed/special needs. Retrieved from http://www.disabilityrights.org/title.htm

United Nations Enable. (n.d.). Article 30: Participation in cultural life, recreation, leisure, and sport. Retrieved from: http://www.un.org/disabilities/default.asp?id=290

CHAPTER 15

Discovering Possibilities

BELINDA STILLWELL

LEARNING OBJECTIVES

1. Identify the four fields of the physical activity relationship (PAR).

2. Describe how culture influences the social world of sport and physical activity.

3. Recognize the roles (i.e., stranger, tourist, regular, insider) an individual may experience within the social world of sport and physical activity, and explain and illustrate how these roles comprise our equation of life.

4. Explain how the PAR can be used to help populations become more physically active.

KEY TERMS

consumption of meanings in physical culture

culture

equation of life

external shape

following of physical culture

insider

internal essence

meanings

personal physical activity

physical activity relationship (PAR)

production in physical culture

regular

social world

stranger

tourist

Case Study: Personal and Cultural Physical Activity

When it came to physical activity, Melvin spent most of his time and energy during his secondary school years competing in baseball, football, and basketball. Melvin had the skill to play college baseball, and in fact got several scholarship offers to do so at a number of in-state and out-of-state universities. Although his parents encouraged and supported his activity choices, Melvin chose not to accept an athletic scholarship. He instead began attending community college to explore his academic interests. One day while on his way to biology class, Melvin took a shortcut through the kinesiology building. In the hallway he heard live music. When he arrived at the doorway, he saw a pianist and several small groups of students leaping, twirling, and bending their way across the floor. Much to his surprise, he enjoyed watching for the few minutes he had to spare and decided to return the next day when he could stay longer.

After the class was over the next day, Melvin talked with some of the students as they exited the dance studio. He was curious about what types of classes were best to take for a person who was new to dance. The students responded in unison, "Ballet!" In this chapter, you will learn how an individual's life can change as his physical activity choices take a new direction.

UNDERSTANDING THE PHYSICAL ACTIVITY RELATIONSHIP

In 2008, Koski, in an attempt to analyze and gain a better understanding of an individual's relationship to sport and physical activity, introduced the idea of the **physical activity relationship (PAR)** as the primary tool for understanding this relationship. The PAR has four fields: (1) personal physical activity, (2) following of physical culture, (3) production in physical culture, and (4) consumption of meanings in physical culture (**FIGURE 15-1**). This perspective includes the concepts of culture, meaning, social world, and the equation of life.

Culture is understood as a web of meanings that consists of four levels: surface level, norms and regulations, values and valuations, and assumptions and beliefs (Kinnunen, 1990; Lundberg, 1985). **Meanings** are the central building blocks that comprise each of the four levels and are combinations that form mainly due to the influences we are exposed to as we function in various social worlds (Koski, 2008). Because Western culture is changing

---

physical activity relationship (PAR)
Tool used to analyze and gain a better understanding of an individual's relationship to sport and physical activity culture.

culture
Dominant and common language, ways of life, roles, and expectations that govern our everyday interactions in the social world.

meanings
Combinations that form mainly due to the influences we are exposed to as we function in various social worlds.

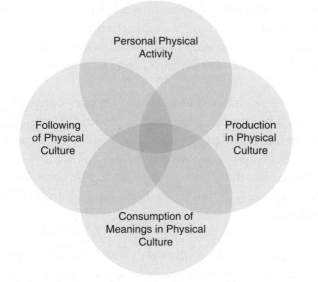

FIGURE 15-1   The four fields of the physical activity relationship (PAR).

Data from Koski, P. (2008). Physical activity relationship (PAR). *International Review for the Sociology of Sport, 43*, pp. 151–163.

rapidly, individuals face more challenges and opportunities than ever before. As a result of this rapid transformation, Unruh (1980) suggests that we live in various social worlds simultaneously, and that one such social world is that of sport and physical activity. Unruh further proposes that we play varying roles within these worlds: stranger, tourist, regular, or insider. The more involved we become in any one world, the more profound our understanding of the meanings of that world. These meanings can be further defined as some type of order of priority, where one thing is more important than another.

LIFE AS A STRANGER

Melvin's first glimpse into the world of dance was that of a **stranger**. He did not understand much about this world or what it meant to him personally, but he was drawn to become involved. He continued to observe a number of different dance classes, looked into joining the dance club on campus, and contemplated taking a ballet class the following semester. While away

stranger
Role where a person does not easily understand much about a new social world or what it means to him or her personally, but is drawn to become involved.

equation of life
A mathematical representation to illustrate the various social worlds we belong to and the level of significance each world holds for us.

social world
Refers to certain areas of life that have their own practices, modes of activity, and ways of thinking—a constellation of meaning structures.

personal physical activity
Physical activity choices that can range from a formal sport experience to general physical activity.

from school, he began to think about how much time, energy, and resources he wanted to devote to this new physical activity. This process of reflection begins to shape his relationship to the world of dance. Koski (2008) helps us conceptualize this process by introducing us to what he calls our *equation of life*.

Koski (2008) illustrated the **equation of life** mathematically: $Aa + Bb + Cc$, and so on. The uppercase letters represent the many social worlds we belong to. The lowercase letters indicate the level of significance that world holds for us. **Social world** refers to certain areas of life that have their own practices, modes of activity, and ways of thinking—a constellation of meaning structures (Strauss, 1978; Unruh, 1979, 1980). Unruh (1979) defines a social world as a:

> unit of social organization which is diffuse and amorphous in character. Generally larger than groups or organizations, social worlds are not necessarily defined by formal boundaries, membership lists or spatial territory … Social world must be seen as an internally recognizable constellation of actors, organizations, events, and practices which have coalesced into a perceived sphere of interest and involvement for participants … (p. 115)

Previously, Melvin's equation of life included many sports and physical activities (e.g., football, basketball, baseball); we can call this social world uppercase "A." We can probably predict that the level of significance it held for him was high, and thus his lowercase "a" would have been heavily weighted at that particular time. Currently, however, Melvin does not participate as often in traditional sports, and he has begun to explore the world of dance. This social world can still be characterized by an uppercase "A," but his lowercase "a" would carry less significance at this point in his life. Koski (2008) reminds us that our life equations are in a state of constant change. Our physical activity choices shift, as well as the intensity at which we approach them. These activities can range in nature from a formal sport experience to general physical activity. Therefore, it is feasible to couple Melvin's current status as a stranger in the world of dance with his low **personal physical activity** level, as illustrated in the first field of the PAR.

LIFE AS A TOURIST

Melvin's experience with dance begins when he enrolls in a ballet class, and it is through this experience that we will explore how an individual's experience with physical activity can change. On the first day of class, he recognizes some of the students he met last semester in the hallway just outside the dance studio. Seeing them helps to eliminate some of his early anxiety about taking this class. As they enter the studio together, others are already spread out across the floor warming up. Some are standing at the barre performing heel raises; many are sitting on the floor stretching their legs; a few are lying down making various formations with their bodies; and the rest randomly move to the music that is playing softly over the speakers.

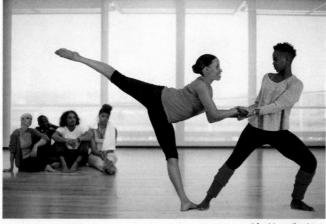

© PeopleImages/Getty Images

Melvin sets his backpack down in the designated area and follows two of his classmates out onto the dance floor as the instructor begins a formal warm-up. Melvin chooses to stand in the back of class as he tries to follow along. He cannot see very well but solves this dilemma by closely following the movements of a classmate positioned in front of him. He begins to relax a bit and starts to feel his body temperature rise, making it easier to bend and flex with each new demand. After the structured warm-up is done, the instructor asks students to form groups of four and get ready to move across the floor. Melvin feels his body become tense and wonders if he can make his way across the floor without embarrassment. With the support of his classmates and the instructor, Melvin makes it through class and manages to enjoy some of the new things he was asked to do. Compared to other sports and physical activities he has experienced, he finds this class as

STOP AND THINK

Using the equation of life ($Aa + Bb + Cc$, etc.) as a guide, reflect on the relationship you currently have with the social world of sport and physical activity. For instance, "A" may collectively represent cycling activities. If you enjoy biking with a club during the week, entering bike races on the weekends, and training for a 50-mile bike race every year, your "a" would carry a significant amount of weight. Using this same process, think back on your relationship with physical activity in high school before coming to college. Compare and contrast these two social worlds. What did you discover about your relationship with physical activity over time?

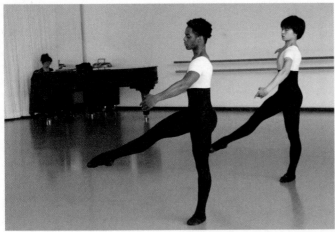

© Buddy Bartelsen/ullstein bild via Getty Images

physically and mentally challenging as baseball practices used to be. He decides to return when the class meets again and promises himself that he will practice the things that proved most difficult for him at home.

Unruh might agree that Melvin has moved beyond his status as a stranger to this new social world and is now operating as a **tourist**. Unruh (1979) defines the *tourist* as such:

tourist
Role whereby a person is curious and interested in the social world in question and might even temporarily participate and test the world.

following of physical culture
Includes being a spectator of competitive sports, but it also involves following physical activities through television, movies, reading, or social media opportunities.

tourists are a little bit curious and interested in the social world in question. They might even temporarily participate and test the social world. The tourist can make some observations about the meanings of the social world, but often the level of significance remains superficial. In short, the tourist's relationship to the social world is momentary (as reported by Koski, 2008, p 157).

The superficial level that Melvin is experiencing is composed of artifacts; that is, observable objects that can be charged with several, often symbolic, meanings (Kinnunen, 1990; Lundberg, 1985). For example, classical music is often associated with ballet as a movement form. Melvin was first drawn toward the dance studio when he heard live piano music playing through the hallway on his shortcut to biology class. Once he arrived at the doorway, he noticed bodies moving across the floor dressed in comfortable, form-fitting clothing that allowed the dancers to move freely. Some wore ballet shoes, whereas others were barefoot. Ballet barres lined the perimeter of the room, with a backdrop of mirrors covering three of the four classroom walls. Soft black flooring allowed each student to land with less impact than that of a wood or cement floor. Taken together, these objects have begun to influence Melvin in ways that allow him to attach meaning to the social world of dance.

In the second field of the PAR, the person follows others' activities, which Koski (2008) refers to as the secondary activity of **following of physical culture**.

Typically, it includes being a spectator of competitive sports, but it also involves following physical activities through television, movies, reading, or social media opportunities. For Melvin, this meant going to dance performances, both on and off campus; watching movies about dancers; reading dance magazines and research; and browsing the Internet for dance information.

Heinilä (1986) suggests that a sporting event has two components: external shape and internal essence. The **external shape** is formed by each sport's purpose, as defined by its unique characteristics and formal regulations. This shape makes the sport recognizable to others. In dance, for example, there is often staging, music, lighting, costumes, and dancers. When we see these things presented together, we know we are watching a dance performance. Also, each dancer is performing movements that abide by formal teachings. For instance, we see dancers executing pliés (bending), pirouettes (spinning), and cabrioles (jumps) while on stage. These movements are specific to the norms and regulations set by the dance world. That is to say that there are standards by which to compare each movement's critical elements (e.g., a pirouette is a controlled turn on one leg with hips and knees commonly turned out). Conversely, a sport's **internal essence** is the subjective experience an individual encounters while watching a performance—in other words, what it means to them. According to Heinilä (1986), a person seeks an event whose essence and meanings best correspond with a particular expectation of experiences. This motivation is what may ultimately explain why we are interested in some sporting events rather than others. For Melvin, the activities and experiences he is exposed to through the world of dance match what he is looking for. This deepens his understanding and serves to accelerate his motivation, which, in turn, strengthens his personal relationship with dance.

external shape
Component of a sporting event that is formed by each sport's purpose, as defined by its unique characteristics and formal regulations.

internal essence
The subjective experience an individual encounters while watching a performance—in other words, what it means to them.

STOP AND THINK

Think about one of your favorite sporting events. Explain why you are drawn to it.

LIFE AS A REGULAR

As the second semester rolls around, Melvin adds an additional dance class (modern) to his schedule and decides to audition for the upcoming spring concert. He is selected as one of many dancers to perform in a group number for the upcoming show. With his added dance course and his participation in the spring concert, Melvin could be considered a regular. **Regulars**, as

regular
Role where a person is relatively committed to the social world and understands much of its meaning.

defined by Unruh (1979), are "integrated into the social world and its activities. They are relatively committed to the social world and they understand much of its meaning. As their commitment continues their understanding becomes deeper" (as reported by Koski, 2008, p 157). At about the same time that Melvin becomes a regular, he is asked by one of his friends in the show if he would like to assist with a dance production he is coordinating at a local elementary school. Melvin takes advantage of this opportunity to learn more about dance movement as it relates to children, dance production (e.g., lighting, music), and the necessary administrative tasks associated with a school production. This involvement illustrates the third field of the PAR, which refers to the **production in physical culture**.

production in physical culture Creation of physical activity opportunities for participants and spectators.

As producers of physical activity, Melvin and his classmate are part of a team that provides dance classes at the elementary school. Parents and caregivers may also be involved in this event as volunteers. Without these producers, there would be no performance. Each individual involved in the dance production will experience it on a different level. Some children will be the dancers; others may help with lighting. Some may handle the publicity; others may contribute the artwork. Just like Melvin, they may also be strangers, tourists, regulars, or insiders (more on insiders later) to this social world of dance. Koski (2008) reminds us that the question is one of how deeply each person will be involved in the meanings of the social world of dance. The more deeply we are immersed in these meanings, the better we understand the language of dance and the more powerful these meanings become. What will these producers and participants take away from this dance experience? Will the experience move them from being tourists to regulars? Their interactions throughout the project will begin to create meaning and expand their internal essence.

As a performer in the spring concert and coproducer of the children's dance show, Melvin begins to appreciate the values embedded in dance on a deeper level. He internalizes the beauty, grace, artistry, and creativity visible in his own performances, as well as in the performances of others. This internalization spreads to a broader appreciation for the world of music and those who produce it, both vocalists and instrumentalists. In turn, Melvin decides to declare himself a dance major and dedicate the next 4 years of his academic life to dance.

If we revisit Melvin's equation of life, we can see that it has changed a great deal. Earlier in the chapter we identified his uppercase "A" as the social world of dance and the lowercase "a" as the level of significance it held for him. As a stranger, this lowercase "a" carried little weight as he was just beginning his dance journey. He had not yet experienced a great deal of personal movement in this area, nor had he been extensively exposed to the language or symbols that represent this world. It is during these 4 years that Melvin rapidly grew in many areas, especially as a performer; follower; and, to a lesser degree, a producer. With his new commitment to becoming a dance major, we witness yet another transformation as Melvin begins to experience this world as an insider.

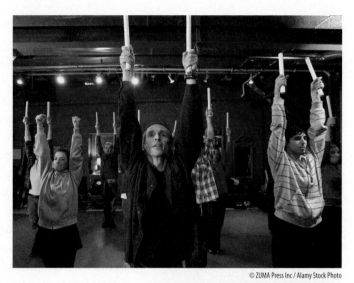

© ZUMA Press Inc / Alamy Stock Photo

LIFE AS AN INSIDER

During his undergraduate years, Melvin lives and breathes dance as a performer, but he also becomes curious about choreography. Koski (2000) and Unruh (1979) characterize **insiders** as those who "are deeply involved in the social world and their life and identity are strongly influenced by the social world and its meanings. They are very committed and act to not only participate but to actively create and maintain the social world and its meanings" (p. 157).

Along with becoming an insider, Melvin's PAR reaches the fourth field, known as the **consumption of meanings in physical culture**. However, this field reaches beyond mere consumption, such as the buying of sporting goods and services related to the social world (e.g., dance fashion, music, performance tickets). It involves the process of *sportization*, or the path through which sport and its meanings have penetrated one's entire way of life (see Elias & Dunning, 1986; Maguire, 1999). It means absorbing the assumptions and beliefs held in a particular social world. For dance, this may include a world governed by self-expression, storytelling through movement, and physical well-being. Dance has shaped Melvin's life by redeveloping his self-image

insider
Person who is deeply involved in the social world and whose life and identity are strongly influenced by the social world and its meanings.

consumption of meanings in physical culture
Involves the process of *sportization*, or the path through which sport and its meanings have penetrated one's way of life.

and personal identity—he is dance, and dance has become his playground. For Melvin, dance now occupies a large proportion of his equation of life. His uppercase "A" remains stable, while his lowercase "a" has magnified to a new power.

After graduating with his dance degree and with his collective experiences as a choreographer for school and community performances, Melvin decides to move to New York City to further develop his professional career. When he first arrives, he seeks out a dance studio that his former instructor told him about so he can continue to practice his ballet and modern dance forms. One day, as his modern class is ending, he notices that a tap class is coming in. He decides to stay and try it out. Because of his former training, Melvin is able to catch on quickly, and he is excited about the new opportunities this type of dance might bring. In fact, it feels to him like a natural fit. Within 2 years of extensive ballet, modern, and tap training, Melvin goes to his first audition for an Off-Broadway show. Although not cast as a lead dancer, he earns a part in two group tap-dancing numbers. The show is successful and brings Melvin's career to a new level. Melvin continues to live and dance in New York City, awaiting his next audition.

STOP AND THINK

Consider your current relationship with sport and physical activity. Are you a stranger, tourist, regular, or insider within this social world? Support your answer with at least three examples. Likewise, reflect on your relationship with physical activity back in high school and do the same. Finally, think about what events and/or persons shaped your role (stranger, tourist, regular, or insider) at each of these times in your life. Write down key points of your life story.

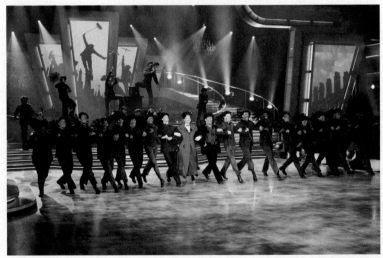

© Adam Larkey/ABC via Getty Images

THE POTENTIAL OF THE PAR

The PAR can be used as a tool to help us not only engage individuals and groups physically, but also cognitively and emotionally. We can find out what other social worlds individuals belong to and attempt to connect physical activity to those worlds. For instance, if someone enjoys traveling, we might encourage that person to enhance his or her travels by incorporating a variety of physical activities while exploring other states and countries. Physical activities could include walking or biking whenever possible; aquatic activities, such as snorkeling, scuba diving, swimming, or surfing; utilizing fitness centers available at hotels; or practicing tai chi outdoors.

For those with a strong connection to a particular sport or physical activity, we might persuade them to attempt similar or brand new activities to broaden their commitment to physical activity. For example, a person who loves to play soccer might also like games with similar tactics. One example is European team handball, which combines the common strategies found in invasion games (requiring one team to invade another team's defense to score) such as soccer, basketball, and hockey. Teams consist of seven players—six field players plus one goalkeeper. It is played on a field

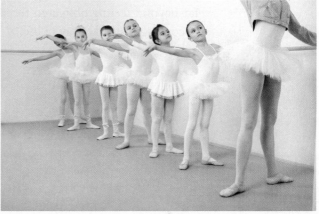

© JoHo/Shutterstock

or court that is 40 × 20 meters. Players dribble (similar to basketball), run, and shoot at a goal measuring 3 × 2 meters in order to score. They may not pass the 6-meter goal line when attempting a shot. This new game presents another movement possibility that may have previously gone unnoticed. Similar to Melvin's experience in dance, this person's skills transferred readily from soccer to handball. Ideally, this game not only builds one's technical skills, but also promotes cognitive and emotional attachment to something new.

Physical activities and sport are an important part of the broader culture. They not only hold value in the educational setting (e.g., physical education), but also in the recreation and leisure industries, the health and well-being policy-making arena, and in the marketplace, where many kinesiologists establish their careers. Culture is a web of meanings that are constructed by individuals through their interactions with various social worlds. The more meaningful the interactions, the stronger the physical, cognitive, and emotional ties to that world.

Professionals in all areas of kinesiology can benefit those they work with by adopting a holistic view of each individual's personal needs and goals. Numerous tools and approaches can aid in accomplishing this, but we must be thoughtful in our selection of these tools in order to appeal to the intellect and emotions of the diverse populations we assist. We can act as guides and facilitators to ensure that individuals internalize sport and physical activities in a positive way, step-by-step. These efforts should reach far beyond feeling obligated to participate (e.g., it is good for my health), becoming instead a way of life.

CHAPTER SUMMARY

In this chapter, the PAR was presented as a tool to assist kinesiologists in helping others develop a positive relationship with sport and physical activity in order to begin or maintain participation levels. The PAR consists of four fields: (1) personal physical activity, (2) following of physical culture, (3) production in physical culture, and (4) consumption of meanings in physical culture. The concepts of culture, meaning, social world, and the equation of life were introduced to further develop this perspective. Additionally, it was proposed that we play varying roles within these worlds as strangers, tourists, regulars, or insiders. Finally, it was emphasized that people are not simply empty vessels moving about during their day, but rather individuals who are composed of a variety of cognitive and emotional experiences. Our life equations are rich with personal meaning, and, depending on those experiences, we may form a positive or negative bond with the social world of sport and physical activity.

DISCUSSION QUESTIONS

1. How do social worlds relate to the equation of life?
2. What role does culture play in the various social worlds?
3. Why is it important to understand the term *sportization*?
4. With regard to your own option area within kinesiology, how can you use the PAR?
5. How can the PAR be used to help people become more physically active?

REFERENCES

Elias, N., & Dunning, E. (1986). *Quest for excitement: Sport and leisure in the civilizing process*. Oxford: Basil Blackwell.

Heinilä, K. (1986). Koripallo penkkiurheiluna [Basketball as a spectator sport]. *Liikuntasuunnittelun laitos, tutkimuksia*, no. 35. Jyväskylä: Jyväskylän yliopisto.

Kinnunen, J. (1990). Terveyskeskuksen organisaatiokulttuuri [Organization culture of the health centre]. *Kuopion yliopiston julkaisuja, yhteiskuntatieteet, alkuperäistutkimukset*, 4.

Koski, P. (2000). Liikunnan kansalaistoiminta kulttuurina: Toiminnan merkityksellisyys ja merkitysrakenteet [Civil activity in sports as a culture: The meanings and meaning structures of the action]. In H. Itkonen, J. Heikkala, K. Ilmanen, and P. Koski (Eds.), *Liikunnan kansalaistoiminta: Muutokset, merkitykset ja reunaehdot* (pp. 135–154). Helsinki: Liikuntatieteellisen Seuran julkaisu nro 152.

Koski, P. (2008). Physical activity relationship (PAR). *International Review for the Sociology of Sport, 43*, 151–163.

Lundberg, C. (1985). On the feasibility of cultural intervention in organizations. In P. Frost, L. Moore, M. Louis, C. Lundberg, & J. Martin (Eds.), *Organizational culture* (pp. 169–186). Beverly Hills, CA: Sage.

Maguire, J. (1999). *Global sport: Identities, societies, civilizations*. Cambridge: Polity Press.

Strauss, A. (1978). A social world perspective. In N. Denzin (Ed.), *Studies in symbolic interaction* (pp. 119–128). Greenwich, CT: JAI Press.

Unruh, D. R. (1979). Characteristics and types of participation in social worlds. *Symbolic Interaction, 2*, 115–29.

Unruh, D. R. (1980). The nature of social worlds. *Pacific Sociological Review 23*(3), 271–296.

CHAPTER 16

Diversity: Sport as Welcoming Space

CAROLE A. OGLESBY

LEARNING OBJECTIVES

1. Identify and describe initiatives that use sport as a vehicle to build peace and good relations in a community.

2. Explain what social rarity is and provide an example.

3. Provide examples of how sport psychology, exercise physiology, and athletic training were all important to the success of Citizen's Fitness.

4. Describe how the suggestions offered by the UN Sport for Development and Peace Working Group can be used for relief in times of disaster.

5. Describe how true competition and decompetition differ.

6. Identify measures a person can take to stop bullying.

7. Describe some of the major changes that have occurred in the last decade with regard to gender and sport.

KEY TERMS

bias	discriminate
bullying	gender diversity
decompetition	human potential approach

institutionalized bias   social rarity
intersectionality   sport for development
marginalization   true competition

Diversity, Safe Space, and Community

The capacity for and need to move is a commonality across humanity. To move is virtually a definition of a living organism. Every culture, every ethnic group, has aspects of a unique character that create the rich vocabulary of sport and physical activity (Schinke & Hanrahan, 2009; Schinke & Moore, 2011). At the same time, commonalities across all physical activity forms enable "playing together" even when there is no common vocal language or cultural familiarity. No rule book is necessary for games of keep away, protecting home base, being the first to run from here to there, or matching movement to rhythm in dance. Additionally, the ever-present nature of social media, television, and film means that there can also be global participation (vicarious and direct) in sport forms such as soccer, basketball, and the Olympic Games.

This chapter uses hypothetical examples to explore one of our paradoxes in kinesiology—valuing and respecting diversity within the context of recognition of our commonly shared humanity. With our world marked by so many divides and so much use of violence to solve problems, both the United Nations (UN) and the International Olympic Committee (IOC) have pledged in the last decade to utilize sport and physical recreation to achieve progress in human relationships. In 2014, UN Secretary-General Ban Ki-Moon stated, "The Olympic spirit sport with fair play, mutual respect and friendly competition, melts away barriers and sets examples for nations" (UN News Centre, 2014).

It is not, however, only for Olympians to benefit from, and contribute to, harmonious development through sport. The United Nations has made a commitment to sport through its Office on Sport for Development and Peace headed by Wilfred Lemke, a Special Advisor to the Secretary-General. As of early 2014, 17 UN agencies or UN-related nongovernmental organizations (NGOs) were spending millions of dollars each year for programming to support **sport for development** and peace goals (**FIGURE 16-1**). Some of these included the United Nations Educational, Scientific and

sport for development
Enhancing an individual or community through well-designed sport/physical activity experiences.

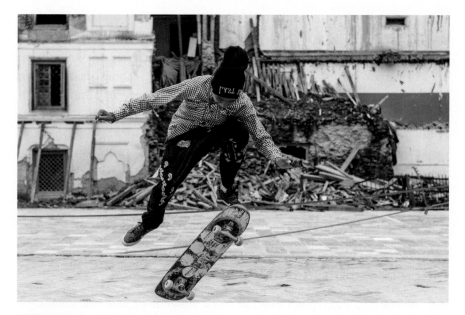

FIGURE 16-1   A step in the return to normalcy.

© Anadolu Agency / Getty Images

Cultural Organization (UNESCO); the United Nations Development Program (UNDP); the United Nations Children's Fund (UNICEF); the World Health Organization (WHO); and the Joint United Nations Programme on HIV/AIDS (UNAIDS).

For its part, the IOC has wholeheartedly endorsed this view of sporting activity as a great hope for enhancing interpersonal peace and respect. In 2013, the IOC proudly announced on its webpage that the UN General Assembly had determined that April 6 of each year would be an International Day of Sport for Development and Peace. This day was selected because it marked the opening day of the first modern Olympic Games in Athens in 1896. IOC then-President Rogge stated, "Sport with values is a gateway to cultural understanding, education, health, economic, and social development" (IOC, 2013).

This discussion is only the tip of the iceberg when reviewing the search for sport strategies to heal divisions between people in schools, communities, countries, and multinational regions. From a kinesiology career

STOP AND THINK

What do you think the effect would be if just 10% of the funding committed to military use globally were budgeted for sport for peace and development projects? Could we make child athletes instead of child soldiers?

perspective, it is well worth noting that sport/physical activity professionals are now able to take their passion and skills on the road globally to utilize sport as an invaluable human resource. In this chapter, we will take on but a tiny piece of this major issue. First, we will review some of our learned human responses that lead us to perceive others as "different"; that is, defining differences in a defensive hierarchal way that closes the doors of communication and creates misunderstanding. We will describe just a few of the key "diversities" that become prominent in movement activity contexts. You will then share in the fictional life stories of five individuals whom you could very likely meet in your kinesiology career. To conclude the chapter, we will explore some of the strategic ways that movement activity settings could greatly enhance these individuals' sometimes-dark journeys.

Difference to Discrimination

discriminate
To categorize individuals or objects on the basis of real or presumed characteristics.

It is interesting, and ironic, that the word **discriminate** has two meanings, and both are crucial to beginning our discussion of the value of diversity. Early in life, one of the fundamentals of a child's cognitive development is the capacity to discriminate. A baby is born to what William James first referred to as "blooming, buzzing confusion." (James, 1890, p. 462). Compared to the relative quiet of the womb, an infant's nursery is a chaos of noise, color, odor, and moving objects. Within a few months, typical development allows the infant to discriminate; that is, to note or observe systematic differences in what was once perceived as chaos (**FIGURE 16-2**).

Child development research has also revealed that in the first 1 to 2 years of life, the infant begins to selectively recognize focal stimuli that embody the essence of a class, or category, of stimuli more quickly and for longer periods (Bauer, Dow, & Hertsgaard, 1995). These recognized differences, once discriminated, become the prototypical basis for the cognition of a group or category. As these first years proceed, the child begins to be strongly influenced by the reactions of those closest to him or her. The child then begins modeling familial responses to groups or categories of things, people, and behaviors. One of the most fundamental of categorizations is the groupings of people and things that are "like me" and "different." Taking note of people different from oneself is certainly a common occurrence in the United States today. In 2011, 31 million U.S. residents had been born in other countries, or about 30% of the total population. Of course, this 30% is not spread evenly across

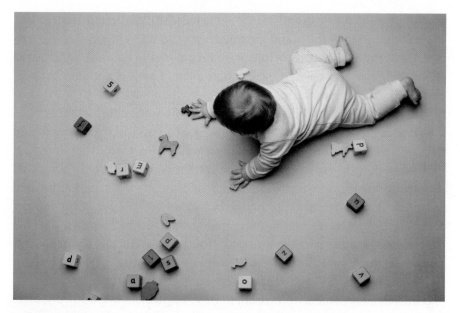

FIGURE 16-2   One path toward the ability to discriminate.

© Image Source Plus / Alamy Stock Photo

the country, and the concentration of diversity is much higher in densely populated urban areas. If you are a boy, roughly 51% of those around you are of a different sex. If you are African American, about 85% of those in United States will be of a different race (Schinke & Moore, 2011). Thus, differences abound. The problem is that all differences are not equal.

The growing young person sees/hears personal bias behavior that creates a hierarchy of category elements: best, good, not good, and bad. The young person often identifies with the biases held by those who are close, and the hierarchy is now fully owned. Additionally, the hierarchical placement is often reinforced by any inability of low-hierarchy groups to both find opportunity for betterment and to gain the necessary resources for betterment (Stein, 1995). When the situation of personal bias, lack of opportunity, and absence of resources all align, the second meaning of 'discrimination' is the result as **institutional bias**.

Here is an example of how this cycle can play out. "Anywhere Park" in Milwaukee, Wisconsin, has a Little League team for 8- to 10-year-olds. The rules may not say "boys only," but only boys have ever played for as long as anyone can remember. Jolene is a girl who really wants to play, and she is

institutionalized bias
Social phenomenon occurring when specific groups gain privileged status and power to control resources.

bias
Perception influenced by relatively stable judgement cognitions.

marginalization
Social disadvantages that result in a group being in a powerless or unimportant position.

intersectionality
Recognition that the course of human events is a result of combinations of factors, such as race, class, gender, language, or religion, and not just one factor.

the same size as the boys and has the same basic skills. She experiences **bias** when all her friends (boys and girls) tell her a girl won't be good enough to play. Her aunt says she wishes Jolene would not try out because "a girl could get hurt" (*bias*). She has not been able to play in any "real games" before, because the boys play after school, and that is when Jolene has to be at home to babysit her younger siblings (*low opportunity*). Some parents hire a coach for a few workouts with their kids before team tryouts just to familiarize the boys with the tryout protocol, but Jolene's family cannot afford anything like that. Also, they do not know about the system that aids skilled young athletes from club teams to move into high school varsity teams and ultimately to college athletic scholarships in baseball or softball (*blocked from human and financial resources*). This combination operates to greatly disadvantage Jolene's chances to make the team. No one is specifically trying to hurt Jolene, but that is how the "ism" (sexism, in this case) works. It is likely there still will not be a girl on the Anywhere Park Little League team this year, and a chance for diversity is missed. In this example, no one knows to care.

In the case of Jolene, sport social scientists would say that her interests (as well as those of other girls who might benefit from the Little League experience) are **marginalized**. Her interests are deemed not important enough to address compared with the interests of the known, and observed, number of boys ready to try out (**FIGURE 16-3**). A relatively new line of research into these kinds of situations, in which there is a linkage of marginalized interest, is **intersectionality**. One might say that this research focuses on the case where 1 + 1 + 1 = more than 3 (Working Group on Women and Human Rights, 2001).

Studies have shown that category membership in marginalized groups based on race, ethnicity, gender, and class are viewed as separate spheres but are in reality more likely to overlap and crosscut. The "traffic" where these influences intersect can be difficult to maneuver and may cause differing types of social and physical injury through resultant disempowerment. The girl in our case study was named Jolene. Did you assume that she was white girl? Not necessarily, but what if her name had been Lawanda or Biara, and she were a black girl? Looking at Jolene's story, we can see that there were class and economic challenges in her quest to be on the Little League team, and that it is quite possible that "Lawanda" would have faced an intersection of race, class, and gender.

As well as being faced with added complexities of finding necessary opportunities and resources as a member of marginalized groups, Jolene also appears

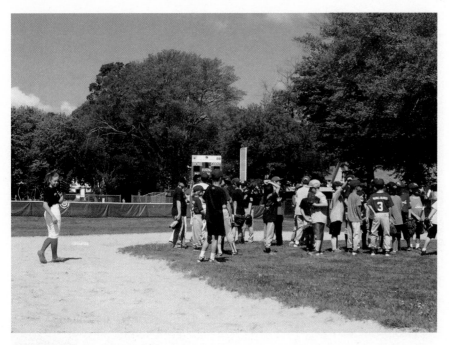

FIGURE 16-3 Marginalization.
© Justine Siegal

as a **social rarity**. More than 30 years ago, Moss-Kanter began investigating what happens when a "different" person enters a group. For example, if Jolene does show up for tryouts, even if a parent comes with her, she will be the only girl among the scores of boys who will be there. She is a *social rarity* in this context, and certain behaviors and reactions are highly probable, not because of any unique characteristics of the people there, but rather due to the rarity phenomenon. A spotlight will seem to highlight Jolene even if she makes every effort to blend in (**FIGURE 16-4**). A level of resentment may be felt by the "boy group" for the extra attention she receives, even when it is obvious she is seeking to avoid it. Moss-Kanter's work with an extensive number of teams and corporations revealed that pressures and tensions emerge in conditions of social rarity no matter what the context (Stein, 1995). This pressure can be overcome, and we will review coping strategies in the last section of this chapter. It is worthwhile for now to realize that all of us have at least some experiences of feeling different, alone, and perhaps even undervalued. It is important to keep that perspective in mind.

social rarity
Being one of a kind in a social group based on one highly visible factor.

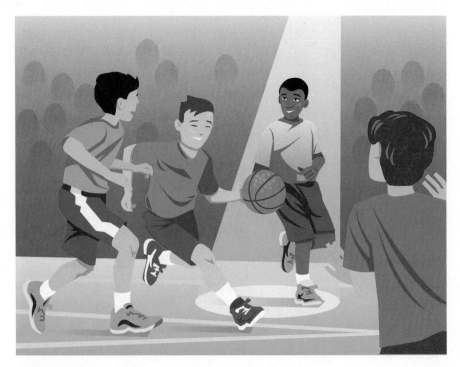

FIGURE 16-4 Want it or not, the spotlight's on YOU.

In movement activity contexts, we often have the opportunity to value each member of a team or class, including all of the individuals' different-ness or diversity. In playing games or exercising together, we have the oppor-tunity to compete with, and against, others from differing races, cultures, religions, sexual orientations, and social classes. These elements of diver-sity can be in our awareness yet not be the focal point. The focal concern is competing well, building skill, or gaining fitness. The common goal stands within the rich uniqueness of the individual.

Individuals on the Margins: The Case of Citizen's Fitness

Renee was the group leader for the Citizen's Fitness project operating 3 days a week at the park in Granville. Granville was a small suburb of Los Ange-les, and a nearby college had a large kinesiology program where Renee and three of her classmates were seniors. All four were bright and motivated to take what they had learned in their classes out into the world to "make a difference." They had enrolled in a practicum that offered the opportunity to take the Citizen's Fitness basic curriculum and conduct a needs assessment with community participants who had signed up for the program. It culminated in delivering a tailored and culturally sensitive activity program that was the hallmark of "Citizen's Fitness."

It was March 2, and the community members were in their appropriate groups and had their individualized routines in place to run until June 1, when season-ending performance days concluded the semester. For more than 90% of the participants, the program ran like clockwork. It would have been easy for a different set of student leaders to view their success rating as a fine record and all that could be expected and move on, but that was not going to happen with Renee and her colleagues (who dubbed themselves the "Fitness Fab Four"). They were meeting today to take up the cases of five individuals who had been identified as either frequently absent, having trouble keeping on target, or markedly alone or avoided by peers. Although each of these participants had a differing self-presentation, the outcome was the same. Each was failing badly in regard to the goals that they had initially accepted.

Renee, as the leader, asked her team to create a sketch of what was known about their challenged participants. Renee, Antonio, D'Andre, and Mai began the descriptions of the clients by owning the context in which the interactions between themselves and client participants took place. Each had, prior to this meeting, thought through the feelings and responses that these particular clients elicited from them. They had all learned the importance of *reflexive practice*; that is, that the student or client is not viewed as an isolated entity, but rather as a person-in-relation to group leaders and other participants (Schinke & Lidor, 2013).

In the challenge group were three boys/young men, a fourth-grade girl, and a woman, all of whom the student leaders felt would benefit from a special set of facilitations that would help them to successfully reach their program goals.

KROMA

Kroma was a woman about 40 years of age from Cambodia. It was difficult to gauge her exact age because her skin was very damaged, which made her appear older. She was rather petite, probably 5 feet tall, but in her demeanor she shrank into herself so deeply that she seemed to become even shorter. Her hair was short, dark, and straight, and her bangs mostly covered downcast eyes.

Cambodia has not yet recovered from the violence of the Vietnam War era, and the fields and countryside are still covered with old, undetonated landmines. The grasses, tree roots, and brush cover them, and each year thousands of people (mostly women) are killed and maimed as they accidently set off the mines when harvesting food or gathering water. Kroma perhaps could be deemed "lucky" as she only lost half of her right arm in such a blast. The wound was never well cared for, and she did not wear a prosthesis, just a long glove that covered (more or less) what was there. This information was never shared with others unless it is had to be, as in the intake procedures for the Citizen's Fitness program. Kroma did not like to be in situations calling for touch, so most of her difficulties with the program arose from not completing activities of a "partner" type, because she would somehow simply disappear when such activities began.

VIKTOR

Viktor was an eighth-grade boy. He was bigger and older than his school peers because he had been held back due to language difficulties when he first moved from Russia to the United States with an aunt and uncle several years ago. No one knew what had happened with his family of origin. Now he spoke both English and Russian very well. He showed leadership abilities, but not in a good way. He tended to act the bully, using his size and strength to intimidate others at school. He belonged to an out-of-school gang of older teens and young men who, in turn, bullied Viktor continually, reminding him he was not yet fully initiated. He could be seen as a developing danger except for one thing: Viktor adored the sport of soccer, and all of its heroes were his heroes. He attended Citizen's Fitness because he wanted to "bulk up and build up" so that as he moved to high school he would be able to try out, make the team, and be a star. The student leaders agreed that this scenario could actually happen. They decided to create strategies to use his motivation toward athletics to enable him to drop his negative gang affiliation and build positive relationships with school peers who might become his teammates.

AODI

Aodi was a 10-year-old boy who had moved from Nepal to the United States with his parents when he was a baby. His parents moved to escape religious persecution, and even today the family kept a very low profile and avoided questions about their background. The student leaders did not know the exact nature of the religious affiliation, but it seemed to share some characteristics with Buddhism. Aodi was extremely averse to hurting anything or anyone. He was very soft-spoken and would not even get close to a friendly bit of rough horseplay. His parents often indulged him with food, and Aodi was approaching the official markers for obesity. For all these reasons, he had become an easy target for behavior from peers and others ranging from well-intended teasing to outright bullying. He seemed to have no friendship group, and the student leaders found that his frequent absences from Citizen's Fitness were matched by his frequent truancy from school. His parents insisted he join Citizen's Fitness due to pressures from school administrators looking for some relief from his issues there. His parents were either unable or unwilling to require Aodi to fully commit.

AKI

The story of Aki, and his situation, seemed to the student leaders to be the most complex and challenging of all. Aki was a premed student at a nearby university. He was tall, very handsome, and athletic. His family was well-off. Aki's father was a South African doctor who had been travelling back and forth to the United States for decades due to his research and practice. Early on, he married an African American woman, Aki's mother, so Aki had dual citizenship. Aki wanted to work on AIDS, and had seen firsthand that HIV/AIDS education, when linked to sport programs, had had spectacular success in Africa, and that was the direction Aki wanted to take. His university was a "private/elite" that did not offer a kinesiology major or minor. Aki had struck bargains with several of the student leaders' professors to allow him to participate in some aspects of Citizen's Fitness and other such programs so he would know more about their operation. You might be wondering how this young man could possibly pose a "problem" within Citizen's Fitness. Aki was gay, and although the student leaders knew that LGBT people are frequently far from stereotypical in appearance, Aki, by choice, was the complete stereotypic gay man. His conversation, dress, and mannerisms were nonstop reminders of his heroes Freddy Mercury, several *Glee* characters, and the gay TV characters in *Modern Family*. In dual and group activities, he was being avoided and shunned by almost all other participants. Aki had one consistent workout partner (Julio), who was also on the "challenge list" for his own reasons. Aki was a treasure and not in need of any special work except that his approach was simply to ignore the cruel and rude behavior of the majority, and thus the issue was not being healed. No one was growing in the positive ways that valuing diversity can foster.

JULIO

Julio was of Cuban ethnicity. His father was a doctor but estranged from the family and resided in Cuba. Four generations of family were living in Julio's house, and several family members were likely undocumented. Julio was a high school dropout and worked nights, although he was attempting to complete a GED. Julio had somehow, perhaps through his friendship with Aki, learned that he most likely was transgender. Julio felt much more comfortable dressing, speaking, and interacting as a woman. He had gotten a job at a local 7-Eleven as "Julia" and looked/acted like a woman when there. At Citizen's Fitness, he was Julio, but was less comfortable as a person and not well accepted by the other participants. Only Aki and some of the women would partner with him for dual exercises.

The student leaders knew that individuals like Julio could, in certain circumstances, undergo reassignment surgery and hormone therapy so they could fully become a person of the other sex. Right now, however, Julio/Julia was managing a "double life" with only makeup, hair, and clothing changes to carry it off. The deception, silence, misunderstanding, and discomfort had a negative impact on the overall program. The student leaders, with the help of faculty and other professionals, were going to do something about it.

Strategies for Positive Inclusion

AWARENESS AND APPRECIATION

Although the student leaders knew each other from the Kinesiology Majors Club and classes they had taken together, they were formed as a team for their specialized areas of expertise. One of the benefits of a comprehensive kinesiology department is that the diverse aspects of movement activity are synthesized and unified in training and coursework. Renee was on the athletic training and adapted physical activity track. Antonio was in teacher professional preparation, and D'Andre was in applied exercise physiology. Mai was minoring in counseling, and her major emphasis in kinesiology was sport and exercise psychology. They utilized training from all of these areas to devise special facilitations for their challenge group (**FIGURE 16-5**).

Their first steps were already underway. As described earlier, the students were versed in what their professional training emphasized as *reflexivity* (Schinke, McGannon, Parham, & Lane, 2012). Past practices were to see one's students or clients as needy or "missing something" to be corrected by the leader. Coming from several fields, but especially cultural sport psychology, contemporary efforts are to view the client as a person with her or his own strengths to be utilized in skill building. The building process is conceptualized as a relationship-building process through which the leader and client both exchange and grow. In such a process, the diversity,

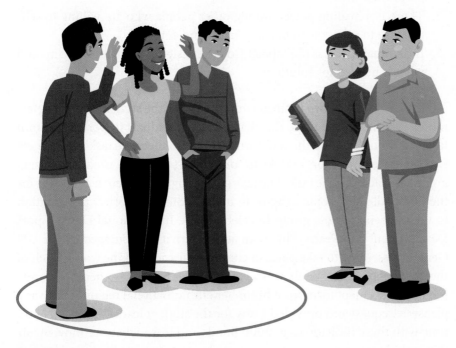

FIGURE 16-5 Practice inclusion.

or "difference," of the student/client is shared to enhance the leader's understanding and background knowledge. The "do what I say and I can fix you" approaches of the past may show a few immediate changes in the student/client, but research has demonstrated that the strength-based process leads to more lasting positive change and a stronger bond between the participant and leader (Giles, 2013). The student leaders (Fitness Fab Four) had worked for several weeks on developing *self-reflexive sensibility*; thus, they were well aware of how their own biases, values, and identities might impact on the Citizen's Fitness participants, and especially the challenge group (Schinke & Lidor, 2013; Schinke & Moore, 2011).

The Fitness Fab Four had experienced a *self-development and sport protocol* in one of their required sport psychology classes and believed that the protocol could be modified and put to work for the challenge group (Oglesby, Beane, Foster, & VanOst, 1985). The self-development model was based on the three principles of the **human potential approach**:

human potential approach
Methods of action based on presumptions of the human capacity to grow, solve problems, and collaborate productively.

1. Individuals are willing to aid others in coping with issues/crises similar to their own.
2. There is a healing power among other people who are willing to self-disclose to others with honesty, trust, and courage.
3. Individuals possess the capacity to have insight into their problems and what is needed for solutions.

Through one or two brainstorming sessions, the student leaders determined a strategy to engage the challenged individuals to perform a joint task that would require them to form a group to meet the task and to meet two times per week for 5 weeks to "organize" (become a problem-solving group) and achieve the task. The task created by the student leaders was for the five challenge people to agree to make a joint (and brief) presentation to the Citizen's Fitness group to celebrate the International Day of Sport Development and Peace. This is an actual activity encouraged by the UN General Assembly to take place in communities around the world. Each of the challenged participants was asked to work with the others to share a popular movement form from his or her ethnic/national region. This was a plausible request and provided a way for the student leaders to spend extra time with these individuals to build bonds and learn whatever movement/dance skill was going to be demonstrated.

The challenged group engaged in the following activities during the 5-week period:

- Made promises to each other in the context of keeping one's word, attending sessions, being honest in feedback, paying attention when other group members spoke, not placing blame, and not telling others their views were wrong.
- Wrote and shared a sport autobiography that recounted how each played from childhood to now.
- Through recounting memories, found their "child" (emotional, having fun), "parent" (caring for self and others), and "adult" (rational, factual self) in their expression of themselves in sport.
- Described the joys/highest highs known in sport, as well as the sorrows (lowest lows).
- Identified patterns they found themselves repeating in different situations, such as when winning, losing, feeling cheated, being bullied.
- Described how they intended to remain active throughout life.

Each session began with one of these activities. This was followed by a light warm-up. Then, at least two people each day would lead the group in the demonstration activity for the International Day. Kroma showed a Cambodian dance. Viktor demonstrated an incredible Russian Bear Dance. A few people volunteered to try the split leaps, and all did some of the easier moves. Aodi led a breathing meditation. Aki showed a South African children's game, and Julio presented a baseball (boys) and softball (girls) eye/hand coordination drill for skill building in fielding.

Many difficulties remain for these challenged individuals, but the participants bonded with each other, and there was a feeling of recognition and acceptance with all the Citizen's Fitness participants as well.

OTHER STRATEGIES FOR FOSTERING UNITY IN DIVERSITY

The case study in this chapter is based on some realistic, yet imaginary, characters. The types of contexts in which diversity creates possibilities for either growth or conflict are as numerous as our population numbers. Let us close this chapter with further examples of meeting diversity challenges.

The UN Sport for Development and Peace Working Group has identified eight situational contexts in which sport programming has been successful as a tool for progress (UN General Assembly, 2003):

1. *Individual development.* Teaching skills and self-efficacy to people who have experienced widespread devastation can aid in recovery. Often such cases are prominent internationally following war, tsunami, earthquake, or floods. Even in countries as developed as the United States, such programming has followed disasters such as Katrina or Hurricane Sandy.

2. *Health promotion and disease prevention programs.* Sport programs incorporating health promotion and disease prevention are utilized with AIDS education and polio prevention. The children and youth participate to enjoy the sport programs and are exposed to extensive supplemental information on the health concerns.

3. *Post-disaster trauma relief and life normalization.* Individuals with sport training and expertise lead sport or play groups (age/stage appropriate) to communicate the normalcy of life before the trauma. These activities are accompanied by guided imagery, meditation, progressive relaxation serving as anxiety-/stress-relieving life skills.

4. *Promotion of gender equity.* Assuring that the same opportunities (equipment, uniforms, coaching) are available for girls and boys is a powerful equity statement.

5. *Social integration and developing social capital.* In the United States and around the world, one of the most common problems is separation, and open conflict, between known social groups. Using sport to "melt down the walls" is perhaps most dramatically seen in the programs in the Middle East for Israeli and Palestinian youth.

6. *Peace building and conflict resolution.* Participation in games and sports with mixed and ever-changing teams so all participants are seen as colleagues and teammates; competitive games are little emphasized. Group exercises are utilized to develop conflict resolution steps that all help develop and agree on. These strategies are formally put into practice if any disagreements are evident.

7. *Economic development.* Governmental and nongovernmental agencies alike are just beginning to discover the innumerable ways that sport and active lifestyles contribute to economic empowerment. This is particularly

evident in regard to progress for girls and women. In many areas of the developing world, women's work is extremely limited to household tasks within the walls of the household. These customs reduce the potential economic contributions to family and community by half the population. An obvious step here in the United States is the growth in the number of girls going to college on athletic scholarships due to Title IX. Women's Sports Foundation data reveal the economic advantages that follow the 'scholarship to college graduation' process (Women's Sports Foundation, 2014.) In the developing world, girls and women perform a great deal of family's physical labor—farming, planting fields, gathering water. Being stronger and more fit is an obvious advantage for boys and girls alike. Additionally, being able to accomplish tasks collaboratively, even without great liking for one another, is just one more of the teamwork learnings from sport that translates to work and economic progress.

8. *Communication and social mobilizations.* Nationally, as well as worldwide, individual and community migrations occur by necessity and by choice. Sport and physical recreation opportunities can offer community building and integration opportunities even before spoken language is possible.

decompetition
Play and sport in which everyone "loses" except the very best players.

true competition
Play and sport in which it is understood that all participants "gain" in some way by having participated and given their best effort.

Nature of Competition

Another valuable source to explore when embarking on efforts to ease tensions and/or build more valuing of diversity is the work of Shields and Bredemeier (2011) in regard to the complex nature of competition. Competition often is viewed as "civilized battle"; someone wins, and everyone else loses. Shields and Bredemeier call this **decompetition** and maintain that it is actually the opposite of what they call **true competition**. See **TABLE 16-1** for a comparison of decompetition and true competition. If you are involved in sport/physical recreation programs with participants from marginalized groups as well as so-called dominant groups, decompetition will emphasize the socioeconomic and cultural barriers that already are firmly entrenched. Taking consistent, incremental, steps to teach true competition can positively impact individuals and communities.

STOP AND THINK

Make a list of words or phrases that come from violent or warlike situations and yet are frequently also used in sport situations (e.g., "My team beat you guys up," "We are going to annihilate you"). Share your list with a few peers and see if they are surprised by any of the words or phrases.

TABLE 16-1   Two Forms of Contesting

Constituent Categories	Competition (Striving *With*)	Decompetition (Striving *Against*)
Deep metaphor	Partnership	Battle or war
Goals	Learning and mastery	Domination/conquest
	Pursuit of excellence	Pursuit of superiority
Primary motivation	Intrinsic: Love of the game	Extrinsic: Use of the game
	Joy of accomplishment	Thrill (at opponent's expense)
View of opponent	Partner or enabler	Enemy/obstacle
View of rules	Rules = Imperfect guides to ethics of fairness and welfare	Rules = Partially tolerated restraints
View of officials	Officials as facilitators	Officials as opponents
Main locus of value	Process (contesting/playing)	Outcome (winning)
Emotional tone	Positive emotions predominate	Negative emotions predominate
	Play and seriousness in balance	Seriousness displaces play
Ideal contest	Closely matched competitors	Opponents outmatched
	Outcome determined late	Outcome determined early

Modified from D. Shields & B. Bredemeier. (2011). Why sportsmanship programs fail and what we can do about it. *Journal of Physical Education, Recreation and Dance, 82,* 7, 24–29.

Bullying

---

bullying
Unwanted, aggressive behavior involving a real or perceived power intolerance.

In situations in which there are individuals or groups who can be marginalized or singled out, conditions are ripe for **bullying** (**FIGURE 16-6**). Most all of us know about bullying because we have most likely experienced it. For people who are perceived as different (e.g., by weight, appearance, language, or dress), bullying can be nonstop, and has even driven individuals to take their own lives.

Researchers and educators are studying this phenomenon very seriously and have developed a complete definition of bullying as being "unwanted, aggressive behavior involving a real or perceived power intolerance" (stopbullying.gov, n.d.). The 2008–2009 School Crime Supplement put the figure for bullying for students in grades 6–12 at 28%. See **TABLE 16-2** to

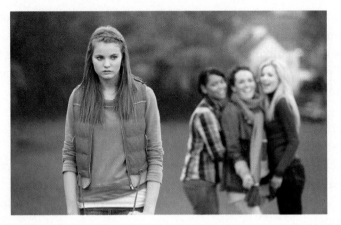

FIGURE 16-6   Bullying is unacceptable.
© iStockphoto/Thinkstock

TABLE 16-2   Forms of Bullying with Special Attention to Athletic Contexts

Bullying is any action that subjects another person to an outcome that is abusing, mistreating, degrading, humiliating, harassing, or intimidating, especially for the purpose of associating on a club or team or to control a younger/weaker person.

Bullying may include physical, mental, emotional, or psychological force or pressure to:
- Drink alcohol or do drugs.
- Ingest a substance.
- Perform an act that is illegal, perverse, or indecent.
- Tamper with or damage property.
- Restrict one's diet in unhealthy ways.
- Be deprived of sleep.
- Paddle, whip, or beat another person.
- Perform stunts.
- Be branded or tattooed.
- Engage in pranks such as stealing or painting property.
- Wear conspicuous or humiliating apparel.
- Engage in morally degrading games.
- Engage in sexual rituals or nudity.
- Perform required chants or rituals.
- Be exposed to deception or threats about losing team opportunity.

Modified from www.Safe4athletes.org.

view the many forms bullying or hazing can take. Athletic programs, athletic teams, sport recreation settings, and physical education classes are all contexts where bullying can, and does, occur. As professionals in training, you will need to be vigilant to make sure it does not occur on your watch. When it happens, here are some steps you can take:

1. Interfere. Stop the behavior on the spot.
2. Separate the parties involved.
3. Check for injury, and address any immediate medical concerns.
4. Be calm and respectful to all involved.
5. Do not interview the parties publically or demand an apology from anyone.
6. Get to the bottom of the problem and take action.

The stopbullying.gov website has a great deal of good advice on how to respond to bullying. In particular, it offers tips to those who have been bullied or feel they are likely targets:

- Talk to a trusted adult; let them know about what is happening.
- Don't get isolated at school or on the way home. Make sure others are around.
- Talk to adults or trusted friend about how to say "stop" and stand up for yourself.

Gender Diversity

gender diversity
The multiple possibilities of gender orientation.

It was not that long ago that **gender diversity**, in the sport context, primarily lent itself to discussions (occasionally heated) about inequitable treatment of females. That was back in the days of "two sexes" and a pink-and-blue world. In 2013, Facebook altered its format to offer users 12 broad categories, and 56 different options, to self-identify in regard to gender. **Box 16-1** provides a starting list of naming suggestions and definitions that we need to become comfortable with as professionals.

Box 16-1 Definitions and Terminology: A Word about Words

Language has immense power to shape our perceptions of others. Using accurate language can help to overcome many of the misperceptions associated with gender and transgender people. Although the vocabulary related to transgender people continues to evolve, the following are some working definitions and examples of frequently used (and misused) terms.

Biological/anatomical sex: The physical characteristics typically used to assign a person's gender at birth, such as chromosomes, hormones, and internal and external genitalia and reproductive organs. Given the potential variation in all of these, biological sex must be seen as a spectrum or range of possibilities rather than a binary set of two options.

Gender identity: One's inner concept of self as male or female or both or neither. One's gender identity can be the same or different than the gender assigned at birth. Most people become conscious of their gender identity between the ages 18 months and 3 years. Most people have a gender identity that matches their assigned gender at birth. For some, however, their gender identity is different from their assigned gender. Some of these individuals choose to live socially as the other gender and may also hormonally and/or surgically change their bodies to more fully express their gender identity. All people have gender identity, not just transgender people.

Gender expression: Refers to the ways in which people externally communicate their gender identity to others through behavior, clothing, hair style, voice, and other forms of presentation. Gender expression also works the other way, as people assign gender to others based on their appearance, mannerisms, and other gendered characteristics. Many transgender people seek to make their external appearance—their gender expression—congruent with their internal gender identity through clothing, pronouns, names, and, in some cases, hormones and surgical procedures. All people have gender expression, not just transgender people.

Transgender: Sometimes used as an umbrella term to describe anyone whose identity or behavior falls outside of stereotypical gender norms. More narrowly defined, it refers to an individual whose gender identity does not match their assigned birth gender. Being transgender does not imply any specific sexual orientation (attraction to people of a specific gender). Therefore, transgender people may additionally identify as straight, gay, lesbian, or bisexual.

(continued)

Sexual orientation: Refers to being romantically or sexually attracted to people of a specific gender. Our sexual orientation and our gender identity are separate, distinct parts of our overall identity. Although a child may not yet be aware of their sexual orientation, they usually have a strong sense of their gender identity.

Genderqueer: This term represents a blurring of the lines around gender identity and sexual orientation. Genderqueer individuals typically reject notions of static categories of gender and embrace a fluidity of gender identity and sexual orientation. This term is typically assigned an adult identifier and is not used in reference to preadolescent children.

Gender nonconforming/gender variant: Refers to individuals whose behaviors and/or interests fall outside what is considered typical for their assigned gender at birth. Someone who identifies as gender nonconforming is not necessarily transgender. To the contrary, many people who are not transgender do not conform to gender stereotypes in their appearance, clothing, physical characteristics, interests, or activities. No one should be treated differently or made to feel uncomfortable or unaccepted because they are gender nonconforming.

Gender fluidity: Gender fluidity conveys a wider, more flexible range of gender expression, with interests and behaviors that may even change from day to day. Gender fluid individuals do not feel confined by restrictive boundaries of stereotypical expectations of girls or boys.

Intersex: An estimated one in 2,000 babies are born with an "intersex" condition, or difference of sex development (DSD), which is defined as reproductive or sexual anatomy and/or chromosome pattern that does not seem to fit typical definitions of male or female. These conditions include androgen insensitivity syndrome, some forms of congenital adrenal hyperplasia, Klinefelter's syndrome, Turner's syndrome, hypospadias, and many others. People with intersex conditions generally identify as men or women, just as people without intersex conditions do. Having an intersex condition does not necessarily affect a person's gender identity.

Transition: The process by which a transgender individual lives consistently with his or her gender identity, and which may (but does not necessarily) include changing the person's body through hormones and/or surgical procedures. Transition can occur in three ways: social transition through changes in clothing, hairstyle, name, and/or pronouns; hormonal transition through the use of hormone "blockers" or cross hormones to promote gender-based body changes; and/or surgical transition in which an individual's body is modified through the addition or removal of gender-related physical traits. Based on current medical knowledge and practice, genital reconstructive surgery is not required in order to transition. Most transgender people in the United States do not have genital reconstructive surgery.

Transsexual: A person whose gender identity differs from the person's assigned gender at birth. Transsexual people do not identify with their birth-assigned genders and desire to live and be treated by others in a manner that is consistent with their gender identity. In addition to transitioning socially, transsexual people may also physically alter their bodies surgically and/or hormonally. This physical transition is a complicated, multistep process that may take years and may include, but is not limited to, cross-gender hormone therapy and a variety of surgical procedures. There is no cookie-cutter approach. The precise treatments required vary from person to person

Transphobia: Fear or hatred of transgender people. Transphobia is manifested in a number of ways, including violence, harassment, and discrimination.

Modified from Gender Spectrum. (n.d.). A word about words. Retrieved from http://www.genderspectrum.org/images/stories/Resources/Family/A_Word_About_Words.pdf

Researchers and scholars who focus on gender and sport use the words *binary* and *dichotomous* to describe how virtually all athletic competition is "sex segregated" (Krane, Barak, & Mann, 2012). The challenges for kinesiology professionals, who are called upon to engage in policy development, fair treatment, and creation of "safe spaces" for all, are enormous and will continue to grow rather than become more simple (Griffin & Carroll, 2010).

This chapter does not even begin to explore all the ramifications of this content area. Here and now, we just want to lay out the basics of the diversity issues that gender identity and expression can present the practicing professional. At birth, doctors, nurses, and parents view the infant and assign the infant's *sex*. The clothing, tastes, and behaviors of the developing child become a *self*, and gender identity is part of the self. The choices of the developing person, particularly around sex and gender, are referred to as *gender expression*.

Today, the majority of people in the United States probably still reflect a complete alignment of sex of assignment and gender identity. Increasingly, however, we are becoming aware of diversities in the area of sex and gender. Traditional notions of attraction and sexual experience suggest males' attraction to females and females' attraction to males. For males attracted fundamentally to males and females to females, the gender identity is described as *gay* (usually men, although the term can describe the class) or *lesbian*, respectively. These are matters of gender identity, and do not necessarily have any impact on the sex-segregated competition regulations of sport. Gender identity does come into focus in sport sociology/psychology when the social norms define sport itself as "masculine" and paint the active women athlete as "lesbian" even when she may not be. The turning of that particular stereotype has occupied a great deal of time in the professional world of kinesiology for the past three decades at least. The other side of the coin comes into play for men and boys who love, and are highly skilled at, grace/strength performance forms such as ballet, figure skating, and water ballet (Griffin & Carroll, 2010).

The material in this chapter makes clear that kinesiology programs are integral to the larger social systems in which they reside, including education, athletics, physical recreation, and rehabilitation. Whatever elements of racism or sexism reside in these larger systems, the chance of tainting or infecting the environment exists (Brooks & Althouse, 2013). We also point out that properly formulated and administered sport/movement programs can act as one small point of "inoculation" to bring growth-enhancing healthy active lifestyle to individuals and communities everywhere (**FIGURE 16-7**).

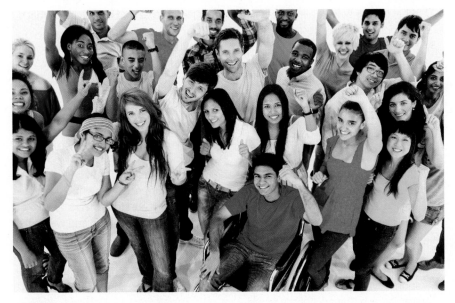

FIGURE 16-7   Sport welcomes everyone.
© Rawpixel.com/Shutterstock

CHAPTER SUMMARY

In this chapter, we reviewed case study of an initiative (Citizen's Fitness) that had the goal of building more enhanced and peaceful communities. The phenomenon of social rarity was described, as well as its effects on group function. You were asked to make distinctions between decompetition and true competition. Bullying was discussed, including how it can occur in sport settings and how we can act to stop it. We also took a serious look at recent changes in our understandings of gender diversity in sport.

DISCUSSION QUESTIONS

1. Identify and describe a situation you faced, or observed, in which a person was motivated to achieve a goal but all the odds seemed to be stacked against him or her. Did any of the obstacles seem to be based on economics, race or ethnicity, or gender? Share your experience with others.

2. What do you believe are the most important factors that lead to bullying? What do you believe are the best steps to stop bullying?

3. Do you feel that sport is a successful way to reduce conflict and build social cohesion in communities around the world? Give reasons to support your view. What barriers exist to having this happen more successfully?

4. Describe to a partner or small group, the worst case of bullying you ever witnessed. How did people handle the situation? Was the leadership flawed or appropriate?

5. Identify and describe to others, a situation where you felt marginalized or ignored. How did it feel? What did others say or do that worsened these feelings? What, if anything, was done or said to allow you to feel included?

6. In a small group, develop a list of characteristics that lead to situations in which people feel excluded. How common are these occurrences? Describe the social, emotional, and financial costs of such exclusions. What are steps that can be taken, especially by professionals, to allow all individuals to feel included and welcome?

7. What career applications can you see for a kinesiology major who wants to specialize in 'sport development', 'peace-building' and/or conflict resolution? Identify any places in the world where you personally would like to become involved in sport development work. Google or use other sources to find organizations that specialize in that area of the world.

REFERENCES

Bauer, P., Dow, G., & Hertsgaard, L. (1995). Effects of prototypicality on categorization in 1- to 2-year-olds: Getting down to basics. *Cognitive Development*, *10*, 43–68.

Brooks, D., & Althouse, R. (2013). *Racism in collegiate athletics* (3rd ed.). Morgantown, WV: Fitness Information Technology.

Gender Spectrum. (n.d.). A word about words. Retrieved from http://www.gender-spectrum.org/images/stories/Resources/Family/A_Word_About_Words.pdf

Giles, A. (2013). It takes several northern communities to raise a reflexive and effective sport researcher. In R. Schinke & R. Lidor (Eds.), *Case studies in sport development: Contemporary stories promoting health, peace and social justice* (pp. 119–134). Morgantown, WV: Fitness Information Technology.

Griffin, P., & Carroll, H. (2010). *On the team: Equal opportunity for transgender student athletes*. East Meadow, NY: Women's Sports Foundation.

International Olympic Committee. (2013, August 23). UN creates International Day of Sport for Development and Peace. Retrieved from https://www.olympic.org/news/un-creates-international-day-of-sport-for-development-and-peace

James, William. (1890) *Principles of psychology*. New York: Henry Holt & Co.

Krane, V., Barak, K., & Mann, M. (2012). Broken binaries and transgender athletes: Challenging sex and gender in sports. In G. Cunningham (Ed.). *Sexual orientation and gender identity in sport* (pp. 13–22). College Station, TX: Center for Sport Management Research and Education.

Oglesby, C., Beane, L., Folzer, S., & VanOst, L. (1985). Helping injured athletes cope. In J. Puhl, C. Brown, & R. Voy (Eds.). *Sport science perspectives for women* (pp. 59–66) Champaign, IL: Human Kinetics.

Schinke, R., & Hanrahan, S. (2009). *Cultural sport psychology*. Champaign, IL: Human Kinetics.

Schinke, R., & Lidor, R. (2013). *Case studies in sport development: Contemporary stories promoting health, peace, and social justice*. Morgantown, WV: Fitness Information Technology.

Schinke, R., McGannon, K., Parham, W. D., & Lane, A. (2012). Toward cultural sensitivity: strategies for self-reflexive sport psychology practice. *Quest, 64*, 34–46.

Schinke, R., & Moore, Z. (2011). Culturally informed sport psychology: Introduction to the special issue. *Journal of Clinical Sport Psychology, 5*, 283–294.

Shields, D., & Bredemeier, B. (2011). Why sportsmanship programs fail and what we can do about it. *Journal of Physical Education, Recreation and Dance, 82*, 7, 24–29.

Starr, K. (2013, November). *Safe 4 Athletes Handbook*. Retrieved from http://www.safe4athletes.org

Stein, B. (1995). *A tale of 'O': A training tool on managing diversity*. Cambridge, MA: Goodmeasure, Inc.

stopbullying.gov. (n.d.). Bullying definition. Retrieved from http://www.stopbullying.gov/what-is-bullying/definition/index.html (This is a Federal Government website managed by Health and Human Services with content provided on a continuing basis by theStopBullying.gov Editorial Board)

UN General Assembly. (2003). Retrieved from www.un.org/ga

UN News Centre. (2014). Sports set a guiding light for international relations to follow, Ban tells Winter Olympics. Retrieved from http://www.un.org/apps/news/story.asp?NewsID=47101#.V4U9aaKfWCg

Working Group on Woman and Human Rights. (2001). Background briefing on intersectionality. Retrieved from http://www.cwgl.rutgers.edu/globalcenter/policy/bkgdbrfintersec.htmc

CHAPTER 17

Promoting Excellence

DOUGLAS W. McLAUGHLIN

LEARNING OBJECTIVES

1. Describe the direct and indirect factors that contribute to achieving excellence.
2. Recognize the role others play, directly or indirectly, in personal achievement.
3. Describe the barriers, both personal and societal, that inhibit excellence.
4. Explain how the subdisciplines of kinesiology make important contributions to achieving excellence.
5. Explain the difference between absolute and relative excellence.
6. Describe how pursuing excellence can contribute to meaningful physical activity experiences.

KEY TERMS

absolute excellence
advocacy
application
community
develop
different treatment

diversity
encouragement and support
give back
honor
leadership
marginalization

membership   role model
personal excellence   sacrifices
priority   shared excellence
relative excellence   transition

Case Study: Personal and Shared Excellence

In anticipation of her enshrinement in her state's track and field hall of fame, Melissa Burt took some time to reflect on her career. Her inclusion in the hall of fame was not a given. As a runner, she never won a championship at any level. As a coach, she never led a championship team. As a contributor, she never hosted the largest events or brought the most attention to the sport. But her running community deemed her worthy of its greatest honor. She was proud and pleased when she learned of her election. However, she questioned how the achievements in her life devoted to running rose to the level of excellence deserving of such honor. Maybe her peers overrated her running career. Maybe she misunderstood what it means to be excellent. Perhaps it is important to reexamine the merits of her career.

Foundations for Excellence

Melissa was born with congenital talipes equinovarus, often referred to as *clubfoot*, in both feet. As an infant, Melissa endured a series of casts. As a toddler, she wore a series of braces and had to complete numerous physical therapy sessions. Melissa's only recollection of her condition was a vague memory of a brace she wore at night during her first years of school. But Melissa's mother always made a point to remind Melissa about the team of nurses, doctors, and therapists that cared for her and allowed her to enjoy running so much. Her dad always told a story of how Melissa's last therapist thought that Melissa was trying to run out of her braces and was encouraged that it meant that she was destined to have a physically active life. If only the therapist knew that she would one day be a hall-of-fame runner.

Upon reflection, Melissa realized that there were many people who had played key roles in her ability to have a successful career. In particular, there were the people she had never met or could not remember meeting because she was too young who had enabled her to live an active life. She never met the medical researchers and biomechanists who developed the treatments, casting methods, and braces that she used. Nor could she remember the doctors who set the casts or the therapists who provided therapeutic massage. If she had been born in an earlier time, she might never have been able to walk normally. But just like most children born with this condition today, she recovered to such a degree that she never thought of herself as being any different from other children. Only now did she realize that it was the efforts of many other people who created the conditions that allowed her to experience the possibility of excellence in her pursuit of running.

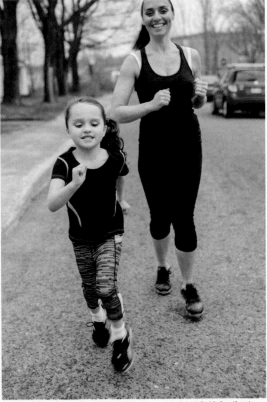

© Louis-Paul St-Onge/Getty Images

When Melissa was 7 years old, she entered her first 5K because she wanted to be like her mother. As the only runner in her age group, she won a first-place trophy. Maybe it was good that she did not know any better, because with that trophy Melissa was hooked. Her mother said that in all her years of running she had never won a trophy and that she could not be prouder of Melissa. From that point on, Melissa's mother encouraged her running ambitions, supported her running, and transported her to races all over the state until she left for college. Even when Melissa was in college, she often traveled to Melissa's meets to support her. Part of Melissa's motivation to run was that it made her mother happy, and it made Melissa happy that her mother was proud of her accomplishments. But she never felt any pressure from her mother. Instead, her mother always tried to make sure that Melissa enjoyed running. Her mother always said that if running wasn't enjoyable, it was time to do something else. All the way through high school Melissa never stopped enjoying running and never wanted to stop competing.

In middle school, Melissa's physical education teacher, Ms. Fry, noticed her passion for running. Ms. Fry had encouraged and supported a number of students over the years to pursue a variety of sports. During winter months when running outdoors was problematic, Ms. Fry would open up the gym

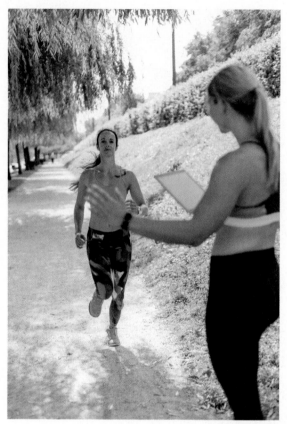

© lovro77/Getty Images

early in the morning so students could train on the indoor track or in the gym. Sometimes she helped develop training programs. She also brought coaches from the high school to encourage athletes to pursue athletics and runners from the community to share their passion for running. At the time, Melissa never knew that students from her middle school had the highest participation rate in athletics among the four middle schools feeding into the local high school. Melissa did not realize at the time that Ms. Fry freely gave her time to make the indoor track available to her and her friends. All Melissa knew was that Ms. Fry was a teacher who cared about the same things she cared about and made a point to share that passion beyond class time.

Ms. Fry introduced Melissa to Coach Kelly in the eighth grade. When Melissa started high school, it was a bit overwhelming because there were so many students and the building was so large that it was intimidating. She was so happy at the end of the day to see a familiar face at cross-country practice. Despite her intense demeanor, Coach Kelly became Melissa's mentor over the next 4 years. Other than her mother, no woman had a bigger impact in influencing the person Melissa would become. Not only did Coach Kelly encourage Melissa to become a better runner, but she also helped Melissa become a leader on the cross-country and track and field teams. Coach Kelly planted the seed in Melissa's mind that she should be thinking about college. Even though her mother had mentioned it as a goal for her, Coach Kelly gave Melissa the confidence she needed to become the first member of her family to attend college.

The **encouragement and support** from her mother, Ms. Fry, and Coach Kelly were just three prominent examples of women who encouraged and supported her running. Thinking back, Melissa realized that she would never have accomplished as much as she had if it hadn't been for their love and support.

encouragement and support
The acts of providing assistance, stimulating development, and promoting confidence on behalf of others in the attainment of a goal.

Sacrificing for Excellence

Melissa enjoyed her daily routine and felt that her habits helped her to **develop** as a runner. Starting in ninth grade, she would wake up at 5:30 a.m. every day to get a run in. Sometimes it was a hard training run; other times it was a short recovery run. But for Melissa, it meant getting her day started on the right track. The first thing she did every day was make a concerted effort to better herself. Running was her first **priority**. Although she often would run again later in the day, that morning run meant that she had taken care of her first priority. She typically finished her daily run, even her long runs, before most of her friends woke up in the morning. Melissa could tackle the rest of the day with the assurance that she had accomplished something important. It oriented and centered her.

Despite the value that she put on her morning run, it often was a source of confusion and ridicule. Melissa would not stay up late because it would negatively impact her morning run. Some of her friends made fun of her because she would not stay out late on the weekends. But her "quirky" habits were also endearing. Her friends knew that she had a passion, and even when they didn't understand why she made the decisions she did or why she cared so much about running, they supported her.

Family vacations were also impacted by Melissa's routine. When they went somewhere that required a stay in a hotel, it was important to Melissa that they stayed at a hotel in a location from which she could safely run. Although it was an inconvenience and sometimes meant spending more money, the family made that commitment to Melissa's pursuit of running.

Family meals were also impacted. When Melissa was younger, family meals were often thrown together at the last minute. It was rare that fresh fruits and vegetables were incorporated into her daily diet. But as Melissa's training intensified, she realized that she needed better fuel. With her encouragement, Melissa's parents made an effort to buy healthier foods and prepare healthier meals.

Melissa recognized that many **sacrifices** were made in her pursuit of running faster. In some ways they did not seem like sacrifices at all because they were in pursuit of her dream of running faster, but these sacrifices impacted

STOP AND THINK

Excellence requires important contributions, directly and indirectly, from other people that set the foundation for achieving excellence.

- Can you identify ways in which professionals in kinesiology can encourage and support people's pursuit of excellence in physical activity?

- Can you identify other factors that contribute to the pursuit of excellence in physical activity?

develop
The process of growth and maturation through directed efforts.

priority
That thing that takes precedence and is deemed more important than other tasks or activities.

sacrifices
Those things that are deferred or abandoned in order to pursue one's own priorities or to support another person's priorities.

her relationships with others. If her friends and family had not understood her passion for running, then perhaps they would not have been as supportive. But in the end, they helped reinforce her own belief that the sacrifices she made to better herself were worth it.

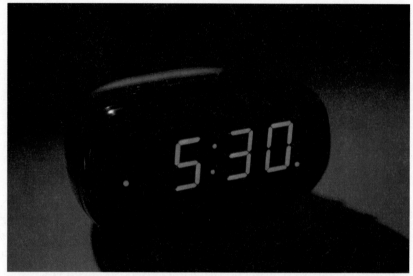

© Hurst Photo/Shutterstock

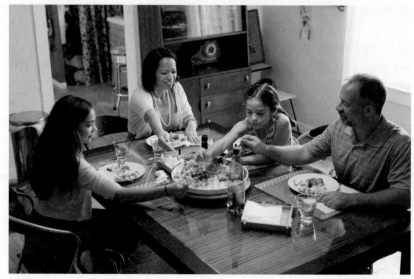

© Image Source / Alamy Stock Photo

Models of Excellence

One of Melissa's favorite events in high school was her local running club's annual women's summer run. It began in 1985, the year after the 1984 Olympics in Los Angeles. The local summer run was a 5K, but the women who started it were inspired by Joan Benoit's gold-medal performance in the marathon. Despite the marathon being the signature event of the first modern Olympics, it was not until 1984 that women were able to compete in the marathon at the Olympics. Melissa enjoyed hearing the organizers tell stories about how they felt when they watched Joan Benoit run into the stadium and the crowd roared in celebration. To them, it was the culmination of many significant achievements in women's sports. Title IX was important in creating the conditions for equality in sport, and Billy Jean King beating Bobby Riggs in the Battle of the Sexes in 1973 was a symbolic event that validated women's participation in sport, but for them it was Joan Benoit's accomplishment that hit home. Perhaps it was because it was the first time they felt they had a woman hero who was a widely recognized long-distance runner. Joan Benoit represented access to the largest sporting mega event, and her accomplishments represented the triumph of fairness over a history of **marginalization**.

Inspired by the performance of Joan Benoit, a group of women in Melissa's community decided that they wanted to run, too. They started running in the fall of 1984. By the spring of 1985, they decided that they wanted to share their new passion with more women. With the help of the local running club, they began to plan a women's run on the first Sunday in August 1985. Their **advocacy** efforts related to promoting running and organizing events for women had a significant impact on the local running community. In 1985, the **membership** of the local running club was 85% male, and the leadership of the club was almost exclusively men. By the time Melissa was a senior in high school, the membership and **leadership** of the running club were almost 50% women. Furthermore, the organizers wanted a race exclusively for women in 1985 to generate interest and participation. Within 10 years, the women's summer run was the club's largest race, and the organizers decided that the increased participation of women runners was so substantial in their community that they could now open the women's run for everyone. After all, they didn't want to exclude the men for as long a time as the men had excluded them.

marginalization
Social disadvantages that result in a group being in a powerless or unimportant position.

advocacy
The act of supporting a cause.

membership
The state of being included in a group or organization.

leadership
The people who provide guidance and direction for an organization.

Melissa was inspired by the organizers' tales of watching Joan Benoit, of being motivated to run, of wanting to share their passion, of organizing the first races, and of opening the race to all runners. While Joan Benoit was a hero and inspiration to Melissa, it was the organizers who were truly her role models. These women were part of her extended running family. Both Ms. Fry and Coach Kelly were part of the early runs. Joan Benoit could never be a **role model** to Melissa in the way that the local organizers were because she would never impact Melissa's running in the same concrete ways as the organizers who provided daily reminders of what a life devoted to running

role model
A person whose behavior and actions in a given context serve as an example for other people.

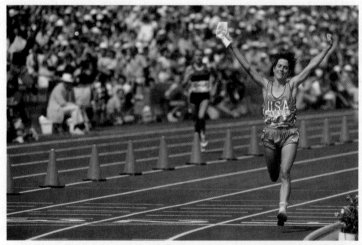

© PCN Photography / Alamy Stock Photo

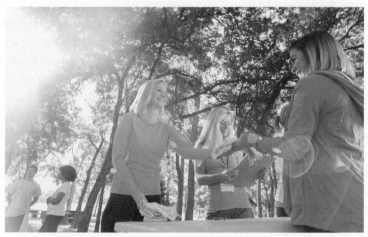

© Steve Debenport/Getty Images

was all about. It was the organizers who brought a generation of women to running, gave them meaningful races,
and educated them on the joys of running. When Melissa
thought about her role models, she couldn't help but think
about how the organizers of the summer run played a piv-
otal role in her life in a direct way. These were women who
lived in her neighborhood and gave so much of themselves
to her and her fellow runners.

Barriers to Excellence

As a sophomore, Melissa regularly ran with a senior named
Alisa who was a strong runner. At the cross-country state
championships, Alisa finished second. That was expected,
because Alisa and a runner from the rival high school had
been first and second the previous year and both had scholarships to elite
Division I track and field programs. Running with Alisa resulted in great
improvements in Melissa's times. Melissa finished eighth at the state meet
as a sophomore. She was ecstatic. She felt like she owed it all to Alisa, who
had taught her to train harder and develop the mental confidence to push
through a wall that seemingly held her back. She was the top nonsenior fin-
isher and was identified as a favorite to win states as a junior.

Unfortunately, the summer before her junior year Melissa tore her ante-
rior cruciate ligament (ACL) while waterskiing. She was so mad at herself.
She would need surgery and miss the entire cross-country season. Much
of the time she had spent running was now spent in physical therapy. She
worked very hard to progress as quickly as she could, but one of the therapists regularly tried to have her take it easy. She noticed this same therapist
often pushed a male athlete from her school much harder. She was frustrated and angry that she was being treated differently because she was a
girl. After a couple weeks, she gained the courage to confront the therapist.
She wanted to know why she received **different treatment** because she was
a girl. The therapist paused to collect his thoughts.

First, he did confide that, historically, therapeutic treatment for female
athletes was very different than that for male athletes. Women were often
held back in an effort to protect them. Men were often encouraged to push
through an injury despite the threat of further injury. But he noted that

different treatment
People being treated in dissimilar ways. If there is no relevant reason for the different treatment, then it is discrimination.

therapy has come a long way since then, and that he didn't think he was guilty of intentional or implicit bias. In other words, he didn't treat Melissa and her male counterpart differently because of their genders, and he didn't unwittingly treat them differently.

Rather, he treated them differently based on valid reasoning. He explained that while they both had similar knee injuries, Melissa had a more severe injury than her male counterpart. Given the difference in severity, they had different restrictions. Also, Melissa was not as far into her treatment plan compared to her male counterpart, so it would be a few more weeks before she started doing some more aggressive exercises. For now, it was important to not push herself too quickly or she might not make a full recovery. The most important difference, her therapist confided, was that Melissa always did more than what was asked of her, which led him to be cautious in determining the appropriate workload because he didn't want her to overdo it. He encouraged Melissa to do no more than 100% of what was asked of her. Soon enough, he promised, her workload would increase to levels similar to that of her male counterpart. Finally, he said that some people do not do 100% of what is asked of them or give 100% effort. In those cases, he needs to make more of an effort to get less-motivated people to work as hard as Melissa does on her own. For Melissa, he has to stress patience to ensure a full recovery, whereas for others he has to stress more effort to ensure full recovery.

Although Melissa appreciated his explanation, she was still frustrated with the rehabilitation process. It was hard to be a patient and have patience when all she wanted to do was run. Missing cross country was bad enough, but the recovery process was taking so long that she felt she would lose the outdoor season in spring, too. Her therapist said that she probably wouldn't be fully ready for the spring, that by the time she could start running again she wouldn't be able to get enough miles in to be as competitive as she was as a sophomore. He encouraged her to start thinking about getting ready for her senior year of cross country. If she could make a full recovery and get more training in, then she could reclaim her place as one of the favorites at states.

Melissa knew what she wanted. Having her therapy contextualized into her goals was helpful. Reinvigorated? That might be an exaggeration, but it helped refocus her efforts and take good care of herself so that she could resume her chase of a state title her senior year.

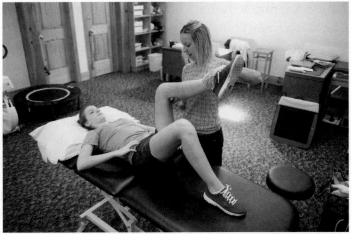

© Blend Images / Alamy Stock Photo

The Contribution of Kinesiology to Excellence

Melissa was able to return to the cross-country team for her senior year, but she suffered from nagging minor injuries unrelated to her prior injury. She tweaked her hamstring. She twisted her ankle. Because of these setbacks, she wasn't able to train as consistently and vigorously as she wanted. Yet she still finished sixth at states. Coach Kelly was so proud of her accomplishments given all that Melissa had to fight through. Melissa's mother cried tears of joy for the same reason. Ms. Fry called to congratulate her. However, Melissa couldn't help but feel disappointed, knowing that she hadn't lived up to her potential. She lost her confidence and, as a result, her outdoor season was a disappointment.

Melissa had several scholarship offers to top programs across the country, but she didn't feel worthy of any them. She considered joining her friend Alisa, who had just transferred to a regional university that was closer to home. The university's cross-country team competed at a Division II level, but was really not much more than a club team. Despite others counseling her that she had better opportunities, she turned them all down in the hopes of capturing the magic she felt when she ran with Alisa as a sophomore.

Melissa couldn't help but feel that she had made the right choice. Running with Alisa was challenging, but it also made

STOP AND THINK

- Identify how professionals in kinesiology can provide treatment and care for people in ways that promote excellence.

- Identify ways bias exists in the treatment and care of people.

- When treating people, what obligations do we have to know people's goals and interests when we design and implement their treatment plans?

running enjoyable again. It was hard, but easy hard because she enjoyed pushing through to reach new limits. That was in stark contrast to how she felt her senior year. She never understood why Alisa left an elite program, but she was glad to be back with her former running partner.

College presented its own challenges. As the first person in her family to attend college, she didn't always know what to expect from school or feel that her family fully supported her. In one sense, she felt supported knowing that her parents wanted her to do well in college, but she didn't think her parents quite understood the challenges she faced or knew how to provide the actual support she needed. One of her hardest challenges was choosing a major. Should she pick a major she was interested in or one that would prepare her for a high-paying job? She didn't know, and felt like her parents couldn't provide good guidance. Because running was what she cared about the most, she decided to major in kinesiology in the hopes that it would give her information to improve her running.

application
The use of one's knowledge and skills in a practical setting.

Melissa couldn't help but interpret every class as pertaining to running. All the new knowledge she gained from her classes had some **application** to her performance. Sport psychology was the psychology of running. Exercise physiology was the physiology of running. Sport philosophy was the philosophy of running. Biomechanics was the biomechanics of running. In each class, she identified strategies and knowledge that she could take directly to her training. In some ways, her major was more of a "coach" to her than the cross-country coach, who was nothing more than a faculty advisor who ran cross country almost 30 years ago. He could provide encouragement, but lacked the knowledge to fully enhance her performance so she could fulfill her potential. If she didn't have Alisa or her major, then she probably wouldn't have improved as a collegiate runner.

STOP AND THINK

- Identify how the subdisciplines of kinesiology can contribute to improved running experiences and promote excellence.

- How can the different subdisciplines be integrated into Melissa's holistic experience of running?

Setbacks and Challenges

Alisa competed as a fifth-year senior during Melissa's junior year. One of the elite runners from their local running club had taken on the role of advisor to the cross-country team. Despite a lack of support from the university, the team finished 11th at the Division II cross-country championships based primarily on the performances of Alisa and Melissa, who both earned All-American honors. For Alisa, it was the end of her competitive running career, but she stuck around town as a training partner for Melissa. For Melissa, now a much stronger runner than Alisa, it was the springboard for her senior season.

The university took notice of their performances and attempted to capitalize on their success. They searched for a coach with more technical expertise. The team lobbied for the advisor from the running club, but the university brought in someone who had more professional coaching experience and was very ambitious. As it turned out, the coach was a little too ambitious. The coach brought some athletes with her. When the team performed well at the beginning of the season, other teams took notice. Some questions and rumors in the running community were raised. An investigation was opened. Midway through her senior season, Melissa's cross-country team was put on indefinite suspension for competing with ineligible athletes. The coach claimed it was an honest mistake despite evidence to the contrary. Based on her early season performance, Melissa was once again a favorite to win a championship, but this time it was the actions of others that prevented her from competing.

Although Melissa was deeply disappointed, it was unlike when she was injured in high school in an important way—she could still run. Now she could take that negative energy and spin it into positive energy through her running. Melissa said she ran harder and meaner during that year because she was more driven than ever before. When she competed in a few regional races, she performed quite well. The running community took notice. Without any more collegiate eligibility, she was offered a sponsorship followed by additional endorsement deals. She was on her way to becoming a professional runner, something she never considered possible for herself. She started running 10K events, but gradually increased her training to compete in longer events. People were telling her that she could become the next great American marathoner.

The life of a professional runner is not glamorous. It affords runners the time to run and keeps them in shoes. There are no luxuries, unless you've won Olympic medals. Even Olympic medals don't guarantee riches. Melissa devoted her life to her training not for riches, but because she truly

STOP AND THINK

- Why do people become so obsessed with winning that they resort to immoral actions?

- How is the pursuit of excellence degraded when it is pursued in immoral ways?

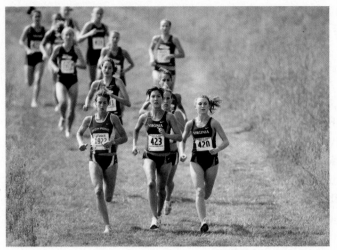

© Jason O. Watson (Sports) / Alamy Stock Photo

loved running. Just 2 years out of college, Melissa finished second at the U.S. national championships in the 10K, and earned the right to represent the United States at the Olympics. She wasn't a favorite to medal, but some considered her a potential dark horse. Melissa considered her training leading up to the Olympic Games as unprecedented and began to believe that maybe she could win a medal.

At the Olympics, she had a disappointing finish. She thought it was largely due to her inexperience at major international competitions. After the Olympics, she gave herself a week to feel bad about her experience. She then focused on the fact that she was an Olympian; maybe not a champion, but still an Olympian. No one could ever take that from her. And so a week after the Olympics was over she began training and designing a plan that would build up her international experience as she prepared for the next Olympics when she would be in her prime.

Just 2 weeks later, she was hit by a car during a training run. It wasn't anything catastrophic. She was knocked down, and the accident seemed relatively minor in the moment. There was no gushing blood or broken bones. She got up, bushed herself off, and ran off. No big deal.

The next morning she woke up sore. She stretched more than usual and did a longer warm-up, but something just didn't feel right. Even though she felt something wasn't right, she wasn't ready to acknowledge that there might be a problem. She put off seeing a doctor. However, after another 2 weeks passed without improvement she realized that she would have to see her doctor. The news wasn't all bad. She would be able to live a long and productive life, but as a runner the news could not have been worse. The accident hadn't caused the problem, but actually led to it being revealed. She had a form of cancer that had a high recovery rate, especially because they diagnosed it at an early stage, but the surgery and resulting treatments would essentially bring her competitive running career to an end. She considered for a day or two trying to keep running and ignore the diagnosis, but running had become too painful. And her family and friends convinced her that there was life after competitive running.

Melissa appreciated all the love and support she received. A popular sports media network profiled her and fans showered her with support. In August, the women's run that had been inspired by Joan Benoit was cobranded to recognize Melissa. But Melissa felt betrayed. She couldn't run away from this frustration like she did with the disappointment in college. Despite all the support she received from the running community, she felt abandoned by running itself. She didn't know what to make of her life if she wasn't a runner. She never dreamed that she would be a professional runner until the moment it happened, but somehow she didn't have any alternative plan for what to do with her life now that she wasn't a competitive runner.

According to her doctors, Melissa made a full recovery. Such a claim only made Melissa angry because for her the only meaningful sense of a full recovery was one that included a path back to the Olympic Games. Despite being cleared to run, Melissa just wasn't interested in running. In fact, for the first time since she started wearing shoes, she didn't own a pair of running shoes. She still saw many friends from the running club, but she wasn't involved in the club, their events, or running.

Almost 3 years had passed when Melissa got a call from one of the organizers of the women's run. She had been diagnosed with cancer and knew that Melissa was a survivor. It didn't matter that it was a different type of cancer with a very different type of survival rate; the woman needed to reach out to someone she knew who had gone through it. Melissa met with the woman on a regular basis and sometimes even took her to her treatments. Summer arrived and the woman continued her fight, but she wasn't strong enough to participate in the women's run. She had helped to organize and had participated in every women's run, but this year she was unable to. She asked Melissa if she would be willing to run for her. Melissa didn't want to run because she felt so disappointed by running so many times before, but the debt she owed this woman far exceeded her disappointment in running. Believing it was more important to **honor** her friend, Melissa reluctantly agreed to run in an organized running event for the first time since she competed in the Olympic Games.

Melissa was nervous. This was the biggest running event in her running **community**, and she was a former Olympic athlete and local running

honor
To respect and hold another person in high regard; acting in a manner that reflects your appreciation of another person.

community
A group of people with a shared interest.

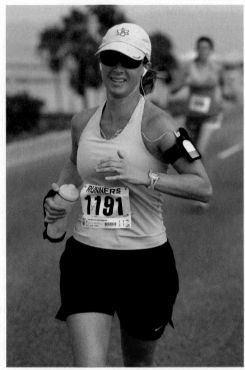

© Peter Weber/Shutterstock

celebrity. She decided to drive across state lines in order to compete in a small 5K race. Competing under an assumed name, she came in second in her division. The trophy only made her angry, because she considered her finishing time pathetic given her prior world-class abilities. Making the **transition** to life after competitive sport was difficult, but at least she had the confidence that she could complete the women's run. It then dawned on her that there might be other forms of excellence associated with running that she hadn't considered before.

transition
A period of change that often requires support and education.

Meaning and Relative Excellence

Melissa ran the women's run. Well, she jogged it with children who were approximately the same age as she was when she first ran. The children didn't know who she was or what she had or hadn't accomplished. All they seemed to care about was the joy of running. They had a playful attitude that she recognized but had not experienced for a long time. After she finished the race, she went to meet up with the race organizer who asked her to run. As she approached her, the woman smiled. All Melissa could do was say, "Thank you!" She finally had a sense of what she needed to do. It was now Melissa's turn to be an organizer and role model and educator and coach and supporter. It was Melissa's turn to **give back** to the community of runners that had given her so much.

Given her status as an Olympian, she was able to encourage running clubs across the country to promote and organize women's runs. She also worked to promote **diversity** in the running clubs, both in membership and leadership, not only in terms of gender, but also in terms of the members of the community who participated. Everybody runs, and therefore everybody should have fun races to run in and a community that fosters a sense of belonging by welcoming all runners. Maybe no single accomplishment in Melissa's life was deserving of hall-of-fame enshrinement, but if she were to identify what she is most proud of it would be how she promoted running to people who had never before belonged to running communities. Although she could not pursue the **absolute excellence** of being an Olympic champion, she could still help others experience **relative excellence**. She continues to devote her time and energies to helping running clubs engage all members of their community so that the running clubs more accurately represent the larger community to which they belong.

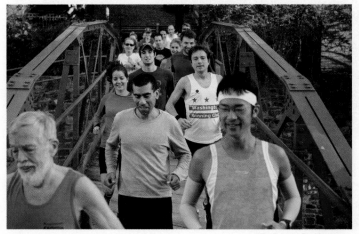

© The Washington Post / Getty Images

give back
Directing one's efforts and resources to an activity or organization that one has previously benefitted from.

diversity
The abilities, interests, and characteristics that differentiate people from one another.

absolute excellence
The condition of being the best compared to all others in a given activity, such as elite sport.

relative excellence
The state of being more excellent in a given, limited context in a given activity, such as recreational sport.

STOP AND THINK

Most of Melissa's life in running was in pursuit of absolute excellence, but at the end it turns toward promoting relative excellence. In what ways can we, as professionals in kinesiology, promote relative excellence and encourage meaningful relationships in and through physical activity?

Excellence as an Unending Quest

On the eve of her induction into the state hall of fame, Melissa is nervous. She realizes that she has demonstrated excellence in her running life in a myriad of ways (Anderson, 2001). Although she never won a championship at any level, she did achieve great success as an All-American collegiate runner and an Olympic athlete. Although those achievements were certainly a form of excellence, she also excelled in the process of devoting her life to running. In one sense, that refers to the many running clubs that have adopted her

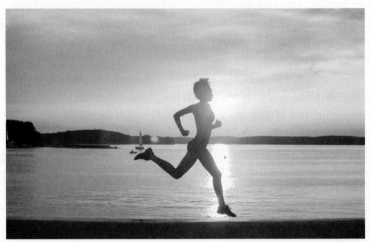

© uzhursky/Shutterstock

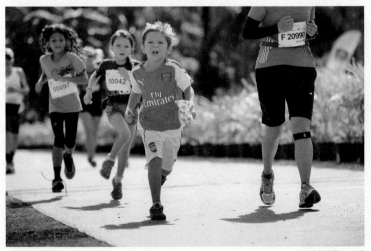

© mooinblack/Shutterstock

training methods or the many All-American and international runners she has consulted with. But in an equally important sense, it refers to the thousands of children she has run with over the past few years as she has become an ambassador for running, modeling to them how running can be a joyful experience. Her career spans the range of excellence from the absolute sense of winning to the relative sense of experiencing running as a meaningful practice.

Melissa has also recognized how excellence can be both **personal** and **shared**. This may reflect her biggest transformation, where she went from being supported in her running to supporting others in their running. Through all the transitions, Melissa has learned that excellence is not a fixed thing. It can be based upon many different factors, including ability, skill level, commitment, interest, age, and gender.

> **STOP AND THINK**
>
> Write an acceptance speech for Melissa that addresses how excellence and meaning have informed her hall-of-fame running career. Or, write an acceptance speech for yourself for a hall of fame of kinesiology (or pick a specific activity or profession).

personal excellence
The pursuit of excellence through achieving one's highest potential.

shared excellence
The pursuit of excellence through the collective efforts of partners toward a common goal.

CHAPTER SUMMARY

In this chapter, the theme of excellence was examined through the running life of Melissa Burt. In devoting her life to running, she has felt that she has lived a life "most worth living" (Suits, 1978, p. ix). It is important to recognize how her pursuit of excellence was not all her own doing. Several people directly and indirectly impacted her pursuit and achievement of running excellence. Achieving excellence also requires hard work and dedication, therefore it is important for people to identify what sacrifices are required to achieve their goals and to determine whether they are willing to make those sacrifices. The subdisciplines of kinesiology provide crucial insights into how to pursue and achieve excellence. Although heroes can be a source of inspiration, it is often role models who are directly involved in supporting and mentoring people's pursuit of excellence. Simon, Torres, and Hager (2015, p. 47) argue that competition is a "mutual quest for excellence through challenge." This not only provides a moral argument for the pursuit of achievement in competition, but it also provides the basis for a morally critical evaluation of the pursuit of excellence. When athletes disregard rules and are disrespectful to the rights of opponents in pursuit of victory, then the overemphasis on winning can no longer be regarded as a mutual quest for excellence.

At some point, most often due to injury or aging, an athlete becomes less competitive. Eventually this leads to a transition to life after sport. Although the pursuit of absolute excellence may no longer be feasible, athletes can still experience relative excellence. In some cases, this can mean competing in a modified way or with modified expectations. It can also mean transitioning to new roles that include promoting physical activity experiences for others (Hochstetler, 2015). In the end, even the importance of individual excellence is meaningful because of a community that values achievement in that particular context. Kinesiology professionals can play an important role in fostering physical activity communities and encouraging their members to maintain humility, express gratitude, and give back in order to promote excellence in participation.

DISCUSSION QUESTIONS

1. What factors contribute to achieving excellence? What role do others play in enabling an athlete to achieve excellence?
2. What barriers, both personal and societal, inhibit excellence? What subdisciplines can help us identify and address those barriers?
3. What are the different forms of excellence? Are they all equally meaningful?
4. Near the end of the case study, Melissa Burt turned her attention from the excellence of her own performance to the excellence of diverse and robust participation in running communities. Describe how kinesiology professionals can impact excellence in participation.
5. In order to achieve excellence, one must personally invest a lot of time and effort. Meaningful activities validate such sacrifices. Identify additional ways people make sacrifices to achieve greatness. How can you, as a kinesiology professional, support these sacrifices?

REFERENCES

Anderson, D. (2001). Recovering humanity: Movement, sport, and nature. *Journal of the Philosophy of Sport, 28*(2), 140–150.

Hochstetler, D. (2015). Narratives, identity, and transformation. *Quest, 67,* 161–172.

Simon, R. L, Torres, C. R., & Hager, P. F. (2015). *Fair play: The ethics of sport* (4th ed.). Boulder, CO: Westview Press.

Suits, B. (1978). *The grasshopper: Games, life, and utopia.* Toronto: University of Toronto Press.

CHAPTER 18

Inclusive Physical Education for Children with Autism Spectrum Disorder

TERI TODD AND MELISA MACHE

LEARNING OBJECTIVES

1. Define *autism spectrum disorder* (ASD), and identify its core characteristics.

2. Describe the motor and balance deficits common to individuals with ASD.

3. Explain the role of the physical educator in addressing the needs of children with ASD in physical education settings.

4. Identify strategies that can be used in physical education classes to address the needs of individuals with ASD.

KEY TERMS

adapted physical education (APE)
autism spectrum disorder (ASD)
balance
evidence-based strategies

gross motor skills
imitation
motor planning

autism spectrum disorder (ASD)
A neurodevelopmental disorder characterized by (1) persistent deficits in social communication and social interactions across multiple contexts and (2) presence of restricted, repetitive patterns of behavior, interests, or activities.

motor planning
The organizational or executive activity of the neural systems that control coordinated movement patterns.

balance
A global term referring to control processes that maintain body parts in the specific alignments necessary to achieve different kinds of mobility and stability. Postural stability, postural control, and postural orientation all play a role in balance.

gross motor skills
Movements that use large muscles and segments of the body, such as arms, legs, or feet, or the entire body.

Case Study: Adapted Physical Education

It was late August, and Mark, an 8-year-old boy, was preparing to enter the second grade. Mark and his father had already taken a trip to meet his new teacher, Ms. Garcia, prior to the first day of school. He was able to check out his new classroom and see where his new desk would be. Despite getting the chance to preview his new learning environment, Mark was still a bit anxious about his first day of school. You see, Mark was not exactly like the rest of his peers, who might be excited about the first day of class, meeting their new teacher, and making new friends. Mark had been diagnosed with **autism spectrum disorder (ASD)** when he was 2 years old. A diagnosis of ASD can mean a wide variety of things; for Mark, it meant that he often struggled with social interactions. Many would describe him as aloof and uninterested in his peers. Mark was very literal with language, and he typically preferred environments and places that were familiar. In addition to these social deficits, Mark also exhibited some deficits in **motor planning** and had trouble with **balance** and coordination. This made **gross motor skills** such as running, jumping, throwing, dribbling, and catching difficult for him to perform with the same ease as his peers. Mark's parents had successfully worked with educators in the past to make Mark's experience in the general education classroom as comfortable as possible. Mark's parents were confident this year would be no different.

Autism Spectrum Disorder in the Physical Education Setting

Despite Mark's anxiety in the days leading up to the first day of school, he had a wonderful first day. He was relieved to see familiar faces, classmates he had met last year in first grade, and he absolutely loved his new teacher, Ms. Garcia. The first week went off without a hitch. During the second week of school, the children were going to begin having physical education class once per week with a physical education specialist. The physical education specialist, Mr. Bryant, was hired by the school district to work across the district on several campuses with first- through fifth-grade students. When Ms. Garcia announced that the children would be going to "play" with Mr. Bryant that afternoon Mark immediately became nervous. So many thoughts began to swirl in his mind: What were they going to do with Mr. Bryant?

Would Mr. Bryant be nice? Mark didn't think of himself as being good at playing games with others. He didn't like being out on the playground. He was convinced this was not going to go well for him.

When the afternoon rolled around, all of the other children were excited to meet Mr. Bryant and get a chance to play on the playground. Mr. Bryant was equally excited, as this was his first physical education teaching job. The weeks leading up to the first day of school had been quite hectic as he tried to become acquainted with the school district, the district's policies, and the campuses where he would be working. Despite the chaos leading up to his first days of teaching, he felt prepared to deliver age-appropriate physical activity and to find meaningful ways for children to enjoy movement. However, Mr. Bryant was aware that this class might not be as easy as some of his student-teaching experiences, as he knew that there was a student in the class with ASD. Immediately before class began, Mr. Bryant started to regret that he did not have time to meet this student and read his Individualized Educational Program (IEP) prior to the first physical education class. There was no time to dwell on this fact now. After Mr. Bryant introduced himself to the children, he told them they were going to do a warm-up activity. Mr. Bryant asked the students to distance themselves so that they were an arms-length away from each of their classmates. Everyone began to spread out on his instruction, and then he proceeded to ask the children to swing their arms in circles. As he did this he noticed one student wandering around and not engaging in the activity. He walked in the student's direction in an attempt to get him to respond to his voice and follow along; however, his attempt was unsuccessful. Mr. Bryant was sure he had now figured out which child was the student with ASD. Indeed, Mark was the child wandering around. As the warm-up continued, with simple hopping, galloping, and running tasks, Mark continued to wander, sometimes so close to other students that he would bump into them.

Upon completing the warm-up, Mr. Bryant told the students that they were going to play a new game called "Red Light, Green Light Dribble" (PE Central, 2013). After reminding the children of the cues for proper dribbling technique that they learned as first graders (i.e., push the ball, use the pads of the fingers, etc.) and providing them each with a ball so that they could practice their dribbling skill for a couple of minutes, he asked the children to walk to the outdoor basketball courts to play a game during which they would practice their dribbling skills (**FIGURE 18-1**).

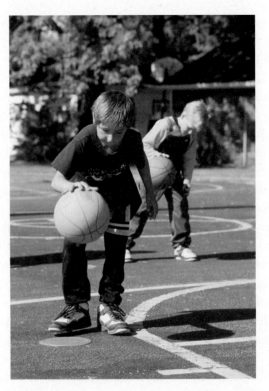

FIGURE 18-1   Children displaying the typical dribbling skills of second graders.

With the children gathered on the two outdoor basketball courts, Mr. Bryant explained that one court would be the blue court and one court would be the red court. On each court Mr. Bryant had set up cones to mark various pathways for the children to follow until they reached the opposite end of the court. Mr. Bryant was going to stand at the opposite end of the court shouting the commands "red light" or "green light" to prompt the children to stop or go while continuing to dribble the playground ball. As the children dribbled they were to move from cone to cone along the pathway that had been laid out by Mr. Bryant. When a child reached the end of the section (e.g., the red section), he or she was to move to the other section (e.g., the blue section) and continue the activity. Mr. Bryant reminded the children that they were to try to keep dribbling throughout the game and that they needed to be aware of the space around them so as to avoid running into their classmates.

Each child was then given a rubber playground ball, and half of the children were sent to the blue section and the other half of the children were sent to the red section. Once the game began, Mr. Bryant was excited to see all of the children engaged and enjoying the activity; all but one child, that is, and that child was Mark. Mark was unable to follow the directions that Mr. Bryant had provided, despite the fact that his classmates seemed to have no trouble following his instructions. When Mark did try to play the game, he appeared clumsy as he moved. Mark was able to dribble, and he could dribble while walking, but only for two or three dribbles. He was not following the pathways and was continually losing the ball and running into his classmates. Mr. Bryant tried to engage him and provide encouragement, but with 24 other students, this was a very difficult task. When the first physical education class had finally come to an end, both Mark and Mr. Bryant were wishing that their 45 minutes together had gone differently. Mark went back to his classroom with a strong desire to never go back to physical education class, and Mr. Bryant left knowing he was going to need to learn more about ASD and how to modify his lessons in ways that would help Mark be successful and enjoy the activities. Mr. Bryant had only completed a single course in **adapted physical education (APE)**; he knew he would need to consult someone with a greater knowledge base and wealth of experience in order to address Mark's needs.

Mr. Bryant and Mark were equally troubled by the first day of physical education class. Mark was frustrated and confused. He wanted to do the activities like everyone else but did not understand what he was supposed to do. Mark wished that Ms. Garcia taught physical education. He planned to ask her if she could please do that.

> **adapted physical education (APE)** Physical education that has been adapted and/or modified so it is appropriate for children and youth with disabilities. This service is federally mandated for all students with disabilities. It includes physical fitness, fundamental motor skills and patterns, and individual and group games and sports, and may also cover aquatics and dance.

> **STOP AND THINK**
>
> Many children affected by ASD are behind their peers in gross motor skills. Identify as many ways as you can how this fact may affect a child's ability to participate in a physical education class.

Overview of Autism Spectrum Disorder

Mr. Bryant decided to meet with the school district's APE specialist, Mrs. Anderson. With Mrs. Anderson's training and resources, Mr. Bryant was confident that she would have all of the answers that he needed to better understand Mark and meet his needs as a student in his physical education class. Mr. Bryant was right about Mrs. Anderson, and here is what he discovered from his meeting with her. First, he learned that ASD is the fastest-growing developmental disability in North America. Recent studies by the Center for Disease Control and Prevention (CDC) revealed that, in 2010, 1 in 68 children was diagnosed with ASD (Baio, 2014). In addition, ASD is five times more common among boys than girls, meaning that 1 in 42 boys has ASD. In practical terms, it is likely that there will be a child with ASD in nearly every classroom, meaning Mr. Bryant was going to encounter many more students similar to Mark throughout his teaching career.

Mrs. Anderson went on to describe when and how ASD is typically diagnosed. ASD is most commonly diagnosed within the first few years of life, often by 2 years of age. Pediatricians are being trained to look for early signs of ASD, because early intervention has been found to be very effective when addressing ASD. Medical, psychology, and speech professionals can be qualified to make the diagnosis. In the state of California, government agencies known as Regional Centers provide free assessment for children suspected of having a developmental delay, including ASD. In addition, the Regional Centers provide services and support to individuals with developmental disabilities and their families. The most common tool used to diagnose ASD is the Autism Diagnostic Observation Scale–Revised (ADOS–R; Lord et al., 2012), coupled with parent questionnaires such as the Vineland Adaptive Behavior Scale (Sparrow, Cicchetti, & Balla, 2005) or the Autism Diagnostic Interview–Revised (Rutter, LeCouteur, & Lord, 2003). The ADOS–R is an activity-based assessment tool designed to evaluate key areas of deficit in people with ASD. The parent questionnaires typically target social characteristics in familiar environments, as well as restricted and repetitive patterns of behavior. When used together, these instruments can help professionals identify those individuals who may be on the autism spectrum.

Mrs. Anderson continued to explain the diagnostic procedure to Mr. Bryant in an effort to help him understand Mark and some of the social and behavioral deficits that he may demonstrate. The diagnostic criteria in the American Psychiatric Association's (2013) *Diagnostic and Statistical Manual of Mental Disorders, Fifth Edition* (DSM-5) recognizes two major areas of deficits: (1) social communication and social interaction and (2) restricted, repetitive patterns of behavior, interests, or activities. Persistent deficits in social communication and interaction can include deficits in social-emotional reciprocity; reduced sharing of interests, emotions, or affect; and difficulty in nonverbal communication behaviors used for social interactions, including eye contact. In addition, individuals with ASD often have problems developing, maintaining, and understanding relationships, which can make it appear that the individual with ASD has an absence of interest in peers. Restricted, repetitive patterns of behavior are characterized, in part, by stereotyped or repetitive motor movements, insistence on sameness and inflexible adherence to routines or rituals, highly restricted and fixated interests, and hyper- or hyporeactivity to sensory input. Although a diagnosis may occur at any age, symptoms of ASD must be present in the early developmental period. Mrs. Anderson explained to Mr. Bryant that each child would not display every symptom. To be diagnosed with ASD, a person has to display a certain number of characteristics. This meant that ASD would likely not manifest in the same way among any two children.

Mrs. Anderson went on to describe the fact that all individuals with ASD will have deficits in social communication and restricted, repetitive behaviors, but that ASD is a spectrum disorder, meaning that the symptoms can range from mild to severe. She explained that some individuals with ASD communicate verbally, like Mark, whereas others are nonverbal. Some children with ASD have cognitive delays, whereas others do not. In fact, data collected at seven different sites in the United States revealed that 46% of 8-year-old children with ASD had IQs in the average to above-average range, 23% were in the borderline range, and 31% were classified as having an intellectual disability (Baio, 2014). From Mr. Bryant's description of Mark, Mrs. Anderson guessed that he would fall among the 46% of individuals with an average to above-average IQ; however, she strongly encouraged Mr. Bryant to read Mark's IEP and meet with Mark's classroom teacher, and perhaps his parents, to learn more about Mark and his presentation of ASD.

Autism Spectrum Disorder and Physical Activity

Due to Mark's high functional abilities, Mrs. Anderson did not believe that Mark would qualify for direct services from her staff of APE specialists. However, she knew that she needed to help equip Mr. Bryant with the tools necessary to address the needs of Mark and other students he would encounter in the future. In order to do this, she felt it necessary to describe some of the motor and sensory deficits that are often present among individuals with ASD, because these may influence an individual's ability to engage in physical activity. For example, researchers have recently shown that the majority of individuals with ASD score below average on tests of motor development (Berkeley, Zittel, Pitney, & Nichols, 2001; Green et al., 2002). Motor behavior, motor development, motor learning, and APE specialists, in addition to biomechanists, continue to conduct research related to these observed motor deficits, because the reasons for the deficits are presently not well understood. Despite an incomplete understanding of motor deficits, an emerging body of research in this area is sufficient to inform educational strategies and evidence-based practices. Physical educators who understand the major areas of motor difficulty among individuals with ASD will more likely be able to prepare to instruct a class that includes children with ASD.

imitation
The act of copying, duplicating, and mirroring. Imitation tasks can be divided into three categories: postural movements, actions on objects, and orofacial movements. Children with ASD show impaired imitation in all areas.

For example, Mrs. Anderson explained that people with ASD often have deficits in **imitation** (Ingersoll, 2008; Williams, Whiten, & Singh, 2004). Imitation is an important component of development and, when absent, can have a pervasive effect on development. Although the existence of an imitation deficit among children with ASD is widely recognized, the reason for the deficit remains unresolved and a subject of controversy (Custance, Mayer, Kumar, Hill, & Heaton, 2014). What is certain is that a lack of imitation has a significant effect on social development and, additionally, may have a large effect on motor development. For example, physical educators often rely on a child being capable of imitating their demonstration to teach a motor skill (**FIGURE 18-2**). Learning this information about imitation helped Mr. Bryant understand why Mark was one of the only individuals in the class who was unable to follow the warm-up activities. It became clear to Mr. Bryant that in order to be a successful physical educator, he was going to need to implement strategies to help Mark understand what he wanted him to do.

Another common area of deficit among individuals with ASD that physical educators should be aware of is balance, or the ability to maintain upright posture (**FIGURE 18-3**). Researchers have assessed balance among individuals with ASD using functional tests such as the Movement ABC (Henderson & Sugden, 2007) and the Pediatric Balance Assessment (Franjione, Gunther, & Taylor, 2003). Biomechanical tools such as the force plate have also been used to measure postural sway, which is an indication of the ability to balance. With each of these measurement tools, children with ASD have been shown to lag behind their peers, and it has been demonstrated that these individuals often do not reach mature levels of balance (Baht, Landa, & Galloway, 2011). Balance is a prerequisite for motor skill development;

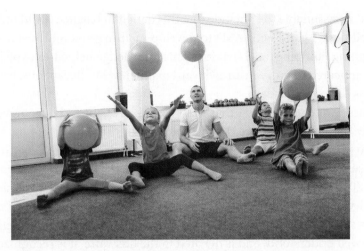

FIGURE 18-2   Physical education teachers often rely on imitation as a means of helping children learn new motor skills. However, children with ASD often have deficits in the ability to imitate.

© BraunS/Getty Images

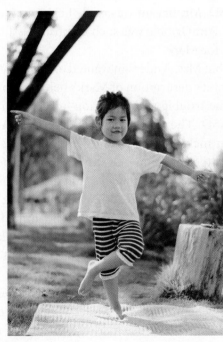

FIGURE 18-3   Deficits in balance are common among children with ASD.
© Krit of Studio OMG/Getty Images

thus, it is reasonable to conclude that this deficit in balance could influence the ability of a child with ASD to develop mature gross motor skills, such as running, jumping, and striking. This knowledge helped to explain why Mark appeared to move in an awkward manner as Mr. Bryant observed him in class the previous day.

Mrs. Anderson agreed that Mark could have appeared to move awkwardly because of balance deficits, but she informed Mr. Bryant that he should also be aware of the fact that many children with ASD also suffer from sensory integration problems and longer movement times (Staples & Reid, 2010). Sensory integration problems may make it difficult for an individual with ASD to effectively use intrinsic information received during motor skill performance. Although the reason for slower movement time is not well understood, and is debated in the literature, it is recognized that deficits in motor planning, executive function, or both, likely affect the child's ability to react quickly to environmental demands (Stolt, van Schlie, Slaats-Willemse, & Buitelaar, 2013). Thus, physical activities that rely on fast responses to a changing environment may prove challenging for children and youth with ASD. Mr. Bryant was really beginning to understand why Red Light, Green Light Dribble was such an unsuccessful and likely unenjoyable experience for Mark.

The last issue that Mrs. Anderson wanted to highlight was that of attention. From Mr. Bryant's description of Mark's behavior in class, she guessed that Mark had some trouble with attention—a common characteristic of individuals with ASD. The majority of children with ASD show atypical attention. This can include impairments in both focused and sustained attention, shifting attention from one stimulus to another, and the inability to selectively attend to pertinent cues, and disregard irrelevant cues, in the environment (Chien, Gau, Chiu, & Tsai, 2013; Ruff & Capozzoli, 2003). Upon learning this information, Mr. Bryant could immediately see how this could be a particularly difficult issue to deal with as his class often met outside where there were endless things in the environment that could potentially interfere with a child's ability to pay attention.

Now that Mr. Bryant had a solid understanding of the deficits that children with ASD may encounter, Mrs. Andersen wanted to take some time to discuss some strategies that he could use to address these deficits and make his physical education class a welcoming, safe, and productive environment for all students.

Evidence-Based Strategies for Inclusive Physical Education for Children with ASD

Mrs. Andersen wanted to provide Mr. Bryant with some effective **evidence-based strategies** for addressing these deficits in children with ASD. Over the past decade, much research has gone into identifying best practices for children with ASD. The National Autism Center (NAC) is continually monitoring research related to ASD interventions in an effort to identify the most promising evidence-based practices for educators and parents to implement with their children. The NAC recently launched the National Standards Project and has authored a comprehensive report outlining interventions that have been shown to be successful for many people with ASD (NAC, 2015). To date, no single evidence-based intervention has been proven to be effective for teaching motor skills to children with ASD. That being said, some of the interventions identified can be used while teaching physical education and are considered best practice in educational settings. Mrs. Anderson suggested that Mr. Bryant visit the NAC website to learn more about each of these interventions.

Now it was time to get to the specifics for which Mr. Bryant had come. Specifically, how was Mr. Bryant going to provide Mark and his classmates with a quality experience in his physical education class? Mrs. Anderson was excited to share her knowledge in this area. First, Mrs. Anderson suggested that it might be helpful for Mr. Bryant to begin by assessing Mark's motor skill level using an instrument such as the Movement ABC (Henderson & Sugden, 2007) or the Test of Gross Motor Development–2 (Ulrich, 2000). Although most of Mr. Bryant's students would come to him knowing many of the basic motor skills that are critical components of physical activities, this may not be the case for children with ASD. Children with ASD may need extra instruction to learn locomotor skills such as running, jumping, skipping, and hopping and basic object-control skills such as throwing, catching, and kicking (**FIGURE 18-4**). Performing an assessment of Mark's motor skills would allow Mr. Bryant to know exactly where Mark's deficits lie and plan lessons and activities accordingly. For example, one possible reason Mark did not participate in Red Light, Green Light Dribble might be that he is not as proficient at dribbling as his classmates. However, Mrs. Anderson

STOP AND THINK

Many children and adolescents affected by ASD have deficits that may inhibit their abilities to interact with others and follow instructions. Write a brief description of the possible deficits that may be experienced by children with ASD.

evidence-based strategies
Strategies that have been tested and evaluated based on data. The evidence is objective, and decisions can be made regarding the effectiveness of the strategy.

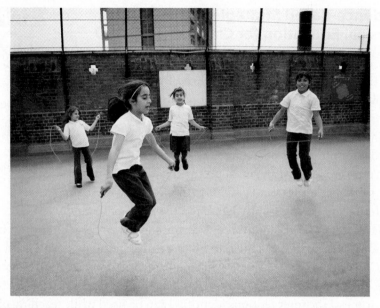

FIGURE 18-4 Children with ASD often exhibit deficits in gross motor skills compared to their peers without ASD.

© roger askew / Alamy Stock Photo

continued, based on recent evidence, it is possible that Mark could develop his dribbling skills sufficiently to be able to engage in such an activity. For example, one study of a fundamental motor skill program for 3- and 4-year-old children with ASD concluded that with proper instruction young children were able to improve their motor skills and eventually use these skills in a free-play setting (Bremmer, Balogh, & Lloyd, 2014). Mrs. Anderson cautioned Mr. Bryant that Mark, and other children with ASD, will likely need more instruction on fundamental motor skills than other children in order to experience success when engaging in games and activities.

Mr. Bryant knew this was going to be a challenge considering the fact that he was teaching a large group of students. However, Mrs. Anderson assured him that he could prepare lessons using a variety of activities so that all children could be engaged in the same motor skill while working at a level that would be beneficial to them. Mr. Bryant thought this sounded like a great idea, but was still not exactly sure how to go about designing the lessons. Mrs. Anderson decided to remind him of something motor learning specialists often turn to when trying to teach a new movement skill—try analyzing the skill you are preparing to teach and recognizing component parts of that skill. This can be done in a number of different ways, but Mrs. Anderson suggested Gentile's (1987) two-dimensional taxonomy of motor skills. This taxonomy provides a useful way to analyze motor skills by taking into account the environmental context and the function of the action. The taxonomy can be a helpful tool in identifying logical sequences when developing a progression of skill instruction.

Gentile (1987) identified two environmental factors that often change in physical activity settings: regulatory conditions and intertrial variability (ITV). *Regulatory condition* refers to objects or other people in the environment, which can be stationary or in motion. *Intertrial variability* refers to change from one trial to the next, and it is either present or absent. The second part of the taxonomy is related to the function of the action. Gentile (1987) recognized two broad categories of action that vary within a task: body orientation and object manipulation. *Body orientation* can range from being still (i.e., body stability) to moving (i.e., body transport). *Manipulation* refers to all action on objects to change or maintain their position, and it is present or absent in a skill (Gentile, 1987). For example, hitting a whiffle ball off a tee requires body stability plus manipulation, whereas running 50 yards requires body transport and no manipulation.

When both of these factors, body orientation (i.e., stable or moving) and object manipulation, are placed into a table, 16 combinations are possible (**TABLE 18-1**). Task difficulty increases as you move from the upper left-hand corner of the taxonomy to the lower right-hand corner. This table can aid teachers in preparing skill progressions and planning a variety of activities to meet multiple skill levels. Categories at the top left-hand side of the taxonomy are generally suitable for beginners and students with low skill level. The framework developed by Gentile is also helpful in sequencing activities to move from a closed environment (e.g., hitting a whiffle ball from a tee) to a more open game situation (e.g., hitting a whiffle ball that has been pitched in an actual organized game). Mr. Bryant was relieved to find a systematic method to increase skill difficulty. He immediately realized that he could implement this idea to ensure that all of his students could become proficient dribblers, including Mark.

Mr. Bryant asked Mrs. Anderson if they could walk through the taxonomy using the skill of dribbling as an example. For dribbling, Mr. Bryant

TABLE 18-1 Gentile's Taxonomy

			Classification of Motor Tasks				
			(Gentile's Taxonomy)				
			Environmental Context				
			Stationary		In Motion		
			No ITV	ITV	No ITV	ITV
Function of Action	Stability	No Manipulation	1A	1B	1C	1D
		Manipulation	2A	2B	2C	2D
	Transport	No Manipulation	3A	3B	3C	3D
		Manipulation	4A	4B	4C	4D

Note: ITV = Inter-trial variability.

Modified from A. M. Gentile. (1987). Skill acquisition: Action, movement, and neuromotor processes. In J. H. Carr, R. B. Shepherd, J. Gordon, A. M. Gentile, & J. M. Held (Eds.). *Movement science: Foundations for physical therapy in rehabilitation,* 111–187. Gaithersburg, MD: Aspen Publishers.

believed that the child could dribble in one spot with no walking, and that this would fall into the first category with an object (1B); the student would then have an opportunity to attend only to how to dribble the ball. As the child becomes more skillful and gains confidence, the environment can be changed to incrementally increase difficulty. For instance, dribbling the ball while walking would fall into the 1D category, whereas dribbling while avoiding an opponent would be category 4D. That skill could be introduced at a higher grade level. Mr. Bryant began to remember these concepts from the motor learning class he had taken, and he felt he could apply this concept when planning his lessons. He could have different activities in the same game and let the children choose which they preferred. Mark might like to dribble while standing still on a poly spot while other children could follow a poly spot trail while dribbling. After listening to Mr. Bryant describe how he might introduce the skill of dribbling next time, Mrs. Anderson's confidence in his ability to meet the needs of all of his students began to grow.

Mrs. Anderson knew that, in addition to analyzing a skill and breaking it into it individualized parts so that he could provide students with varying abilities an opportunity to learn, Mr. Bryant was going to need some strategies that he could use to deliver this instruction in a meaningful and helpful manner. She was happy to suggest a few instructional strategies for Mr. Bryant to try.

Finding ways for Mark to overcome potential deficits in imitation was going to be a challenge for Mr. Bryant because he often relied on imitation as a means of teaching new motor skills to children. Mrs. Anderson told Mr. Bryant that she knew that children with ASD imitated actions better if the actions were meaningful (Zachor, Ilanit, & Itzchak, 2010). Mrs. Anderson suggested that it might be a good idea for Mr. Bryant to chat with Mark as they walked to class and tell him what they were going to do that day and why they were going to do that particular activity. Mrs. Anderson believed that this might give the activity specific meaning for Mark, thus creating a better chance for success in that day's activities.

Mr. Bryant and Mrs. Anderson discussed ways to modify the outdoor teaching area and teaching strategies to address some of the issues that Mark may have with an unfamiliar environment and imitation. This would help Mark to feel less overwhelmed and distracted. She explained that providing physical boundaries for children with ASD can be very helpful; something as simple as providing a poly spot on the floor so the child knows where to stand can completely change how a child is able to engage in the activity. Other helpful tools might include boundary lines, targets, and goals. Yoga mats, hula hoops, and cones can also be great tools to help children identify the boundaries of their personal space and the personal space of those around them during activities (**FIGURE 18-5**).

Mrs. Anderson went on to explain that visual schedules, pictures, and video-modeling have been found to be effective when teaching new skills to individuals with ASD (Fittipaldi-Wert & Mowling, 2009). Fortunately, a variety of programs (some low cost or even free) are available online that can be useful for providing such information. Classroom teachers often use such schedules to present the order of the different activities during the day; for instance, story time, recess, lunch, spelling, and math might be shown to a student with ASD using a series of illustrations (**FIGURE 18-6**). Because of a strong need for visual information, Mrs. Anderson suggested that Mr. Bryant prepare a visual schedule for Mark before each physical education

STOP AND THINK

How could you use Gentile's two-dimensional taxonomy of motor skills to break down the task of striking a ball? How would the progression from using a ball stationary on a T-ball stand to a game situation drill aid a child affected by ASD?

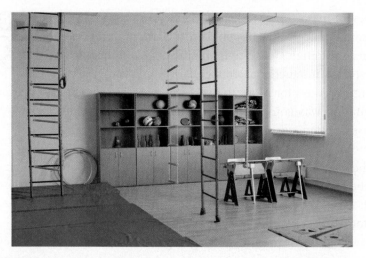

FIGURE 18-5   Common physical education equipment can be used to modify the environment to assist with focus and reduce distractions for children with ASD.

© Lauren Cameo/Shutterstock

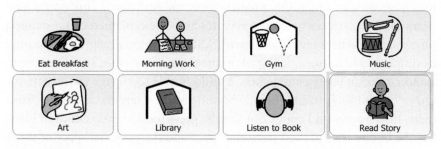

FIGURE 18-6   An example of a visual schedule for an elementary school child with ASD.

© SET – Special Education Technology British Columbia, "Daily Schedule Picture Cards," 2014.

lesson and directed him to the Autism Classroom website to learn how to create a visual schedule.

Mrs. Anderson knew that Mr. Bryant would also need to work on developing instructional strategies that enhance attention and decrease distractions in the environment so that Mark could thrive in the physical education setting. Mrs. Anderson stressed that he would need to emphasize relevant instructional

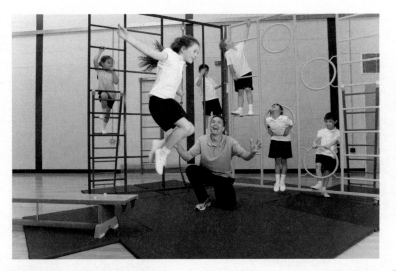

FIGURE 18-7   A loud, noisy gymnasium is a poor learning environment for a child with ASD who may feel overwhelmed or distracted in such a setting.
© Echo/Getty Images

cues, employ short instructional periods interspersed with frequent breaks, and teach self-monitoring techniques to stay on task. Unfortunately, the often active and noisy environment of gymnasiums and playgrounds are a poor fit for children with ASD (**FIGURE 18-7**). Although completely eliminating sensory stimuli and distractions from the physical education environment is rarely possible, Mrs. Anderson was able to provide a few simple suggestions:

- Put away any equipment not presently in use.
- Store equipment that is not in use in opaque, closed containers so it is not visible to students.
- If indicated by the child's IEP, noise-canceling earphones might be offered to the child to minimize noise that the child might find distracting or upsetting (**FIGURE 18-8**).
- Use short, concise instructions.
- If possible, choose quiet times to use the playground or gymnasium.

Lastly, Mrs. Andersen warned Mr. Bryant that children with ASD may become easily upset during transitions or if a new activity or routine is introduced. Preparing the child in advance can decrease anxiety

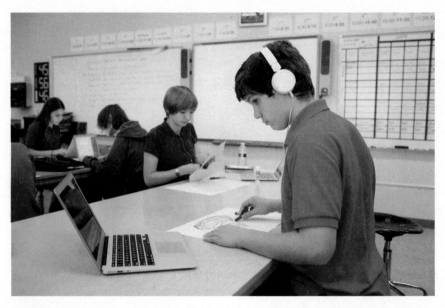

FIGURE 18-8 Noise-canceling headphones may be helpful in reducing distractions for some children with ASD.
© Blend Images / Alamy Stock Photo

STOP AND THINK

Identify strategies a physical educator might use to improve the experience of a child affected by ASD. What are some of the obstacles a teacher in a large, contemporary urban school might face in implementing these strategies? How can these obstacles be overcome?

and help the child transition with ease. This is where the visual schedules she had previously suggested can be very helpful. In addition, she mentioned that simply letting a child know that an activity will finish in 3 minutes may be enough to ensure a smooth transition to the next activity. Mrs. Anderson again suggested that Mr. Bryant become familiar with Mark's IEP so that he can find out how his other teachers, including Ms. Garcia, are providing schedules to Mark.

Before they ended their meeting, Mrs. Anderson reminded Mr. Bryant that knowing that a child has ASD is helpful but that there is a large amount of variability within the disorder. It is likely that Mark portrays many of the symptoms listed discussed earlier, and it is equally likely that Mark does not exhibit some of the characteristics. The key point to remember is that all individuals with ASD will have deficits in the core areas.

Understanding Mark and Addressing His Needs

After reading Mark's IEP, Mr. Bryant immediately set up a meeting with Ms. Garcia and Mark's parents during which he was able to gather some valuable information. First, Mr. Bryant learned that Mark was considered to have mild ASD, but that he struggled with many of the issues that Mrs. Anderson had described to him as affecting children with ASD. Mark was not comfortable with new environments, he did not do well with transitions, and he struggled with imitation and attention, although he did not have any particular issues with noise sensitivity. Mr. Bryant also learned that his physical education class during the second week of school was Mark's first experience in this sort of environment. Ms. Garcia explained that she had been successfully using visual schedules with Mark in the classroom and offered to provide Mr. Bryant with an example of such a schedule. Mark's parents offered that they often relied on visual schedules at home. Mr. Bryant confidently showed Ms. Garcia and Mark's parents a visual schedule that he had been working on for Mark using information that he had found on the Autism Classroom News website (Reeve, 2014). This action increased everyone's confidence in Mark's ability to potentially enjoy physical education. All parties agreed that Mr. Bryant would conduct a motor skills assessment with Mark prior to the next physical education class. Mr. Bryant walked away from the meeting feeling confident that he could find ways to address Mark's needs.

Mark's parents went home and explained the meeting they had with Mr. Bryant to Mark. They explained to him that tomorrow during school he was going to go with Mr. Bryant to play. They told him that he would get to run, jump, skip, throw, and strike and that he would be the only person who got to play with Mr. Bryant. Mark was nervous, but his parents were confident he would be okay because they had given him enough warning to prepare for the event.

The next day when Mark arrived at school, Ms. Garcia shared his visual schedule with him (**FIGURE 18-9**). The schedule included his "play" time with Mr. Bryant. When Mr. Bryant arrived to take Mark with him for the motor skills assessment, he gave Mark a visual schedule of all of the activities they would be doing. Mr. Bryant completed the assessment while trying to incorporate many of the suggestions he had received from Mrs. Anderson. For each motor skill that Mark was to be tested on, Mr. Bryant showed Mark

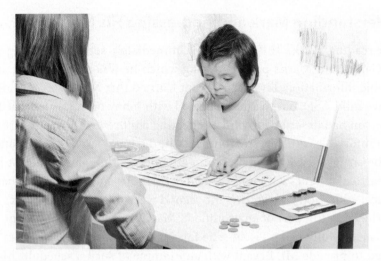

FIGURE 18-9   A visual schedule is often a helpful means of helping a child with ASD navigate a busy school day and transition from task to task.
© SerrNovik/Shutterstock

a picture of a child performing the skill. Mr. Bryant then performed the skill so that Mark could see the skill. Lastly, he gave very short, concise instructions for each skill. Mr. Bryant used poly spots to show Mark where to stand, where to start, and where to stop for each skill. Mark appeared to enjoy attempting to perform the skills, and by the end of their time together, it was clear that Mr. Bryant had developed a rapport with Mark. As expected from his conversation with Mrs. Anderson, Mark did perform below average on the motor skills assessment; however, he was able to perform a few of the skills at a level that was typical for a child of his age. Mr. Bryant was now better prepared to present lessons in a manner that would address Mark's specific deficits.

Red Light, Green Light Dribble Revisited

Mark's physical education time with Mr. Bryant and his classmates became an enjoyable time for him as the year progressed. Ms. Garcia included physical education on Mark's visual schedule every Tuesday so he was prepared for this activity. Mr. Bryant moved their physical education class to the courts and fields as far as possible from the chaos of other physical education classes to minimize distractions in the environment. When they performed

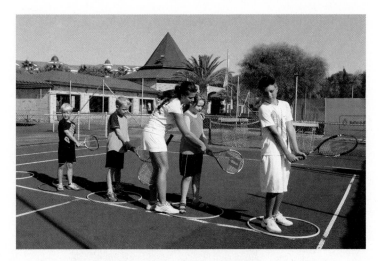

FIGURE 18-10   Poly spots can be used to provide guidance for children with ASD in an open environment such as the playground.

© Juergen Hasenkopf / Alamy Stock Photo

warm-ups, each child was given a poly spot. The poly spot helped Mark know where to stand and helped him to learn to understand and respect his classmates' personal space (**FIGURE 18-10**). Although this did not always go perfectly, Mark's behavior and interactions during the warm-up period improved greatly over the course of the year.

A couple of months after the first attempt at Red Light, Green Light Dribble, Mr. Bryant felt that Mark and his classmates were ready to attempt the game again. After completing the motor skills assessment, Mr. Bryant knew that Mark was capable of dribbling and running. He realized the game would just take a few simple modifications to make it enjoyable for all of his students. First, Mr. Bryant began by visually defining the boundaries of the red and blue courts with blue and red canvas strips that he laid on the ground. Next, rather than using cones to mark pathways, he opted to use poly spots so that Mark could physically stand on each poly spot as he moved through the pathways. Also, at the end of each court, Mr. Bryant posted signs indicating that students should move to the opposite court (i.e., if they just finished the red court to move to the blue court, and vice versa). Lastly, rather than just shouting the commands "red light" and "green light," Mr. Bryant planned to hold up signs that depicted a red light and a green

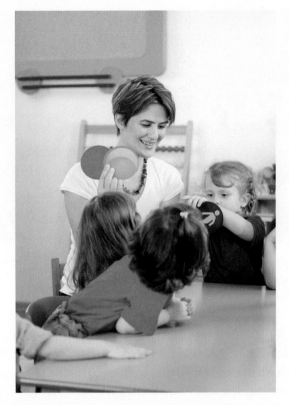

FIGURE 18-11 Visual cues can help children with ASD actively engage in playground games.

© fatihhoca/Getty Images

light (**FIGURE 18-11**). After reintroducing the game to the students, play began. Although Mark still did not move with the same ease as his classmates, with these new visual cues Mark was able to actively engage in the game with his peers. Mr. Bryant had successfully created an environment that helped Mark and his classmates enjoy physical activity and develop age-appropriate motor skills.

Conclusion

Physical activity is an important part of a healthy lifestyle. Unfortunately, recent statistics confirm that adults with ASD rarely meet recommended levels of physical activity and are at risk for secondary conditions such as obesity, diabetes, and cardiovascular disease (Srinivasan, Pescatello, & Bhat, 2014). It is important that research continues so that we may develop a better understanding of motor deficits and effective strategies to teach motor skills and encourage participation in physical activity in children with ASD. Physical activity during the early years and childhood are strong indicators of future behaviors, including educational attainment, physical activity levels, health, and happiness (ukactive, 2014). Ms. Garcia, Mrs. Anderson, and Mr. Bryant are all working hard to lay a foundation of motor skills and provide positive, enjoyable physical activity experiences for everyone, including Mark. Learning to enjoy physical activity in a healthy and meaningful physical education environment will, hopefully, prepare Mark for a lifetime of being physically active.

STOP AND THINK

Identify as many ways as possible that physical education classes and intramural activities can contribute to children with ASD feeling that they are included, and valued, as schoolmates. What do you believe are the red flags that indicate that inclusion is *not* occurring on the school grounds and play areas?

CHAPTER SUMMARY

In this chapter, autism spectrum disorder (ASD) and the core characteristics of the disorder were introduced. Special attention was given to the fact that many individuals with ASD exhibit deficits in gross motor skills and balance compared to their peers without ASD. Evidence-based strategies were identified to address the needs of children with ASD in a physical education setting, including assessing a child's motor abilities, using visual schedules, and providing visual cues to complement verbal instruction. Lastly, successful implementation of some of these strategies was illustrated using the dribbling game of red light, green light. Most important, it is important to remember that ASD is a spectrum and that the characteristics of the disorder will present differently for each individual. With this in mind, it is essential to assess the needs of each child on an individual basis and develop means of addressing these needs in a physical education setting so that an individual can learn to enjoy physical activity.

DISCUSSION QUESTIONS

1. What is autism spectrum disorder (ASD)? What are the core characteristics of ASD?
2. How does ASD impact physical activity?
3. What role do physical educators have in addressing the needs of children with ASD in a physical education setting?

4. What strategies can physical educators use to address the needs of children with ASD in a physical education setting?
5. What challenges do physical educators face when addressing the needs of children with ASD in a physical education setting?

REFERENCES

American Psychiatric Association. (2013). *Diagnostic and statistical manual of mental disorders* (5th ed.). Arlington, VA: American Psychiatric Publishing.

Baio, J. (2014). Prevalence of autism spectrum disorder among children aged 8 years: Autism and Developmental Disabilities Monitoring Network, 11 Sites, United States, 2010. *Morbidity and Mortality Weekly Report, 63*(SS02), 1–21.

Berkeley, S. L., Zittel, L. L., Pitney, L. V., & Nichols, S. E. (2001). Locomotor and object control skills of children diagnosed with autism. *Adapted Physical Activity Quarterly, 18*, 405–416.

Bhat, A. N., Landa, R. J., & Galloway, J. C. (2011). Current perspectives on motor functioning in infants, children, and adults with autism spectrum disorder. *Journal of the American Physical Therapy Association, 91*, 1116–1129.

Bremmer, E., Balogh, R., & Lloyd, M. (2014). Effectiveness of a fundamental motor skill intervention for 4-year-old children with autism spectrum disorder: A pilot study. *Autism, 19*, 980–991.

Chien, Y., Gau, S. S., Chiu, Y., & Tsai, W. (2014). Impaired sustained attention, focused attention, and vigilance in youths with autistic disorder and Asperger's disorder. *Research in Autism Spectrum Disorders, 8*, 881–889.

Custance, D. M., Mayer, J. L., Kumar, E., Hill, E., & Heaton, P. F. (2014). Do children with Autism reenact object movements rather than imitate demonstrator actions? *Autism Research, 7*, 28–39.

Fittipaldi-Wert., J., & Mowling, C. (2009). Using visual supports for students with autism in physical education. *Journal of Physical Education, Recreation and Dance, 80*(2), 1–58.

Franjione, M. R., Gunther, J. S., & Taylor, M. J. (2003). Pediatric balance scale: A modified version of the Berg Balance Scale for the school-aged child with mild to moderate motor impairment. *Pediatric Physical Therapy, 15*(2), 114–128.

Gentile, A. M. (2000) Skill acquisition: Action, movement, and neuromotor processes. In J. H. Carr & R. B. Shepard (Eds.), Movement science: Foundations for physical therapy (2nd ed., pp. 111–187). Rockville, MD: Aspen Publishers.

Green, D., Baird, G. Barnett, A. L., Henderson, L., Huber, J., & Henderson, S. E. (2002). The severity and nature of motor impairment in Asperger's syndrome: A comparison with specific developmental disorder of motor function. *Journal of Child Psychology and Psychiatry, 43*(5), 655–668.

Henderson, S. E., Sugden, D., & Barnett, A. (2007). Movement Assessment Battery for Children–Second Edition (Movement ABC–2). San Antonio, TX: Pearson Clinical.

Ingersoll, B. (2008). The effect of context on imitation skills in children with autism. *Research in Autism Spectrum Disorders, 2*, 332–340.

Lord, C., Rutter, M., DiLavore, P. C., Risi, S., Gotham, K., & Bishop, S. L. (2012). ADOS-2: Autism Diagnostic Observation Schedule. Los Angeles, CA: Western Psychological Services.

National Autism Center. (2015). National Standards Project. Retrieved from http://www.nationalautismcenter.org

PE Central. (2012, May 12). Red Light, Green Light Dribble. Retrieved from http://www.pecentral.org

Reeve, C. (2014). Schedule Visuals for PE. Retrieved from http://www.autismclassroomnews.com

Rogers, S. J., Hepburn, S. L., Stackhouse, T., & Wehner, E. (2003). Imitation performance in toddlers with autism and those with other developmental disorders. *Journal of Child Psychology and Psychiatry and Allied Disciplines, 44*, 763–781.

Ruff, H. A., & Capozzoli, M. C. (2003). Development of attention and distractibility in the first 4 years of life. *Developmental Psychology, 39*(5), 877–890.

Rutter, M., LeCouteur, A., & Lord, C. (2003). Autism Diagnostic Interview- Revised (ADI-R). Los Angeles: Western Psychological Services.

Sherrill, C. (2004). *Adapted physical activity, recreation, and sport: Crossdisciplinary and lifespan* (6th ed.). New York: McGraw-Hill.

Sparrow, S. S., Cicchetti, D. V., & Balla, D. A. (2005). Vineland Adaptive Behavior Scales-Second Edition (Vineland™-II). San Antonio, TX: Pearson Clinical.

Srinivasan, S. M., Pescatello, L. S., & Bhat, A. N. (2014). Current perspectives on physical activity and exercise recommendations for children and adolescents with autism spectrum disorders. *Physical Therapy, 94*(6), 875–889.

Staples, K., & Reid, G. (2010). Fundamental movement skills and autism spectrum disorders. *Journal of Autism and Developmental Disorders, 40*, 209–217.

Stolt, A. M. B., van Schlie, H. T., Slaats-Willemse, D. I. E., & Buitelaar, J. K. (2013). Grasping motor impairment in autism: Not action planning but movement execution is deficit. *Journal of Autism and Developmental Disabilities, 48*, 2793–2806.

ukactive. (2014). *Start young stay active: Childhood physical literacy report.* London: Author. Retrieved from http://www.ukactive.com/downloads/managed/Start_Young_Stay_Active.pdf

Ulrich, D. (2000). Test of Gross Motor Development, Second Edition. Austin, TX: Pro-Ed.

Williams, J. H. G., Whiten, A., & Singh, T. (2004). A systematic review of action imitation in autism spectrum disorder. *Journal of Autism and Developmental Disorders, 34*, 285–299.

Zachor, D. A., Ilanit, T., & Itzchak, E. B. (2010). Autism severity and motor abilities correlates of imitation situations in children with autism spectrum disorders. *Research in Autism Spectrum Disorders, 4*, 438–443.

CHAPTER 19

Kinesiology and the Public's Health: Collaboration Imperatives

STEVEN LOY

LEARNING OBJECTIVES

1. Explain the actions that are required in order to apply the concept of *controlling your destiny* to kinesiology and your career.

2. Describe the steps required to create a successful and meaningful network of professionals.

3. Differentiate between an advisor and a mentor, and describe the importance of identifying a mentor early in college preparation.

4. Describe the potential relationships between the subdisciplines of kinesiology and the public's health through the promotion of physical activity, thus creating opportunities for collaboration.

5. Explain why many believe that the public health arena represents the greatest opportunity for employment of kinesiologists in the future.

6. Describe the value of being passionate about one's career, and explain how one's personal life and professional life can be successfully integrated.

7. Identify that the most successful professionals are those who continue to be relevant and seek excellence throughout their career and that it is your responsibility to establish relationships with these professionals in your department and in the community.

KEY TERMS

letter of recommendation	professional goals
mentor	professional network

Reaching Your Destination

You might be asking yourself, "How do I know I should study this discipline of kinesiology if I don't know where it might lead?" Conversely, "How do I know what I may want to do with *my life* if I don't know what I must learn and need to know for this career?"

One of the first questions students often ask is, "What can I do with this major?" Ironically, the majority ask this after they've already declared kinesiology as their major. Some take the introductory class and find out that there are multiple options or directions they can take. Unfortunately, many students we have met still lack clarity following their introduction to the major. For others, the next question has a higher degree of specificity: "What can I do with this option or subdiscipline?" My experience tells me that the majority of students do not conduct the significant exploration necessary given the number of years they hope to be working in their chosen field. I suggest a minimum investment of 1 year in career exploration for what is hoped will be 30 or more years of dedication and enjoyment. This is not a lot to ask given the alternative of blindly choosing the wrong career.

Setting the Course

Being in the introductory class is a great first step. By now you have identified some possibilities for your area of focus, and, hopefully, you have taken the initiative of visiting the faculty members in your department who are engaged in the subdisciplines that you have found to be most interesting. Depending on the size of your department, you may have one or more faculty in your main area of interest. Note, and this is an important point, that they represent only a glimpse of the possibilities in the subdiscipline. The reality is that some may have a very narrow perspective based on their own experiences. This brings me to a statement that I believe should govern your professional life—"Control your destiny!" *You* are responsible and must take the necessary steps to ensure that the right decision for you is made. Again, *you* are responsible.

Strategic Planning for Success

STOP AND THINK

- What is your area of focus?

- Who are the first two faculty in your department that you should speak to regarding your interests? If you don't know, how can you find out?

As mentioned earlier, it is important to meet with the faculty who are involved in your area of interest. During this process, it is important for you to consider identifying a **mentor**. It is likely you have been assigned an advisor in your area of interest, and this individual might be your mentor, though oftentimes, it is someone else. What is the difference between a mentor and an advisor? An advisor is usually responsible for academic advice, providing guidance through the major, and completing paperwork all of which may be rather generic. By contrast, a mentor *knows* you and invests time and energy in your present and your future. A mentor will provide advice and guidance with your best interest in mind with an eye to the impact of each step on future career goals and typically has maintained a high level of professional involvement. Finding a mentor is very valuable if not critical for your future.

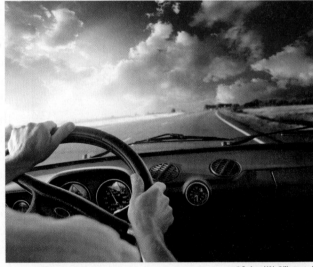

© Dudarev Mikhail/Shutterstock

mentor
An individual who will guide and support you on various aspects of your life journey.

professional network
A group of people you are prepared to collaborate with to generate positive action for yourself and others.

As you meet faculty, do this with both an open mind and a questioning attitude. This means that you should listen to the possibilities each faculty member will describe, yet recognize that this is only one person's opinion and experience. Inquire of your faculty the names of other professionals you might speak to (asking for a personal or email introduction to someone in their network) or local conferences you might attend to learn of additional possibilities. This is a way of expanding your **professional network** and increasing the breadth and depth of the information you can acquire. Follow up on the suggestions or referrals and report back what you learned to the original faculty contact. If the faculty see that you are insightful and attentive, they will view you as being responsible and diligent, and this may persuade them to provide you with other opportunities. At a minimum, reaching out and speaking with professionals in the field improves your communication skills and enables you to acquire good networking habits, which will benefit you in the future.

When you meet other professionals, they become a part of your professional network. You should note their name and contact information and write them a brief thank-you note (snail mail is better than email and memorable given the rarity of the practice today), which most students will not do, and this will elevate your status in the mind of the professional you have recently met. Consider every contact an interview for your next position. You will find that the world of kinesiology is a very small, very connected, place, and that all of the "small," but right, things you do can lead to new opportunities. Are you seeing and understanding how you are controlling your destiny? This is particularly important, because even though the rest of your class is reading this chapter, my experience is that the majority will not act upon these strategies. You might be in the distinct minority, which is a good thing for you!

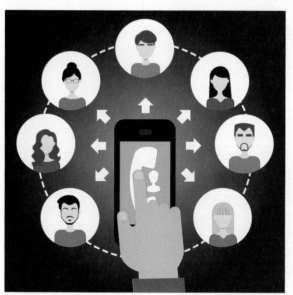

© Fedorenko Kateryna/Shutterstock

Personal and Professional Goals

Each person you meet will be helpful to you in defining your goals. Consider the following strategy whenever you do anything new, such as buying a used car. You know "nothing." You seek the advice of friends, the Internet, and your family, and with each contact you make you add to your knowledge, and your questions become more specific and have greater depth. So it is with every person with whom you discuss your future. Through your discussions, what you are seeing as a possibility for yourself is becoming clearer; that is, you like this, or you don't like that. Perhaps you want to work with an older population, especially those with disabilities, and your ability to speak another language is an advantage. A portrait of your career is beginning to form. As you engage in thinking about your future, you will begin to think about what is important to you as a person with regards to financial security, family life, and where you want to live. In a related fashion, questions will begin to arise regarding what kind of professional you want to be: How will you spend your days? Do you want to be a hands-on person or a supervisor? Do you have great communication skills, or are you best in the background or in support roles?

Many of these questions regarding your personal and **professional goals** will not arise until you begin the journey described above. It is easy to get caught up in the quizzes, midterms, and assignments, thinking only that it is important to get good grades and that you will think about the rest later. The reality is that if you do this, when you graduate, who will know you? Nobody! You do not have a professional network. You have not even given thought to the direction in which your education is going to lead!

Remember the suggestion of a 1-year minimum of exploration? You are to do this concurrently with being in school. Consider it another class you are taking, and your objective is to meet one new person each week. Impossible, you think? Each time you meet a new person, you should ask for a new contact. Then, it is up to you to make the time to follow up with that contact. This is your homework! If you find you do not like the direction you are going in, go back to your faculty or someone in your broadening network and ask them about a different direction. Remember, you are exploring!

As you speak with more people, your vision will become clearer—a future will begin to crystallize. Some of the professionals you encounter will begin to represent the career you envision. Now your questions will become "How did you get here?" "What steps/education do I have to engage in to be you?" "Would you consider being my mentor?" or "Do you know of any projects I could engage in that would improve my skills?" Note that the question of projects

professional goals
Identifying what you would like to accomplish or produce with your education and career.

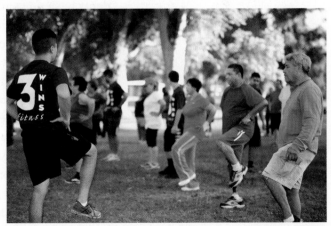

© Carmen Anthony Photography

STOP AND THINK

- During the past month, how many times have you talked to someone, in some depth, about your future career? Who were these people, and what key messages did you gain from the conversation?

- If your answer to the question above was "never," see if you can identify one person with whom you *could* have had such a conversation. Why didn't it happen? Do you think you might have a pattern of letting opportunities pass by? If yes, how can you change that?

- What aspects are important to you in a career? What are you seeking with regard to financial security, family, or location? What would you like your daily routine to look like? Do you think you would be more comfortable in a hands-on role or a supervisory role?

letter of recommendation
A letter that identifies your strengths and qualifications for a particular post; the quality and power of the letter varies based on many factors.

you could engage in could include internship (volunteer or paid) experiences that you could find out about from the individuals in your expansive network. One of the best steps might be going back to your faculty to inquire about project possibilities. This is because you may require a letter from a faculty member for your next position.

Assessing Your Progress

By the end of your junior year (even better at the end of your sophomore year), it is time to *honestly* assess your current standing by answering the following questions:

1. Have I identified my career area of focus?
2. Have I created a network of professionals related to my focus?
3. Have I acquired significant experiences related to my focus?

If your answer to any of these questions is "no," what does this say about you controlling your destiny?

In senior-level classes, many students ask a faculty member for a **letter of recommendation**, hoping it will be an excellent letter. In my experience, the majority of students have *no* faculty member they are really comfortable with asking for a letter. The majority of students who do request a letter know only teaching assistants or part-time faculty members who, by virtue of their experiences and professional standing in the field, may not be able to write as convincingly as a full-time, tenure-track faculty member. If you have just read the prior sentence and are unaware that there are differences in faculty levels, now would be a good time to discuss this with your advisor, even if this is the very first time you will meet your advisor.

With regard to letters of recommendation, recognize that there are *excellent* letters and that there are *perfunctory* letters (check out the synonyms for perfunctory!). Excellent letters come from faculty who know you and who have worked with you at a significant level of interaction and for whom you have also done well in classes. This is a letter that allows the faculty member to write a letter describing you as "the whole package"; that is, a student who has been immersed in her or his career pursuits while continuing to perform well in the classroom. That being said, excellent letters may also be written for students who have not done exceptional classroom work because the position they are applying for requires a skill set in which they *do* excel, and this fact is known by the aware faculty mentor based on extensive experiences and interactions with such a student.

From this discussion, you should now recognize that everyone you meet is a potential lead that can important to your future career. Earlier, I suggested that each person you meet could be your next interview. It is also true that "someone" is always watching your actions and performance. Be a professional in all your actions and seek quality in all you do every day and every class. Someone is always watching.

Facing Uncertainty: The Promising Future of Kinesiology

In the United States, and indeed around the world, people are experiencing increasingly poor health, and physical inactivity has been described as a pandemic. The negative effects of physical inactivity impact an exceptionally high proportion of the population, covering a wide geographic area, with corresponding health, economic, environmental, and social implications (Kohl et al., 2012). However, in kinesiology we are positioned to provide solutions for physical inactivity, obesity, type 2 diabetes, and the many chronic diseases associated with physical inactivity, which together are considered the world's fourth leading cause of death (Kohl et al., 2012). This is our time, and if we do not *control our destiny*, then kinesiology will lose the opportunity to lead. That said, it is uncertain where the future will be for our discipline. It is up to you, the reader of this text, to be a leader, to create programs, and to be involved in the solving of the problem and not think that someone else will do it!

STOP AND THINK

- Did you really look up the synonyms on your computer for the word *perfunctory*? (In other words, do you follow through on suggestions?)

- What does perfunctory mean? What are some synonyms?

- Have you engaged in career-related activities, and is your faculty mentor (who will eventually receive that request for a letter) aware of your activities? Perhaps even better, do your activities involve working with this faculty?

- What are some specific aspects of excellent letters?

- What are some specific aspects of perfunctory letters?

- What are the different faculty levels? Which provide the most valuable letters and why?

- How have you interacted with faculty outside of the classroom?

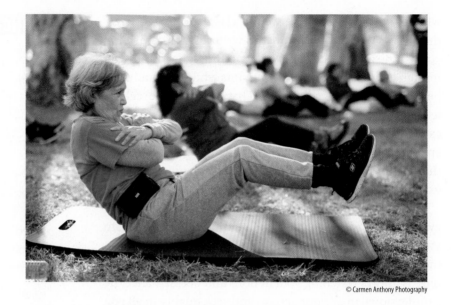

© Carmen Anthony Photography

THE QUESTION WE MUST ASK

Our field has multiple subdisciplines. However, the common thread in kinesiology is the art and the science of human movement. If low physical activity is pandemic and human movement is what we are about, then the question we must ask is, "What are we, as professionals within a discipline, going to do about providing solutions for physical inactivity and preventing the development of the related chronic diseases?" We often say we must not just talk the talk, we must walk the walk, and isn't that appropriate for this question?

THE METHODS WE USE, THE ANSWERS WE OFFER, AND THE OPPORTUNITIES WE SEEK AND DEVELOP

I suggest that every kinesiology subdiscipline or option should be able to address the question above by offering multiple solutions, because there is seldom a one-size-fits-all answer. You, as a student, must challenge yourself and your faculty members to develop workable solutions to pandemic physical inactivity that are affordable, accessible, and sustainable. Yours is the first generation projected to die at an earlier average age than your parents, so you must take this personally. You are positioned to see that while the generation of kinesiology/physical education professionals before you have identified the problem, we have failed to develop the solutions that meet the above criteria. Challenge your faculty to teach you, to show you, and to involve you so that you can understand what you need to do as a problem-solver in this critical matter, regardless of your area of study within kinesiology.

As you explore these issues in your classes, ask your faculty how you can collaborate and combine methods with other subdisciplines and, of equal importance, with colleagues across the campus. What we have here is a concern that crosses many disciplines. It affects every person in the university, but at this very moment, kinesiology is the only major on campus directly focused on physical activity. We may be one of the fastest-growing majors in the university system, but we are a small number in the global picture, so we must come up with meaningful solutions that are socially and culturally sensitive, accessible to all, and sustainable. Together, we can provide the variety of programs and solutions that can slow and perhaps even reverse the health decline we are presently facing.

We must do the research, gather the evidence, and publish our answers, not only in scientific journals, but also in the ever-expanding print and social media to which we have access. We must change the mindset of traditional faculty that "publicity is not what we do." In fact, if you have a solution, should you keep it as the best-kept secret? You are part of a new generation of kinesiology professionals, and you can *control your destiny*. I cannot say this enough, because there are those who do not understand this concept; thus, you must lead the way by example. Work with others, collaborate, and expose the public to what kinesiology has to offer. This will include raising awareness at your own university. Help your university community understand what kinesiology is through newsletters, social media, and program development. *Be innovative in the community and establish relationships with new nontraditional partners.* In a case study exemplar program called 3 WINS Fitness at California State University Northridge, we have partnered with city officials and have integrated Spanish-speaking journalism students into our diabetes prevention program so they can provide first-person and reporter perspectives on a Spanish–English blog. We created a Twitter and Facebook presence that will continue to evolve. As upcoming professionals, you can introduce new means of communication to your faculty who may not be as media savvy as you. Be a partner in your education. Don't wait to be led; take the lead!

The Long Run

Recognize that we must evolve as a profession. We must be nimble, because change is coming ever faster. This means that how we do things as faculty and as students is going to change. To not change is to become obsolete. We have a health problem in front of us that is the responsibility of *everyone* in kinesiology to address. The beauty of it is you get to select where you want to make your mark.

ACHIEVING YOUR PERSONAL AND PROFESSIONAL GOALS

And so here we are, back to the beginning of "What brings you here?" Is it what you thought? If you have a passion for movement, then you are in the right place. Apply what you will learn in your classes and *let your personal and professional goals intertwine and integrate.* Live your profession. Enjoy your profession. Make it your passion!

BE AN ADVOCATE FOR MEANINGFUL PHYSICAL ACTIVITY

As mentioned earlier, don't keep your solutions secret. Make them known. Make them relevant. Seek to create programs of excellence and relevance. This is how your career will become your passion. You will be making a difference for many, not just a few. You need to think big, to think that what you and your colleagues can develop can change the world. Embrace excellence and avoid mediocrity. Be a leader and create a following. Challenge yourself and challenge others and ensure that everything you do makes a difference in the lives of others. If what you develop is meaningful to your participants, they will become lifelong participants. Seek professional leadership roles in your profession so you can touch others who will touch the thousands you cannot reach. Don't be afraid of change. Meet change head on, because if you don't you will cease to be relevant. The very best thing about kinesiology is

STOP AND THINK

- What can we, as kinesiology professionals, do about providing solutions for inactivity and the development of related chronic diseases?

- How can the different options/subdisciplines within kinesiology each contribute to the development of solving the problem of physical inactivity?

- What does it mean to make a solution accessible, and why is this important?

- What does it mean to make a solution sustainable, and why is this important?

STOP AND THINK

"Let your personal and professional goals intertwine and integrate."

- What does this statement mean, and why is it important?

- What are some possible consequences of not letting your personal and professional goals intertwine and integrate?

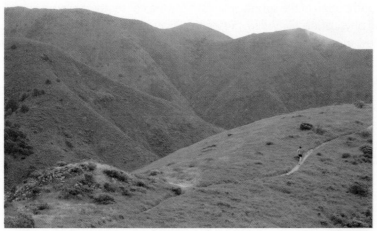

© Martin Sundberg/Getty Images

that it is about movement, and people were made to move, but you have to discover what kind of movement will resonate with your particular population—and with you.

STOP AND THINK

How can you control the destiny of your family? The community? The world around you?

A Journey Without End: Lifelong Learning

As mechanical and technological developments continue, it will become increasingly challenging to have people move sufficiently and effectively. Your challenge is to grow in your knowledge, to anticipate the challenges, and to create programs that will be successful. To fail to engage people in movement will result in a decrease in longevity and quality of life. You have the power to create change. Not only can you control your own destiny, but you can control the destiny of your family, community, and the world around you. Learn today, tomorrow, and continue to learn. Our health, and future, depend on you.

CHAPTER SUMMARY

The chapter emphasized the many ways that kinesiology majors have the opportunity, and responsibility, to control their own destiny, for their own good and that of others. Suggestions were provided on how to build a diverse and expansive professional network. The differences between an advisor and a mentor were pointed out, along with the importance of identifying a mentor early in the academic career. The contribution of the subdisciplines in solving contemporary problems of widespread physical inactivity were presented. Encouragement was offered for students to follow their hearts and deepen their professional commitment to guide lifelong career development.

DISCUSSION QUESTIONS

1. What is the minimum amount of time you should invest in exploring your career options? Describe some specific things you can do to find career information.
2. What does *control your destiny* mean to you? What are some specific examples of how you can control your destiny?
3. How can you find professionals in your field of interest to talk to?
4. What are some specific ways you can expand your professional network?
5. How can you acquire significant experiences related to your focus?
6. How can kinesiology share answers and solutions in print and through social media?

REFERENCE

Kohl, H. W., Craig, C. L., Lambert, E. V., Inoue, S., Alkandari, J. R., Leetongin, G., & Kahlmeier, S. (2012). The pandemic of physical inactivity: Global action for public health. *The Lancet*, 380(9838), 294–305.

Prelude to Your Career

CAROLE A. OGLESBY, KIMBERLY HENIGE,
DOUGLAS W. McLAUGHLIN, AND BELINDA STILLWELL

Congratulations! You are about to complete your formal introduction to kinesiology. You are now ready to pursue more advanced classes that address more complex information and have more direct applications. We hope that you are eagerly looking forward to the challenges ahead. But before you embark on your next steps, we encourage you to take some time to reflect upon what you have learned in this introduction to kinesiology.

First, you learned important information about the field of kinesiology. In Part I, you learned about the field of kinesiology's history, purposes, and paradoxes. In Part II, you learned about the different subdisciplines, their key issues, and possible related careers. In Part III, you learned from the case studies a number of different ways that kinesiology can make a difference in people's lives. However, be advised that the field of kinesiology continues to grow and develop. You need to always be alert to the changes and developments in the field of kinesiology that will impact you and your professional interests. This is both a joy and a challenge of being part of the future of a field that consists of so many dynamic professions. For example, some scholars are beginning to identify exercise psychology as a distinct subdiscipline, separate from sport psychology. Despite significant overlap, the psychology of exercise differs from the psychology of sport performance in several important ways. How exercise psychology and sport psychology develop, whether staying unified or becoming more distinct areas of study, will have an impact on what core knowledge kinesiology students will be expected to know.

Second, you learned important information about yourself. In Part I, you were encouraged to accept three guiding principles: developing competencies, becoming learner-centered, and maintaining a holistic perspective. Throughout the text, you had opportunities to develop your competency skills, such as being attentive, completing tasks, and communicating clearly. Hopefully, you have made improvements in your competency skills and have identified areas for continued development. The text also provided a number of resources to facilitate your taking responsibility for your own learning. If you took the time to develop your competency skills and learner-centered habits, then you are better prepared for your future coursework.

The text also provided examples of how the field of kinesiology is better approached in a holistic manner. Each subdiscipline chapter identified a number of ways that the subdiscipline was related to other subdisciplines. The case study chapters provided examples of addressing the issues facing kinesiology from holistic perspectives. Hopefully, you will continue to identify and comprehend the myriad ways that the subdisciplines are intertwined and mutually informing. You will continue to recognize the value of a holistic approach to kinesiology. If you do so, then you are better prepared to understand the complex problems in your chosen career and identify complex, holistic solutions.

Finally, you should begin to develop a sense of how you see yourself fitting into the field of kinesiology. Perhaps some subdisciplines stood out to you as particularly interesting. Perhaps some career possibilities stood out to you as particularly enticing. Perhaps some of the case studies have you thinking about how you can put your strengths to good use and how you can derive significance in a career devoted to the field of kinesiology. There will be plenty of time to rethink and refine your thoughts on your future, but in order to be prepared for the future you should be thinking about what you want to do and how you need to prepare to do it. Your development of competency skills and a learner-centered focus should help you seek out mentors and engage in opportunities that are not only interesting but that will also best prepare you for what lies ahead.

So, as your introduction to kinesiology comes to an end, a prelude to possibilities exists. A *prelude* is often thought of as an event that introduces you to something even more important. That is hopefully what this introduction has done. But also note that *ludus* is Latin for "play," and play is often thought of as an intrinsically valued activity. Our hope is that this introduction serves as a motivating factor in your intrinsically valued engagement with the study of kinesiology and the importance of physical activity. Our hope is that you will find delight in the challenges that await you.

We leave you with two parting gifts. The first gift comes in the form of a guiding question: What difference will you make? We are not asking you to justify yourself to us, but rather invite you to think about what contributions to the field of kinesiology you would like to make. Are you interested in addressing existing problems by implementing current solutions? Are you interested in acquiring new skills in the process of developing new solutions? Are you interested in experiencing new challenges? Are you interested in advancing new lines of research? Are you interested in seeking out the next horizons in the field of kinesiology? You are embarking on a journey with an open future. Take the time to discern what you want to do and why you want to do it. Take time to discover what steps you need to take to prepare for a successful journey and career. And take time to ask yourself what difference you are making, because there are so many rewarding career paths available to graduates of kinesiology programs. Make sure you pick the one that is right for you.

The second gift is our own guiding principles. Remember in Chapter 2 that we said that the principles guiding us, as authors, involved being rigorous mentors who, in a shared voice, conveyed our passion for physical activity and kinesiology. It is our good fortune to have a front-seat view of the current state of the field of kinesiology. But we fully recognize the inheritance we received from our teachers, advisors, and mentors. They held us to high standards, but they also supported our development so that we could achieve those standards. They shared their love for physical activity itself and the wonder of discovery and innovation that came from the careful and thoughtful study of it. They saw in us the future, and they empowered us to develop the field in new and interesting ways.

Now we see in you the future of the field of kinesiology. Remember to be guided by the principles that ensure the integrity and viability of kinesiology. Be rigorous in your study. Be a mentor and trusted advisor to others. Promote an abiding love for physical activity experiences and their meanings. And become part of the collective chorus that sings a unified song praising the value an active lifestyle. Through hard work, determination, and passion, great rewards await you!

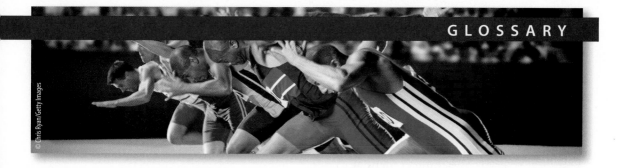

absolute excellence   The condition of being the best compared to all others in a given activity, such as elite sport.

academic discipline   A branch of knowledge designed to produce and disseminate expert knowledge.

academic learning time–physical education (ALT–PE)   Time during class when students are successful and actively engaged in accomplishing the goals of a lesson.

achievement goal theory   Theory of motivation that states that individuals tend to create their own goals based on either task or ego orientations, which subsequently influence motivation.

action research   Type of research typically undertaken in a school setting by teachers who are looking for ways to improve instruction and increase student achievement. Also referred to as *action participatory research*.

activities of daily living (ADLs)   The basic personal tasks individuals perform on a daily basis.

acute exercise effects   Sudden and immediate responses to exercise.

acute physiological responses   The immediate effects on the body's systems in response to the stress of exercise.

adaptation   Something that is changed or modified to suit new conditions or needs.

adapted aquatics   Aquatic activities that have been modified for people with special needs.

adapted physical activity (APA)   A field of study of physical activity that is modified for people with special needs to promote healthy and active lifestyles.

433

adapted physical education (APE) Physical education that has been adapted and/or modified so it is appropriate for children and youth with disabilities. This service is federally mandated for all students with disabilities. It includes physical fitness, fundamental motor skills and patterns, and individual and group games and sports, and may also cover aquatics and dance.

added authorization   Additional subjects that can be added to an existing teaching credential.

adenosine triphosphate (ATP)   The body's fuel source.

advocacy   The act of supporting a cause.

aerobic capacity   The ability to perform prolonged, large-muscle, dynamic exercise at moderate to high levels of intensity.

aesthetic sports   Sports that rely on agility, fluidity, beauty, and precision to showcase excellence. Aesthetic sports often include aspects of subjective judging where competitors compete in a parallel fashion, as seen in figure skating, diving, gymnastics, and synchronized swimming.

aesthetics   The branch of philosophy that is concerned with the nature and appreciation of beauty.

allied health professional   A professional involved with the delivery of health or related services pertaining to the identification, evaluation, and prevention of diseases and disorders; dietary and nutrition services; and rehabilitation and health systems management; among others.

American Kinesiology Association (AKA)   Professional organization whose mission is to promote and enhance "kinesiology as a unified field of study and advances its many applications."

American Physical Therapy Association (APTA)   First professional organization to publish a broad research agenda for the allied health professions.

Americans with Disabilities Act (ADA)   Federal law that extended the broad protections of the Civil Rights Act of 1964 to people with disabilities.

analytic knowledge techniques   Research techniques that focus on the cultural meaning and values related to sport and physical activity; methods may include ethnography, including interviews.

analytic research   Research conducted in the field of sport humanities, which includes sport history, sport philosophy, and sport literature.

application The use of one's knowledge and skills in a practical setting.

Article 30 Article in the United Nations Convention on the Rights of Persons with Disabilities that asserts human rights for persons with disabilities.

attribution theory Theory of motivation that focuses on the factors that individuals use to explain their successes and failures.

autism spectrum disorder (ASD) A neurodevelopmental disorder characterized by (1) persistent deficits in social communication and social interactions across multiple contexts and (2) presence of restricted, repetitive patterns of behavior, interests, or activities.

axiology The branch of philosophy that is concerned about the nature of values or the good.

balance A global term referring to control processes that maintain body parts in the specific alignments necessary to achieve different kinds of mobility and stability. Postural stability, postural control, and postural orientation all play a role in balance.

bias Perception influenced by relatively stable judgement cognitions.

biomechanics The application of the methods of mechanics to the study of the structure and function of biological systems.

blood pressure The force of blood on the blood vessel walls.

body Any collection of matter that is being examined.

body composition The proportion of total body weight made up of fat mass and fat-free mass.

bone density The amount of bone tissue within the bones.

braking force A force that causes a body to slow down.

bullying Unwanted, aggressive behavior involving a real or perceived power intolerance.

cardiovascular disease A disease of the heart and blood vessels, sometimes referred to as heart disease; a chronic disease.

case study evaluation (CSE) An evaluation to assess an individual's current abilities to determine if he or she qualifies for special education services.

chronic exercise effects Gradual and long-term responses to exercise.

chronic health problems/chronic disease Health problems or diseases that begin gradually and last for an extended period of time.

classical mechanics   The study of the motion of bodies under the action of a system of forces.

clinical biomechanics   Examination of the causes of musculoskeletal disorders and evaluation of various treatment methods.

clinical sport psychology   Branch of sport psychology that focuses on personality factors that influence performance and/or team interactions.

cognitive-behavioral orientation   Sport psychology approach that posits that behaviors stem from individuals' thoughts and beliefs (i.e., cognitions).

cohesion   The total field of forces that act on members to remain in a group.

Commission on Teacher Credentialing (CTC)   State agency that regulates the issuance of teaching credentials to those who qualify.

communication   The ability to write, compose emails, give presentations, and have conversations with people across the generations.

community   A group of people with a shared interest.

competency approach   An emphasis on skill development that will help you become an exceptional professional.

competency skills   The set of skills required to efficiently and successfully participate in a professional setting.

Comprehensive School Physical Activity Program (CSPAP)   Goal that all schools provide a physical activity program with the following five components: (1) physical education, (2) physical activity during school, (3) physical activity before and after school, (4) staff involvement, and (5) family and community involvement.

concentric action   Action whereby the MTC length is shortening and generating energy.

conceptual clarity   When concepts are presented in a coherent, intelligible, and straightforward manner to support deeper insight.

consumption of meanings in physical culture   Involves the process of *sportization*, or the path through which sport and its meanings have penetrated one's way of life.

corrective physical education   An early name of APA that came from the medical root of physical education designed mostly for World War II veterans with amputation or spinal cord injury.

critical inquiry   The use of sound reasoning and clear arguments to identify concepts and principles.

cultural conditions   Ideas behind human actions and societal norms that inform our beliefs and practices, often before we are even aware of their existence.

cultural theories   Theories that attempt to explain the core values and collective meanings assigned to human interactions.

culture   Dominant and common language, ways of life, roles, and expectations that govern our everyday interactions in the social world.

curriculum   What will be taught (e.g., nontraditional games, dance, educational gymnastics).

decompetition   Play and sport in which everyone "loses" except the very best players.

demand   Amount of resources needed; for example, the need for ATP to do the required work.

descriptive research   Uses description, classification, measurement, and comparison to describe a population or phenomenon.

desired skills   The ability to do something through practice or training that is highly valued in professional settings.

develop   The process of growth and maturation through directed efforts.

diabetes   A disease in which blood sugar is high; a chronic disease.

diastolic blood pressure   Pressure in the blood vessels when the heart is relaxed and refilling with blood.

different treatment   People being treated in dissimilar ways. If there is no relevant reason for the different treatment, then it is discrimination.

disability   An umbrella term that encompasses impairments, activity limitations, and participation restrictions.

disciplinary specialization   The fragmenting of the components of a discipline into multiple subdomains.

discretionary income   The amount of money left over after an individual or family pays for necessities such as shelter, food, and clothing. Sport competes with other brands of entertainment, such as movie theaters, for this segment of money.

discriminate   To categorize individuals or objects on the basis of real or presumed characteristics.

diversity   The abilities, interests, and characteristics that differentiate people from one another.

domains of learning   The fundamental motor (psychomotor) skills, social (affective) skills, and thinking (cognitive) skills necessary to promote lifelong health and well-being.

dualistic interpretation of a person   The view that body and mind are separate and distinct parts of human beings and that we can isolate one aspect from the other within a person.

due process   The legal requirement that the state must respect all legal rights that are owed to a person.

dynamics   The study of things that are moving.

eccentric action   Action whereby the MTC length is increasing and absorbing energy.

educational sport psychology   Branch of sport psychology that focuses primarily on cognitive factors in performance enhancement.

embryonic period   The first stage of the development of kinesiology (1880–1900) in the United States.

emergent sport   Activities that involve participants in new ways of exercise and sport, often including competition.

empowered learner   A learner who can take responsibility for preparing for course requirements and distinguish between being adequately prepared and being underprepared.

encouragement and support   The acts of providing assistance, stimulating development, and promoting confidence on behalf of others in the attainment of a goal.

energy   The state of matter that makes things change or has the capacity to make things change.

epistemology   The branch of philosophy that is concerned with the nature of knowledge.

equality   A concern for the equal rights, access, and opportunities of all people.

equation of life   A mathematical representation to illustrate the various social worlds we belong to and the level of significance each world holds for us.

ethics   The branch of philosophy that is concerned about the nature of right and wrong conduct.

evidence-based principles   Principles that have been developed based on sound and objective scientific research.

evidence-based strategies   Strategies that have been tested and evaluated based on data. The evidence is objective, and decisions can be made regarding the effectiveness of the strategy.

exercise   A specific type of physical activity that is planned and structured with the explicit purpose of improving physical fitness.

exercise physiology   The study of how the body responds and adapts to physical stress.

exercise prescription   The details of an exercise program, including frequency, intensity, duration, and exercise mode.

exercise psychology   The application of psychological principles in exercise settings, usually not involving competition.

experience   Knowledge, skills, and mastery of an activity that is developed through participation.

experience knowledge techniques   Research techniques where the goal is to learn about the actual experiences of people involved in sport and physical activity settings; methods may include surveys, in-depth interviews, and focus groups.

experiences of physical activity   The variety of ways that people participate in physical activity that are coherent, complex, diverse, and meaningful.

extension pattern   A multijoint pattern whereby two segments are rotating in opposite directions and the distance between the beginning and end of the chain is increasing.

external shape   Component of a sporting event that is formed by each sport's purpose, as defined by its unique characteristics and formal regulations.

extreme sports   Countercultural, nature-based, or other sports that involve elements of personal danger. Examples include freestyle skiing, parasailing, cliff diving, and slacklining.

extrinsic motivation   Motivation that comes from external factors outside of the individual.

fair play   Appropriate behaviors in sport that respect the rules and opponents.

Fitts's law   The label for the observed, and exceedingly robust, relationship between speed and accuracy in motor tasks.

flexibility   The ability of the joints to move freely through their normal range of motion.

flexion pattern   A multijoint pattern whereby two segments are rotating in opposite directions and the distance between the beginning and end of the chain is decreasing.

focus   Directing sustained attention toward an area of interest.

following of physical culture   Includes being a spectator of competitive sports, but it also involves following physical activities through television, movies, reading, or social media opportunities.

force   A push or pull by one body on another body.

forensic biomechanics   Examination of accidents and failures.

formative assessment   Assessment that is used as a checkpoint to evaluate student learning from day to day.

free, appropriate public education (FAPE)   Right of children with disabilities to have access to education, as guaranteed by the Rehabilitation Act of 1973 and the Individuals with Disabilities Education Act (IDEA).

functional capacity   A person's ability to participate in physical activity, including basic daily tasks.

fundamental movement skills   Building blocks of human movement upon which sport skills are based, including catching, hopping, jumping, kicking, skipping, running, throwing, twirling, and walking.

game   A voluntary attempt to overcome unnecessary obstacles that is a form of intrinsically valued problem-solving.

games-based approach   Approach to learning that allows students to discover what to do in a game and then how to do it.

gender diversity   The multiple possibilities of gender orientation.

give back   Directing one's efforts and resources to an activity or organization that one has previously benefitted from.

good life   A form of living that consists of personal well-being, fulfillment, and meaning.

gross domestic sport product (GDSP)   The financial (monetary) measurement of all sport-related goods and services produced in a country over a year.

gross motor skills   Movements that use large muscles and segments of the body, such as arms, legs, or feet, or the entire body.

group norms   Levels of performance, behavior patterns, or the belief systems held by the group.

group role   The set of expected behaviors required of someone occupying a certain position within the team.

guiding principles   Core ideas and concepts that direct and influence a plan of action.

health-related components of physical fitness   The components of physical fitness that are associated with good physical health, including body composition, muscular strength, muscular endurance, aerobic capacity, and flexibility.

historical context   The circumstances of a given time period.

holistic approach   View that different course experiences and practical applications are parts of a whole, with each part interacting with and influencing the others.

holistic interpretation of a person   The view that we must take seriously and account for all aspects of a person's experience, realizing that mind, body, and spirit are interconnected.

honor   To respect and hold another person in high regard; acting in a manner that reflects your appreciation of another person.

human movement   The change of position of the individual in time-space resulting from force developed from expending energy in interaction with the environment.

human potential approach   Methods of action based on presumptions of the human capacity to grow, solve problems, and collaborate productively.

hypertension   High blood pressure; a chronic disease.

imitation   The act of copying, duplicating, and mirroring. Imitation tasks can be divided into three categories: postural movements, actions on objects, and orofacial movements. Children with ASD show impaired imitation in all areas.

impact exercise   Physical activity that places stress on the bones.

impairment   Something that causes a limitation in performance, such as a deficit in range of motion, strength, power, endurance, etc.

in silico   An investigation using computer simulation.

in vitro   An investigation using cadaveric or animal tissues.

in vivo   An investigation of a living person.

inclusive fitness trainer   Fitness trainer who can assist people with special needs in an inclusive fitness setting.

Individualized Education Program (IEP)   A legal document that defines a child's special education plan.

Individuals with Disabilities Education Act (IDEA)   Federal law that outlines the rights and regulations for students with disabilities in the United States who require special education.

information processing   A focus on the brain and nervous system in the control of movement; views the brain as a computer.

insider   Person who is deeply involved in the social world and whose life and identity are strongly influenced by the social world and its meanings.

Institute of Medicine (IOM)   Federal institute tasked with helping those in government and the private sector make informed health decisions by providing science-based evidence.

institutionalized bias   Social phenomenon occurring when specific groups gain privileged status and power to control resources.

instruction   How the curriculum is delivered (e.g., instructional formats, curriculum models, teaching strategies).

instructional time   Time students spend watching or listening to the teacher.

instrumental activities of daily living (IADLs)   Daily activities involved in maintaining a household.

internal essence   The subjective experience an individual encounters while watching a performance—in other words, what it means to them.

International Federation of Adapted Physical Activity (IFAPA)   An international, cross-disciplinary professional organization of individuals, institutions, and agencies concerned with promotion and dissemination of knowledge and information about adapted physical activity, disability sport, and all other aspects of sport, movement, and exercise science for the benefit of persons who require adaptations to enable their participation.

interpersonal skills   The ability to effectively relate to and communicate with other people in a given context.

intersectionality   Recognition that the course of human events is a result of combinations of factors, such as race, class, gender, language, or religion, and not just one factor.

intrinsic motivation   Motivation that comes from within the individual.

intrinsic reasons   Explanations or justifications that rely on the thing itself rather than on something else.

isometric action   Action whereby the length is not changing and the MTC is transferring energy.

kinematics   The study of motion without consideration of the cause of the motion.

kinesiology administrative location   The place where kinesiology is housed within the organizational structure of a university.

kinesiology   The study of the art and science of human movement.

kinetic energy   The energy of motion.

kinetics   The study of the causes of motion (i.e., forces).

knowing how   Practical knowledge that is demonstrated through application and performance.

knowing that   Propositional knowledge that is demonstrated through abstractions and theories.

landscape knowledge techniques   Research techniques that provide important information about different populations; includes surveys of large populations, community case studies, and census surveys.

leadership   The people who provide guidance and direction for an organization.

learner centered   Information exchange and knowledge enhancement produced through the shared effort of the professor, student, and classmates.

learner-centered strategies   Activities and behaviors that enable you to take responsibility for and maximize your learning.

learning skills   Skills such as time management, study skills, and computational skills that facilitate engagement with course content to expand one's knowledge base.

least restrictive environment (LRE)   A student who has a disability should have the opportunity to be educated with peers without disabilities, to the greatest extent appropriate.

letter of recommendation   A letter that identifies your strengths and qualifications for a particular post; the quality and power of the letter varies based on many factors.

longitudinal study   Observational research method where data are gathered from the same subjects repeatedly over a long period of time.

major life activities   Functions such as caring for one's self, performing manual tasks, walking, seeing, hearing, speaking, breathing, learning, and working.

managerial time   When students are involved in tasks that are not related to the lesson objectives, such as time spent taking roll, getting into groups, or putting away equipment.

marginalization   Social disadvantages that result in a group being in a powerless or unimportant position.

materialistic interpretation of a person   The viewpoint that people are reducible to physical matter and can be fully understood through the disciplines of physics and chemistry.

meanings   Combinations that form mainly due to the influences we are exposed to as we function in various social worlds.

mechanopathology   Mechanics that cause injury.

medical gymnastics   The first organized school activities involving human movement in the United States. The most popular types were those based on German, Danish, and Swedish programs.

mega events   Large-scale sporting events or festivals that occur infrequently or on a scheduled basis. Examples include the NFL Super Bowl, the FIFA World Cup, the Summer and Winter Olympic Games, and the Boston Marathon.

membership   The state of being included in a group or organization.

mental toughness   Being motivated, dealing with pressure, having confidence, and maintaining concentration.

mentor   An individual who will guide and support you on various aspects of your life journey.

metaphysics   The branch of philosophy that is concerned with the nature of things.

moderate-to-vigorous physical activity (MVPA)   Moderate-intensity physical activity is when a person is working hard enough to raise his or her heart rate and break into a sweat; vigorous physical activity is when a person is breathing hard and fast and his or her heart rate has increased significantly.

motivation   The direction and intensity of effort.

motor activity   Activities that cause or produce motion.

motor behavior   Study of how humans move, including control, acquisition of skills, and change throughout the lifespan.

motor control   Study of motor performance at a given point in time.

motor development   Study of the change of performance over time, including growth and development factors as well as practice.

motor learning   Study of the acquisition of skills for effective movement over time and with practice.

motor performance   Observable actions that humans make when performing a task.

motor planning   The organizational or executive activity of the neural systems that control coordinated movement patterns.

multidisciplinary conference (MDC)   The follow-up meeting after a school district has completed a case study evaluation of a child. The purpose of the meeting is to inform the parents of the results of the school's evaluation and the multidisciplinary team's recommendations.

muscle-tendon complex   The muscle (belly) and all of the elastic components (tendon, fascial layers, etc.).

muscular endurance   The ability of skeletal muscles to generate force, repeatedly.

muscular strength   The ability of skeletal muscles to generate force.

National Collegiate Athletic Association (NCAA)   Organized into three separate divisions, the NCAA overseas intercollegiate sport contests and championships for American institutions of higher education. Currently, it has more than 1,200 member institutions from all 50 states.

National Physical Activity Plan (NPAP)   A plan to create a national culture that supports physically active lifestyles by improving health, preventing disease and disability, and enhancing quality of life.

national standards   Five standards developed by SHAPE America that define a physically literate person and are intended to guide teachers in planning the curriculum and instruction for their students.

nature versus nurture   Study of the effects of genetic predisposition on performance versus the effects of environmental factors.

North American Society for Sport Management (NASSM)   The main sport management governing academic association in North America. Founded in 1985 by a group of sport scholars, NASSM hosts an annual conference and publishes the *Journal of Sport Management*.

obesity-related disease   A disease for which obesity is a possible contributing risk factor.

observational research   A technique used to observe and record behaviors that occur in a participant's natural setting.

occupational biomechanics   Examination of the interactions of workers with their tools, machines, and materials.

osteoporosis   A disease in which bone density is reduced, increasing the risk of bone fracture.

pathomechanics   Mechanics that are a result of an injury.

pedagogy   The art, science, or profession of teaching.

person-first attitudes and language   More appropriate and empowering way to refer to someone with a disability by focusing on what the person can do instead of solely on his or her disabilities.

personal excellence   The pursuit of excellence through achieving one's highest potential.

personal physical activity   Physical activity choices that can range from a formal sport experience to general physical activity.

philosophical orientation   A particular perspective on how learning occurs.

philosophy of kinesiology   The subdiscipline of kinesiology that uses philosophical methods to examine various aspects of kinesiology.

physical activity (PA)   Any bodily movement that requires the use of energy by the individual.

physical activity relationship (PAR)   Tool used to analyze and gain a better understanding of an individual's relationship to sport and physical activity culture.

physical culture   A social, organized way of life that promotes the physical development in persons.

physical education   A planned, sequential program of curricula and instruction that helps students develop the knowledge, skills, and confidence needed to adopt and maintain a physically active lifestyle.

physical fitness   Physiological attributes that reflect the ability of the systems of the body to support physical activity.

physiological mechanisms   Interacting processes within the body that bring about one or more effects.

physiological training adaptations   Long-term changes within the systems of the body in response to the stress of exercise.

play   An activity that is pursued intrinsically and for its own sake.

popular sport media   The host of media outlets that televise, broadcast, and report on sport issues. These outlets are widely available to the general public and are not peer-reviewed by sport scholars. Examples include ESPN, CNN, *Sports Illustrated*, the Bleacher Report, CBS Sports, NBC Sports, and countless other networks and individuals that cover sport topics.

potential energy   The energy of position.

power and performance sports   Sport or athletic contests that involve direct physical contact between athletes or participants in order to secure the primary goals of the activities. These sports generally favor athletes who are bigger, faster, and stronger, rather than displaying the flexibility and artistry required in aesthetic sports.

prepared   Making an organized effort to skillfully or knowledgably engage in an activity.

principle of overload   The body must be stressed to a level beyond that to which it is normally accustomed in order to stimulate physiological training adaptations.

principle of progression   As the body adapts to exercise, the exercise intensity must be increased in order to continue to stimulate physiological training adaptations.

principle of reversibility   When an exercise stress is removed, the physiological training adaptations to that stress are lost.

principles of exercise training   Foundational guidelines for planning an exercise program that successfully leads to the desired physiological adaptations without causing undo stress and/or injury.

priority   That thing that takes precedence and is deemed more important than other tasks or activities.

production in physical culture   Creation of physical activity opportunities for participants and spectators.

profession of physical education   The second stage of the development of kinesiology that occurred in the 1920s and 1930s, when *physical education* became the dominant title for the field.

professional goals   Identifying what you would like to accomplish or produce with your education and career.

professional network   A group of people you are prepared to collaborate with to generate positive action for yourself and others.

professionalism   The demonstration of conduct, behavior, and qualities that are expected in a professional setting.

propulsive force   A force that causes a body to speed up.

psychological skill development (PSD)   The systematic and consistent practice of mental/psychological skills for the purpose of enhancing performance, increasing enjoyment, or achieving greater sport and physical activity self-satisfaction.

psychophysiological orientation   Sport psychology approach that posits that the best explanation for sport and exercise behavior lies within the physiological processes that are happening within the brain and body.

Public Law 94-142   The Education for All Handicapped Children Act of 1975, which guarantees a free, appropriate public education to children with disabilities.

qualitative research   Data collected and analyzed are expressed in the form of words or images to examine how people make sense of their world and the experience they have in the world.

quantitative research   Research that generates numerical data and seeks to establish causal relationships between two or more variables by using statistical methods to test the strength and significance of the relationships.

reasonable accommodation   A school is required to take reasonable steps to accommodate a student with a disability unless it would cause the school undue hardship.

reflective scrutiny   Critical analysis of a position to determine if it is supported by compelling arguments and reasons that are consistent and unbiased.

regular   Role where a person is relatively committed to the social world and understands much of its meaning.

relative excellence   The state of being more excellent in a given, limited context in a given activity, such as recreational sport.

role model   A person whose behavior and actions in a given context serve as an example for other people.

"rolling-out-the-ball" methods   Physical activity programs focused only on play rather than on planned human movement using scientific methods.

sabermetrics   Term coined by Bill James to describe the quantitative study of baseball to predict player and team performance. Sabermetrics gained mainstream popularity with the release of the book, and subsequent movie, *Moneyball*.

sacrifices   Those things that are deferred or abandoned in order to pursue one's own priorities or to support another person's priorities.

Section 504 of the Rehabilitation Act of 1973   Civil rights law that prohibits discrimination against individuals with disabilities and ensures that children with disabilities have equal access to an education.

sedentary   Participation in very little physical activity.

self-assessment   An activity that allows you to reflect on how well you are learning and identify what learning-centered strategies work best for you.

shared excellence   The pursuit of excellence through the collective efforts of partners toward a common goal.

skill-related components of physical fitness   The components of physical fitness that are associated with good sport and motor-skill performance.

social cognitive theory   Theory of motivation developed by Alfred Bandura that views behavior as being influenced by the combination of personal, environmental, and behavioral factors.

social currents   The short-term but deeply influencing "feelings" in a collective setting that shape the same everyday roles.

social facts   A fixed institution or civil governance structure that may influence how one performs their everyday roles as student, parent, worker, etc. This fixed governance takes the form of laws and public policy and even penalty for breaking such public contracts.

social rarity   Being one of a kind in a social group based on one highly visible factor.

social world   Refers to certain areas of life that have their own practices, modes of activity, and ways of thinking—a constellation of meaning structures.

social-psychological orientation   Sport psychology approach that posits that behaviors are the result of an interaction between environmental and personal factors.

sociological imagination   Framework used by C. Wright Mills to think about the world around us, taking into account how the individual is connected to the "bigger picture."

sociology of sport, exercise, and physical activity   Academic study of sport as a social phenomenon.

sound philosophical arguments   Statements that present consistent and impartial reasons for accepting a conclusion.

sport and exercise biomechanics   Examination of the cause-and-effect mechanisms of sport movements and exercises.

sport for development   Enhancing an individual or community through well-designed sport/physical activity experiences.

sport   Games that test and contest physical skills and abilities.

sport management   The business-related aspects of producing, managing, or organizing spectator events or sport-specific products.

sport pedagogy   Pedagogy that encompasses school programs of physical education as well as community-based club programs of sport and fitness.

sport physiology   The application of exercise physiology principles to guide training and enhance sport performance.

sport psychology consulting   Role where sport psychologists apply principles learned from research, and perhaps personal experience, to help individual athletes, teams, coaches, and sport organizations develop the psychological skills necessary to be successful in their endeavors.

sport psychology   The study of the psychological factors that come into play before, during, and after sport performance situations and the application of that knowledge.

statics   The study of loads applied to a stationary body.

status quo   The typical way of being in the everyday (i.e., the "way things are").

stranger   Role where a person does not easily understand much about a new social world or what it means to him or her personally, but is drawn to become involved.

stress   Response of the body to a stressor that interferes with normal physiology.

stretch-shortening cycle (SSC)   A concentric MTC action that is immediately preceded by an eccentric MTC action.

stroke   Reduced blood flow to the brain that causes cell death; a chronic disease.

structural components   Major spheres of social life that offer stability and transmit traditions.

structural theories   Theories that attempt to explain broad societal systems and pose questions about how the systems work to meet the needs of societal members, or not.

subdiscipline   Field within a discipline. Kinesiology has a number of subdisciplines, including biomechanics, exercise physiology, neurophysiology of performance, and others.

summative assessment   Assessment that is used to determine what students have learned at the end of a learning segment.

supply   Amount of resources made available; for example, the production of ATP.

supply equals demand   When the amount of resources needed are matched by the amount made available; for example, when the amount of ATP needed is matched by the amount of ATP produced.

swing pattern   Multijoint pattern whereby two segments are rotating in the same direction at submaximal speed.

systolic blood pressure   Pressure in the blood vessels while the heart is contracting and ejecting blood.

teacher movement   Where the teacher goes within the activity area.

teaching behaviors   Verbal or nonverbal actions the teacher performs, such as instructional time or teacher movement.

teaching credential   A state-issued license to teach in public schools.

teamwork   The ability to work with other people to accomplish a shared task.

torque   The turning effect of a force.

tourist   Role whereby a person is curious and interested in the social world in question and might even temporarily participate and test the world.

transition   A period of change that often requires support and education.

traumatic brain injury (TBI)   Brain dysfunction caused by an external mechanical force; usually results from a violent blow or jolt to the head or body.

true competition   Play and sport in which it is understood that all participants "gain" in some way by having participated and given their best effort.

unprofessional qualities   A failure to demonstrate conduct and behavior that is expected in a professional setting.

waist circumference   Measurement of waist size, usually in inches.

wait time   When students do not have any task to do; that is, they are simply standing around.

weight-bearing exercise   Physical activity that requires an individual to support their body weight.

whip pattern   Multijoint pattern whereby two segments are rotating in the same direction at maximal speed.

work   The process by which energy is either added to or subtracted from a body.

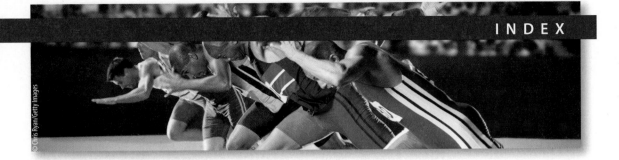

Note: Page numbers followed by '*f*', '*t*' & '*b*' represent figures, tables and boxes respectively.

A

AAAPE (American Association for the Advancement of Physical Education), 43, 43*t*
Absolute excellence, 387
Academic discipline
defined, 46
of physical education (1960–1980), 46–49
Academic journals, sport management, 265–266*t*
Academic learning time in physical education (ALT-PE), 196, 197
Accommodation, reasonable, 306
Achievement goal theory, 101
Acoustic energy, 68
ACSM. *See* American College of Sports Medicine (ACSM)
Action research model, sport pedagogy, 198
example, 199–200*b*
Active-learning strategies, 27
Activities of daily living (ADLs), 126, 127*f*, 129
Acute exercise effects, 120
Acute physiological responses, 128
ADA. *See* Americans with Disabilities Act (ADA)
Adams, Jack, 145

Adaptation. *See also* Adapted physical activity (APA)
defined, 239
Adapted aquatics, 245
Adapted aquatics instructor, 248–249, 249*f*
Adapted fitness business owner, 250
Adapted fitness trainer, in recovery exercise program, 251
Adapted physical activity (APA), 315–320
adaptation, defined, 239
adapted aquatics instructor, 248–249, 249*f*
adapted fitness business owner, 250
adapted fitness trainer in recovery exercise program, 251
adapted wellness program director at retirement community, 251–252
adaptive ski programs, 244–245, 244*f*
aging and disability and, 240–241
APA coordinator in the public sector, 250
APA researcher in university, 251
APA service program director at community college, 250–251
APA specialist at medical center, 249
APE teacher, 247–248, 248*f*

appropriate language in, 239–240
concept map, 233, 234*f*
courses available in, 241–242
cross-disciplinary nature, 235
defined, 233–235
history of, 235–238
medical roots of, 235–236
research activities in, 246*f*
research areas in, 254–257
   administrative and
      epidemiological approach,
      254–255
   biomechanical approach, 255
   motor behavioral approach,
      255–256
   pedagogical approach, 256
   physiological approach, 256
   psychological approach, 256–257
service programs, 242–245, 243*f*,
   244*f*
training in, 245–254
   Aquatic Therapy and
      Rehabilitation Institute
      Certified (ATRIC), 253–254
   Certified Adapted Physical
      Educator (CAPE) certification,
      252–253
   Certified Inclusive Fitness Trainer
      (CIFT) certification, 253
   credentials/certifications, 252–254
   working designations, 247–252
university-based APA program,
   243–244, 243*f*
Adapted Physical Activity Council
   (APAC), 238, 252
Adapted physical education (APE),
   235, 311, 395
   case study, 392
   defined, 235, 236, 309, 395
Adapted Physical Education National
   Standards, 252
Adapted Physical Educators (APE),
   188, 312–315, 313*t*

Adapted Therapeutic Exercise
   Center, 244
Adapted wellness program director, at
   retirement community, 251–252
Adaptive ski programs, 244–245, 244*f*
Added authorizations, 312
Adenosine triphosphate (ATP), 128, 129
ADLs. *See* Activities of daily
   living (ADLs)
Administrative and epidemiological
   approach, APA research,
   254–255
ADOS–R (Autism Diagnostic
   Observation Scale–
   Revised), 396
Advocacy, 377
Aerobic capacity, 292
Aesthetics, 172–174
   defined, 162
Aesthetic sports, 263
Aging, APA and, 240–241
Agon, role of, 160
AKA. *See* American Kinesiology
   Association (AKA)
Allied health, issues in, 324–326
Allied health professionals, 321–322,
   323–324*t*
ALT-PE (academic learning time in
   physical education), 196, 197
Alzheimer's disease, 240
Amateur sport, 268–269
American Academy of Physical
   Education, 46, 50
American Alliance for Health, Physical
   Education, Recreation, and
   Dance (AAHPERD), 202
American Association for the
   Advancement of Physical
   Education (AAAPE), 43,
   43*t*, 121
American Association of
   Cardiovascular and Pulmonary
   Rehabilitation (AACVPR), 125

American Association on Mental
    Deficiency, 236
American College of Sports Medicine
    (ACSM), 61, 123, 124, 125,
    253, 290
    Exercise Is Medicine (EIM)
        initiative, 125, 126
    exercise prescription, 296–297
    on responsibilities of professional
        exercise physiologists, 126, 128
    website, 290
American Federation of College
    Women, 186b
American Journal of Physiology, 121
American Journal of Sports Medicine, 61
American Kinesiology Association
    (AKA), 20
American Orthopaedic Society for
    Sports Medicine, 61
*American Physical Education Review
    (Research Quarterly for Exercise
    and Sport)*, 43
American Physical Therapy
    Association (APTA), 61, 325
American Physiological Society (APS),
    123, 125
American Psychiatric Association, 396
American Society of Biomechanics,
    59, 60
American Society of Exercise
    Physiologists (ASEP), 125
Americans with Disabilities Act
    (ADA), 253, 316
    Article 30, 316, 317t
Analytic knowledge technique, 218,
    219, 221–223
Analytic research, sport pedagogy, 200
Anatomical/biological sex, 363b
Anatomical period, biomechanics, 58
*Anatomy, Physiology, and Physical
    Training*, 121
Anatomy and Physiology, 121
Andrews, David, 223

Ankle plantar flexors, 75
Anxiety, 92
    as stressor, 128
APA. *See* Adapted physical activity
    (APA)
APA coordinator, in public sector, 250
APA researcher, in university, 251
APA service program director, at
    community college, 250–251
APA specialist, at medical center, 249
APE. *See* Adapted physical education
    (APE)
APE teacher, 247–248, 248f
Application, defined, 382
Applied Physiology Study Section, 124
Appreciation, positive inclusion and,
    354–357, 355f
Appropriate instruction, in sport
    pedagogy, 190–193
    instructional time, 192–193
    managerial time, 192–193
    meaningful feedback, 192, 192t
    teacher movement, 190–191
    wait time, 192–193
Appropriate language, in APA,
    239–240
APS (American Physiological Society),
    123, 125
APTA (American Physical Therapy
    Association), 325
Aquatic Therapy and Rehabilitation
    Institute Certified (ATRIC),
    253–254
Aristotle, 58, 59
Arthrometers, 87
Article 30, ADA, 316, 317t
ASD. *See* Autism spectrum disorder
    (ASD)
Association for Applied Sport
    Psychology (AASP), 95
Association for Intercollegiate
    Athletics for Women (AIAW),
    186b

Association for the Advancement of
    Physical Education, 43
Athletic Conference of American
    College Women (ACACW),
    185, 186*b*
ATP (adenosine triphosphate), 128, 129
ATRIC (Aquatic Therapy and
    Rehabilitation Institute
    Certified) exam, 253–254
Attribution theory, 101–102, 102*f*
Autism Classroom, 406
Autism Diagnostic Interview–
    Revised, 396
Autism Diagnostic Observation Scale–
    Revised (ADOS–R), 396
Autism spectrum disorder (ASD), 240
    case study, 409–410, 410*f*
    defined, 392
    diagnosis, 396
    evidence-based strategies, 401–408,
        402*f*
    Gentile's taxonomy, 403, 404*t*
    overview, 395–397
    and physical activity, 397–400, 399*f*
    in physical education setting,
        392–395, 394*f*
    "Red Light, Green Light Dribble"
        game
        393, 401-402, 410-412, 411*f*, 412*f*
Awareness, positive inclusion and,
    354–357, 355*f*
Axiology, defined, 162

B
Balance, 392
Balance of power, learner-centered
    approach, 25–26
Ball Four, 210
Bancroft, Jessie, 183
Bandura, Alfred, 100
Ban Ki-Moon, 344
Barriers, to excellence, 379–380
Baseball, throwing, 72–73

Basic movement skills, 12, 13*f*
Beck, Charles, 183*b*
Beecher, Catherine, 183*b*
Behavior change, transtheoretical
    model of, 298–299, 298*t*
Benoit, Joan, 377, 378, 385
Berger, Bonnie G., 110–112*b*
Bernstein, Nicholas, 145
Bernstein, Nikolai, 60
Bias
    defined, 348
    institutional, 347
Big choices, 4, 4*f*
The Biggest Loser, 225
Big Ten Body-of-Knowledge
    Symposium, 46–47
Biological/anatomical sex, 363*b*
Biological principles, biomechanics,
    74–83
    MTC action(s), 74–78, 75–77*f*, 79*f*,
        81–82
    MTC force, factors affecting,
        79–83, 80*f*
    MTC length, 79–80, 81*f*
    stretch-shortening cycle, 83
    velocity, MTC and, 82–83, 82*f*
Biomechanical approach, APA
    research, 255
Biomechanics, 10–11, 11*t*, 21, 34,
    56–88
    areas of application, 57
    areas of research in, 87–88
    biological principles, 74–83
    careers in, 84–87, 84*t*, 85*t*
    defined, 57
    equipment, 62
    evaluation and diagnosis, 86
    history of, 58–61
        anatomical period, 58
        experimental period, 59–60
        modern period, 60–61
        theoretical period, 59
    intervention, 86–87

mechanical principles, 63–69
multisegment principles, 69–74
objectives, 62
observation, 85
overview, 56–57
for performance improvement, 62, 63*f*
principles, 63–83, 64*f*
reasons to study, 61–63
Bissinger, H. G., 222
Blood pressure, 290–291
diastolic, 290–291
high (hypertension), 291–292
systolic, 290
"Blooming, buzzing confusion," 346
Body, defined, 64
Body composition, 292
Body orientation, 403
Bolt, Usain, 208
Bone density, 297
Borelli, Giovanni Alfonso, 59
Bouton, Jim, 210
Braking force, defined, 65
Braune, Wilhelm, 60
British Philosophy of Sport
Association, 161
Brown Aquatic Therapy Center, 244
Bucciere, Robert A., 112–114*b*
Bullying, 360–362, 361*t*
Burchenal, Elizabeth, 183
Byford, William H., 121

C
California State University (CSU)
system, 6, 20
Calisthenics, 42
CAPE (Certified Adapted Physical
Educator), 252–253
Cardiovascular disease, 293
Careers/career opportunities, 429–431
APA, 245–254
Aquatic Therapy and
Rehabilitation Institute
Certified (ATRIC), 253–254

Certified Adapted Physical
Educator (CAPE) certification,
252–253
Certified Inclusive Fitness Trainer
(CIFT) certification, 253
credentials/certifications,
252–254
working designations, 247–252
applications, 14
biomechanics, 84–87, 84*t*, 85*t*
exercise physiology, 134–138,
135–136*t*
motor behavior, 149–151
coaching, 149–150
opportunities for, 151
physical education, 150
physical/occupational therapy,
150–151
philosophy of kinesiology, 174–176
prelude, 430–431
restorating function, 320–321
sociology of sport, exercise, and
physical activity, 227
sport management, 276, 277*t*
Case study evaluation (CSE),
304–305
Cassidy, Rosiland, 184*b*
Cecil, Brittanie, 275
Centers for Disease Control and
Prevention (CDC), 220, 396
Certified Adapted Physical Educator
(CAPE), 252–253
Certified Inclusive Fitness Trainer
(CIFT), 253
Chemical energy, 68
Childhood obesity, 240
Children, ASD in. *See* Autism
spectrum disorder (ASD)
Chronic exercise effects, 120
Chronic health problems, 287
Chronophotograph, 60
CIFT (Certified Inclusive Fitness
Trainer), 253

Cinematography, 60

Citizen's Fitness project (case study), 350–354

Classical mechanics, 63–64
areas of, 64–65, 64f
Newton's second law, 74
rules of, 65

Clinical and health psychology, educational backgrounds of specialists in, 111–112b

Clinical biomechanics, 57, 84t, 85t

Clinical Biomechanics, 61

Clinical sport psychology, 97

Clinical training, exercise psychology, 113b

Closed-loop theory, of motor learning, 145

Clubfoot, 372

Coach, functions, 35

Coaching, career in motor behavior, 149–150

Cognitive-behavioral orientation, in sport psychology, 99

Cohesion, 107f
defined, 106
factors influencing, 106–108
and performance, relationship between, 106
types of, 106

Cold War, 45

Collective conscience, 215

Collins, Jason, 172

Color Runs, 225, 226

Combe, A., 121

Commission on Intercollegiate Athletics for Women (CIAW), 186b

Commission on Sport Management Accreditation (COSMA), 265

Commission on Teacher Credentialing (CTC), 312

Committee on Adapted Physical Education, 236

Communication
defined, 20
and social mobilizations, 359

Community, 344–346, 385

Community college, APA service program director at, 250–251

Competencies, 21–22

Competency approach
defined, 21
implementation, 35–36
popularity of kinesiology and, 20–21
skills and competencies, 21–22
surveys reports and, 20–21

Competency skills, 21–22
defined, 19
development, 36

Competition, 225
nature of, 359, 360t

Comprehensive School Physical Activity Program (CSPAP), 202–203

Computational skills, 23

Conant, James B., 45–46, 123

Conant Report, 124

Concentric actions, MTC, 76, 82, 83

Conceptual clarity, defined, 156

Concurrent patterns, 72

Conflict resolution, 358

Consulting, sport psychology, 96

Consumer behavior, sport, 271–272, 272f

Consumption of meanings in physical culture, 337

Contesting, forms of, 359, 360t

Continuing education units (CEUs), 252

Cooper, Kenneth, Dr., 224

Cooper Institute, 224, 225, 227

Core scientific domains, 10–11, 11t

Corrective physical education, 236

Corrective Physical Education, 236

Co-twin control studies, 144

Course, setting, 418–419

Credentials/certifications, in APA, 252–254
Critical inquiry, defined, 156
CrossFit, 166, 175, 221, 222, 224–225, 226
CSE (case study evaluation), 304–305
CSPAP (omprehensive School Physical Activity Program), 202–203
Cultural conditions, 212, 225–226
Cultural norms, 208
Cultural physical activity. *See* Personal and cultural physical activity
Cultural theories, sociology of sport, exercise, and physical activity, 217–218
Culture, 207, 330, 340
Cureton, Thomas K., 123
Curriculum, PE, 181
Cybex Total Access weight machine, 247*f*

D

Dart, throwing, 72, 73
Data generation techniques, 223
da Vinci, Leonardo, 58
Davis, Ronald, 125
Decision-making, 418
  about learning, 26
Decompetition, 359
Demand, 128
De Motu Animalium (On the Movement of Animals), 58, 59
Descriptive research, in sport pedagogy, 195–196
Desired skills, 20
Develop, defined, 375
Developmental disabilities, 240
Diabetes, 293
Diagnostic and Statistical Manual of Mental Disorders, 5th edition (DSM-5), 113*b*, 396
Diastolic blood pressure, 290–291
Different treatment, 379

Dill, David Bruce "D.B.", 122, 122*f*
Direct teaching approach, 197
  vs. games-based approach, 197*t*
Disability(ies). *See also* Person with a disability
  APA and, 240–241
  defined, 239–240, 306
  developmental, 240
Disabled person. *See* Person with a disability
Disciplinary specialization, 47
Disciplinization, 47. *See also* Academic discipline
Discretionary income, 271
Discrimination
  defined, 346
  from difference to, 346–350
Disease, as stressor, 128
Disease populations, physical activity needs of, 113–114*b*
Diversity, 5, 344–346
  bullying, 360–362
  Citizen's Fitness project, as case study, 350–354
  defined, 387
  difference to discrimination, 346–350
  gender, 362–366
  nature of competition, 359, 360*t*
  strategies for positive inclusion awareness and appreciation, 354–357, 355*f*
  for fostering unity, 357–359
Division for Girls' and Women's Sports (DGWS), 186*b*
Document analysis, 220
Domains of learning, 180
Dorsiflexion, MTC during, 75, 77*f*
Drinkwater, Barbara, 125
Dual-energy x-ray absorptiometry (DXA), 87
Dualism, 163, 164, 168
Dualistic interpretation of a person, 32, 163, 164

Due process, 307
Durkheim, Emile, 214–215
Dynamic pattern perspective, motor
    behavior, 145
Dynamics, defined, 64–65

E

Eccentric action, MTC, 77, 81, 82, 83
Economic development, 358–359
Education
    historcal perspectives, 44
    interprofessional, for exercise
        psychology students, 114b
Educational sport psychology, 97–98
Education for All Handicapped
    Children Act of 1975, 311
The Education of American Teachers,
    45–46
Edwards, Harry, 210
Einstein, Albert, 64
Eisenhower, Dwight D., 45, 123
Eitzen, Stan, 206
Electromagnetic energy, 68
Electromyography (EMG), 87
Embryonic period (1880s–1900s),
    42–44
Embryonic years, 122, 124
Emergent sport, 224–225
Empowered learner, 26
Encouragement and support, 374
Energy
    defined, 66, 68
    exchange of, 66, 68–70, 70f
    types of, 68f
Epistemology, 168–169
    defined, 162
Equality, 171–172
Equation of life, 332, 333
Equipment, 62
Ergonomics, 61
Espenscade, Anna, 145
ESPN, 267, 274
Ethics, 162, 170–172

defined, 162
    sport management, 274–275
Ethnicity, 207, 223
European Sport Management
    Quarterly, 274
Evaluation and diagnosis, in
    biomechanics, 86
Evidence-based practice/strategies,
    324–325
    defined, 401
    for inclusive physical education for
        children with ASD, 401–408
Evidence-based principles, 290
Excellence
    absolute, 387
    barriers to, 379–380
    contribution of kinesiology to,
        381–382
    foundations, 372–374
    meaning, 386–387
    models of, 377–379
    personal, 372, 386
    relative, 386–387
    sacrificing for, 375–376
    setbacks and challenges, 382–386
    shared, 372, 389
    as unending quest, 388–389
Exercise, 120. See also Sociology of
        sport, exercise, and physical
        activity
    defined, 126
    discovering joys of, 110–111b
    as playful, 166
    vs. physical activity (PA), 128–129
Exercise in Education and Medicine,
    236
Exercise Is Medicine (EIM) initiative,
    125, 126
Exercise physiology, 21, 33
    areas within, 128–130
    career areas, 135–136t
    careers in, 134–138, 135–136t
    defined, 120

degree in, 134–138
embryonic years, 122, 124
formative years, 124
history of, in United States, 121–125
principles, 128–130
reasons to study, 126–128
recognition years, 125
research areas, 136–138t, 139
Exercise prescription, 21, 287, 296–297
Exercise programs, 12–13, 13f
Exercise psychology. *See also* Sport
        psychology
    Berger on, 110–112b
    clinical training, 113b
    defined, 92
    educational backgrounds of
        specialists in, 111–112b
    future directions, 110–114b
    hedonic experience, 110–111b
    interprofessional education for
        students, 114b
    vs. sport psychology, 93t
Exercise science, educational
        backgrounds of specialists
        in, 111b
Exercise training, principles of,
        132–134
Experience, defined, 158
Experience knowledge techniques,
        218, 219, 220–221
Experiences of physical activity,
        31–35
Experimental period, biomechanics,
        59–60
Experimental research, in sport
        pedagogy, 196–198
Extension pattern, 70, 71, 73
    joint motions associated with,
        71–72, 71t, 72f
External shape, 335
Extreme sports, 263
Extrinsic motivation, 99
Extrinsic values, 169

F

Facility(ies), sport, management of,
        272–274, 273f
Fair play, defined, 157
FAPE (free, appropriate public
        education), 306, 311
Fatigue, 144
Fédération Internationale de Football
        Association (FIFA), 276
Federation of American Societies for
        Experimental Biology (FASEB),
        123, 125
Feedback, meaningful, 192, 192t
FIFA World Cup, 262
Fischer, Otto, 60
Fishburne, Laurence, 56
Fitness. *See* Physical fitness
Fitness assessment, 292–293, 294t
Fitness program, 297–300
Fitts's law, 144
Fitz, George W., 121
Flexibility, 292
Flexion pattern, 70, 71
    joint motions associated with,
        71–72, 71t, 72f
Focus, defined, 36
Focus groups, 221
Following of physical culture, 334–335
Force
    defined, 65
    and exchange of energy, 66,
        68–70, 70f
    and torque, 65–66, 66f, 67f
    work–energy concepts, 68–69, 70f
Force-velocity relation, MTC, 82f
Forensic biomechanics, 57, 84t
Formative assessment, 193
Formative years, 124
Forms of movement, 9
Foundations, excellence, 372–374
Fraleigh, Warren, 160
Framingham Heart Study, 220

Free, appropriate public education
    (FAPE), 306, 311
Friday Night Lights, 222
Functional capacity, 287
Function of the content, learner-
    centered approach, 25, 27
Function restoration. *See* Restoration,
    function
Fundamental movement skills, 12, 13*f*

G

Gait, study of, 59–60
Gait & Posture, 61
Galen, 58
Galilei, Galileo, 58, 59
Game
    defined, 167
    features, 167
Games-based approach, 196–197
    vs. direct teaching approach, 197*t*
Gay, 366
Gender, 223
Gender diversity, 362–366. *See also*
    Diversity
Gender equity, promotion of, 358
Gender expression, 363*b*, 366
Gender fluidity, 364*b*
Gender identity, 363*b*
Gender nonconforming/gender
    variant, 364*b*
Genderqueer, 364*b*
Gentile's taxonomy, 403, 404*t*
George Williams College (Illinois), 123
Gerontology, educational backgrounds
    of specialists in, 112*b*
Gesell, Arnold, 144
Give back, 387
Glassow, Ruth, 145
Goals, personal and professional,
    420–421, 426
Goal setting, health and wellness,
    293–297
Good life, defined, 157

Google, 216
Great Depression, 184
Greendorfer, Susan, 210
Griffith, Coleman, 93
Griffith era, 93
Gross domestic sport product
    (GDSP), 267
Gross motor skills, 392
Group dynamics. *See* Team/group
    dynamics
Group norms, 106
Group roles, 106
Groups, formation of, 105–106
Guiding principles, 18–20
Gulick, Luther, 183, 184*b*
Gulick, Luther Halsey, 43
Gymnastics, 42

H

Handicap, 240
Hanna, Delphine, Dr., 182–183,
    182*f*, 184*b*
Hartwell, Edward, 184*b*
Harvard Fatigue Laboratory,
    122, 123
Health and wellness (case study),
    286–301
    common problems, 288
    fitness assessment, 292–293, 294*t*
    fitness program, 297–300
    goal setting and exercise
        prescription, 293–297
    health evaluation, 290–292, 291*f*
    physician clearance, 292
    post-assessment, reevaluation, and
        revision, 300, 301*t*
    solution of problems, 289–290
Health evaluation, 290–292, 291*f*
Health promotion and disease
    prevention programs, 358
Health questionnaire, 290, 291*f*
Health-related components of physical
    fitness, 131, 131*t*, 292

Healthy balance restoration, care for (case study), 304–309

Healthy People 2020, 203

Healthy population, physical activity needs of, 113–114*b*

Hedonic exercise experiences, 110–111*b*

Heinrich, Ernst, 59

Hemenway, Mary, 184*b*

Henderson, L. J., 122

Henry, Franklin, 46, 94, 145, 209

High blood pressure, 291–292

Hill, A. V., 60

Historical context, 212

History, of kinesiology, 41–50
  academic discipline of physical education (1960–1980), 46–49
  embryonic period (1880s–1900s), 42–44
  1990–present, 49–50
  overview, 42
  profession of physical education (1900–1960), 44–46
  sport history, 48–49

Hitchcock, Edward, 121, 183*b*

Holism, 163–164

Holistic approach, 19–20, 30–31
  commitment to, 35
  defined, 19, 30
  development, 37–38
  experiences of physical activity, 31–35
  implementation, 37–38
  in kinesiology, 33–35

Holistic interpretation of a person, 32, 163–165

Homans, Amy Morris, 184, 184*b*, 235–236

Honestly, 422

Honor, 385

Hopping, MTC during, 78

Hot war, 45

"Human Adaptation to Environmental and Exercise Stress," 124

Human and functional anatomy, 21

Human gait, study of, 59–60

Human movement
  core scientific domains, 10–11, 11*t*
  defined, 8
  sociocultural-based forms, 11–12, 12*t*
  specialized movement forms, 12–13, 13*f*
  study of, 8 (*See also* Kinesiology)

Human potential approach, 356

Hypertension, 291–292

I

IADLs. *See* Instrumental activities of daily living (IADLs)

IDEA. *See* Individuals with Disabilities Education Act (IDEA)

IEP. *See* Individualized Education Program (IEP)

IFAPA. *See* International Federation of Adapted Physical Activity (IFAPA)

Illness, as stressor, 128

Imitation, 398

Impact exercise, 297

Impairment(s), 86. *See also* Disability
  defined, 239–240

Inclusion, positive, strategies for
  awareness and appreciation, 354–357, 355*f*
  for fostering unity, 357–359

Inclusive fitness trainers, 245

Individual development, 358

Individualized Education Program (IEP), 307, 393
  contents of, 310*t*
  extra content for youth with disabilities, 309–326
    adapted physical activity, 315–320
    adapted physical education, 311
    adapted physical educator, 312–315

allied health professions,
321–322, 322–324*t*
career possibilities, 320–321
therapeutic exercise and allied
health, issues in, 324–326
postsecondary goals, 310
Individuals with Disabilities Education
Act (IDEA), 307
IEP contents, 310
Industrial Revolution, 225
Information processing, 145
Information processing perspective,
motor behavior, 145
Injury(ies), decreasing risk of
mechanical principles application,
69, 70*f*
Injury mechanics, 87–88
In-phase patterns, 72
Insiders
defined, 337
life as, 337–338
In silico investigations, 88
Instagram, 216
Institute for Ergonomics and Human
Factors, 61
Institute of Medicine (IOM), 203, 324
Institutional bias, 347
Institutional housing of kinesiology,
6, 7*f*, 7*t*
Instruction, PE, 181
Instructional time, 192–193
Instrumental activities of daily living
(IADLs), 126, 127*f*, 129
*The Integrative Action of the Nervous
System*, 143
Intercollegiate Athletic Association
of the United States (IAAUS),
184–185
Intercollegiate Conference of Faculty
Representatives, 186*b*
Intercollegiate sport, 268–269
Interdisciplinary kinesiology, 50
Internal essence, 335

International Association for the
Philosophy of Sport, 161, 174
International Federation of Adapted
Physical Activity (IFAPA), 233,
236, 238, 316–318
*International Journal of Sport
Management and Marketing*, 271
*International Journal of Sports
Biomechanics*, 61
International Olympic Committee
(IOC), 344, 345
*International Review for the Sociology
of Sport*, 210
International Society of
Biomechanics, 60
International Sociology of Sport
Association (ISSA), 210
International Special Olympics, 236
International Sports Organization for
the Disabled, 236
Interpersonal skills, defined, 36
Interprofessional education, for
exercise psychology
students, 114*b*
Interscholastic sport, 268–269
Intersectionality, 348
Intersex, 364*b*
Intertrial variability, 403
Intervention, in biomechanics, 86–87
Intrinsic motivation, 99
Intrinsic reasons, PA, 165–166
Intrinsic values, 169
In vitro methods, 88
In vivo investigations, 87
IOM. *See* Institute of Medicine (IOM)
Isokinetic dynamometry, 87
Isometric action, MTC, 78, 81, 82, 83
Itard, Jean-Marc, 236

J

James, Bill, 278
James, William, 346
Johnson, Warren, 94

Joint motions, associated with flexion/
    extension pattern, 71–72,
    71*t*, 72*f*
Joint United Nations Programme on
    HIV/AIDS (UNAIDS), 345
Journal for the Philosophy of Sport, 275
Journal of Amateur Sport, 269
Journal of American Medicine, 225
Journal of Applied Biomechanics, 61
Journal of Applied Physiology, 123
Journal of Applied Sport Psychology, 95
Journal of Athletic Training, 61
Journal of Biomechanics, 60
*Journal of Electromyography and
    Kinesiology*, 61
*Journal of Issues in Intercollegiate
    Athletics*, 269
Journal of Legal Aspects of Sport, 275
*Journal of Orthopaedic and Sports
    Physical Therapy*, 61
*Journal of Physical Education,
    Recreation, and Dance*,
    209–210
*Journal of Sport Management, Sport
    Marketing Quarterly*, 272
Journal of Sport Psychology, 95
Journal of Sports Economics, 272
*Journal of Strength and Conditioning
    Research*, 61
Journal of the Philosophy of Sport,
    160–161
Joys of exercise, discovering, 110–111*b*

K

Kaepernick, Colin, 215
Karpovich, P. V., 123
Kelso, J. Scott, 145
Kinematics, 65
Kinesiology. *See also* Philosophy of
    kinesiology
    background, 8–9
    challenges, 11–12
    contribution to excellence, 381–382
    core scientific domains, 10–11, 11*t*
    defined, 5
    diversity, 5
    educational backgrounds of
        specialists in, 111*b*
    future of, 423–425
    guiding principles, 18–20
    history of (*See* History, of
        kinesiology)
    institutional housing, 6, 7*f*, 7*t*
    interdisciplinary, 50
    methods in career applications, 14
    as multidisciplinary, 50
    paradoxes, 5–8
    popularity of, 20–21
    public health and (*See* Public
        Health)
    sociocultural-based forms of
        movement, 11–12, 12*t*
    specialized movement forms,
        12–13, 13*f*
    strata of, 10–13
    subdisciplines, 10–11, 11*t*, 21, 33–34,
        50 (*See also specific entries*)
    terminological meaning, 49
    values, 169–170
Kinesiology administrative location, 6
Kinesiology home, 7*f*
Kinetic energy, 68
Kinetics, 65
Kiphard, Ernst, 239
Knowing how, 168
Knowing that, 168
1953 Kraus-Weber tests, 45

L

LaLanne, Jack, 225
Landscape knowledge techniques, 218,
    219–220
Language, appropriate, in APA,
    239–240
Laws of motion (Newton's laws),
    69–70, 74

Leadership, 377
Learner awareness, 27
Learner-centered approach
    balance of power, 25–26
    decisions about learning, 26
    focus for students, 28–30
    function of the content, 25, 27
    implementation, 36–37
    principles, 24–28
    purpose and processes of
        evaluation, 25
    responsibility for learning, 25
    role of teacher, 25
    teacher's role, 28
    vs. teacher-centered, 23–24, 25*t*
Learner centered skills
    defined, 19
    development, 36–37
Learner-centered strategies, 28
Learning, lifelong, 427
Learning skills
    defined, 23
    examples, 23
Least restrictive environment, 307
Legislation
    restoring function and, 306–309
    supporting individuals with
        disabilities, 311*t*
Lemke, Wilfred, 344
Length, of MTC, 79–80, 81*f*
Lesbian, 366
Letter grades, learner-centered
    classrooms, 29
Letter of recommendation, 422
"Life is a game. Live accordingly," 167
Lifelong learning, 427
Life-span human development, 235
Ling, Per Henrik, 235
Longitudinal study, 149, 220
Lower extremity(ies), motions
        associated with flexion and
        extension patterns of, 70–72,
        71*t*, 72*f*

M

Madison Square Garden (New York
    City), 273*f*
Magnetic resonance imaging
    (MRI), 87
Major life activities, 306–307
Managerial time, 192–193
Manipulation, 403
Marey, Etienne-Jules, 60
Marginalization, 348, 349*f*, 377
Marketing, sport, and revenue
    generation, 269–271
Mason, James, Dr., 264
Materialistic interpretation of a
    person, 163, 164
Materials science, 65
The Matrix (movie), 56, 57*f*
Matrix of difference, 224
Mayo, G. E., 122
McGraw, Myrtle, 144
McKenzie, R. Tait, 236, 237*f*
McNamee, Mike, 161
MDC (multidisciplinary conference),
    304, 305
Meaningful content, in sport
    pedagogy, 189–190
Meaningful feedback, 192, 192*t*
Meaningful questions generation, 26
Meanings, 330–331
*Meat on the Hoof: The Hidden World
    of Texas Football*, 210
Mechanical energy, 68
Mechanical principles, biomechanics,
    63–69, 64*f*
*The Mechanics of the Human Walking
    Apparatus*, 59
Mechanopathology, 62
Medical center, APA specialist at, 249
Medical gymnastics, 8–9, 235
    defined, 8
*Medicine and Science in Sports and
    Exercise*, 61, 124

Mega events, 275
Membership, 377
Mental consultant, 98
Mental skills, 104, 105f. *See
        also* Psychological skill
        development (PSD)
Mental toughness, 103
Mentors, 18, 419
Metaphysics, 163–167
    defined, 161–162
Mills, C. Wright, 206, 211–212
Miracle (film), 45
Moderate-to-vigorous physical activity
        (MVPA), 196
Modern period, biomechanics, 60–61
Moment of force, 65
Moneyball (movie), 278
Mortality, 287
Motivation, 92
    achievement goal theory, 101
    attribution theory, 101–102, 102f
    defined, 99
    extrinsic, 99
    intrinsic, 99
    social cognitive theory, 100–101, 100f
    in sport psychology, 99–102
    tips for increasing, 103t
Motor activity, 196
Motor behavior, 142–151
    as area of inquiry, contemporary
        history of, 143–145
    building blocks of study,
        142–143, 143f
    in career, 149–151
        coaching, 149–150
        opportunities for, 151
        physical education, 150
        physical/occupational therapy,
            150–151
    defined, 142
    dynamic pattern perspective, 145
    information processing
        perspective, 145

motor control, 147–148
motor development, 148–149
motor learning, 148
nature *versus* nurture, 144
outside-in approach, 146, 146f
research
    motor control, 147–148
    motor development, 148–149
    motor learning, 148
    during World War II, 144–145
subdisciplines, 147–149
time frames of, 143f
Motor behavioral approach, APA
        research, 255–256
Motor control, 60, 142–143, 147–148
    research on, 147–148
Motor development, 21, 33, 143
    research on, 148–149
Motor learning, 21, 33, 143
    research on, 148
Motor performance, 142
Motor planning, 392
Movement, 49
Movement ABC, 401
MTC. *See* Muscle–tendon complex
        (MTC)
Multidisciplinary conference (MDC),
        304, 305
Multisegment principles,
        biomechanics, 69–74
Muscle mechanics, 60
Muscle model, 60
Muscle–tendon complex (MTC)
    action(s), 74–78, 75–77f, 79f, 81–82
    concentric actions, 76, 82, 83
    defined, 74
    during dorsiflexion, 75, 77f
    eccentric action, 77, 81, 82, 83
    force, factors affecting, 79–83, 80f
    force-velocity relation, 82f
    function of, 75–76, 78
    during hopping, 78
    isometric action, 78, 81, 82, 83

length of, 79–80, 81*f*
during plantar flexion, 75, 77*f*
principle of, 74–75, 75*f*
stretch-shortening cycle, 78, 83
velocity and, 82–83, 82*f*
Muscular endurance, 292
Muscular strength, 292
Muybridge, Eadweard, 59–60
MVPA (moderate-to-vigorous physical
       activity), 196
Myths, about PSD, 103–104

N

NAK. *See* National Academy of
       Kinesiology (NAK)
Nash, Jay, 183
NASSM (North American Society for
       Sport Management), 263, 265
National Academy of Kinesiology
       (NAK), 50
   evolution of, 50*t*
National Association for Girls'
       and Women's Sport
       (NAGWS), 186*b*
National Association for Physical
       Education for College Women
       (NAPECW), 186*b*
National Athletic Trainers'
       Association, 61
National Autism Center (NAC), 401
National Center on Health, Physical
       Activity and Disability
       (NCHPAD), 253
National Collegiate Athletic
       Association (NCAA), 268–269,
       269*f*, 276
National Consortium for Physical
       Education and Recreation for
       Individuals with Disabilities
       (NCPERID), 238, 252
National Football League (NFL) Super
       Bowl, 262
National Hockey League (NHL), 275

National Institutes of Health
       (NIH), 124
National Intramural Association, 186*b*
The National Physical Activity
       Alliance, 201
National Physical Activity Plan
       (NPAP), 201–202
National standards, 181
National Standards Project, 401
National Strength and Conditioning
       Association (NSCA), 61,
       125, 290
Nature *versus* nurture, 144
NBC Sports, 267, 274
NCAA. *See* National Collegiate
       Athletic Association (NCAA)
NCAA Division I athletics, 276
NCAA Division III athletics, 276
NCAA March Madness, 269
Neuroscience, 60
Newell, Karl, 48, 49
New physical education, 187. *See also*
       Physical education (PE)
Newton, Sir Isaac, 59, 64, 69
Newton's laws, 69–70, 74
Newton's second law, 74
Nike, 225
1990–present, 49–50
Nissen, Hartvig, 183*b*
North American Federation of
       Adapted Physical Activity
       (NAFAPA), 238
North American Industry
       Classification System, 266–267
North American Society for Sport
       History, 49
North American Society for Sport
       Management (NASSM),
       263, 265
North American Society for
       the Psychology of Sport
       and Physical Activity
       (NASPSPA), 94

North American Society for the Sociology of Sport (NASSS), 210
Note-taking, 27
NPAP (National Physical Activity Plan), 201–202
NSCA. *See* National Strength and Conditioning Association (NSCA)
Nuclear energy, 68

O

Obama, Barack, 124
Obesity
   childhood, 240
   prevalence of, 240
Obesity-related disease, 293
Observation, in biomechanics, 85
Observational research, in sport pedagogy, 196
Occupational biomechanics, 57, 84*t*, 85*t*
Ogilvie, Bruce, Dr., 94, 94*f*
Olympic Games, 160, 172, 208, 209, 227, 344, 345, 384, 385
Olympic Project for Human Rights, 210
O'Malley, Walter, 263, 264, 264*f*
Opportunity to learn, in sport pedagogy, 189
Orientations, in sport psychology, 98–99
   cognitive-behavioral, 99
   psychophysiological, 98
   social-psychological, 98
Osteoporosis, 287
Outside-in approach, motor behavior, 146, 146*f*
Overload, principle of, 133

P

PA. *See* Physical activity (PA)
PAR. *See* Physical activity relationship (PAR)
Paradoxes, kinesiology, 5–8

Paralympic athlete, 34
Paralympic Games, 172
Paralympic National Committees, 321
Paralympics, 188
Parent disciplines, 10
Parkinson's disease, 233, 240, 244
PAR-Q (Physical Activity Readiness Questionnaire), 290, 291*f*
Participatory action research, 198
Pathomechanics, 62
Paul, Joan, 42
PE. *See* Physical education (PE)
Peace building and conflict resolution, 358
Pedagogical approach, APA research, 256
Pedagogy, 48. *See also* Sport pedagogy
   defined, 180
Performance, 62
   biomechanics for improvement of, 62, 63*f*
   and cohesion, relationship between, 106
   measurement, 144
   team, factors influencing, 106–108, 107*f*
Perrin, Ethel, 183
Personal and cultural physical activity (case study), 330–340
   life as an insider, 337–338
   life as a regular, 335–337
   life as a stranger, 331–332
   life as a tourist, 333–335
   physical activity relationship, 330–331, 331*f*
potential of, 339–340
Personal excellence, 372, 386
Personal goals, 420–421, 426
Personal physical activity, 332
Person-first attitudes and language, 239
Person with a disability, 239, 240
   extra IEP content, 309–326

adapted physical activity, 315–320
adapted physical education, 311
adapted physical educator, 312–315
allied health professions, 321–322, 322–324*t*
career possibilities, 320–321
therapeutic exercise and allied health, issues in, 324–326
federal laws supporting, 311*t*
PETE (physical education teacher education) program, 312
Philosophiae Naturalis Principia Mathematica (Mathematical Principles of Natural Philosophy), 59
Philosophical orientations, 187–188, 187*t*
Philosophical Society for the Study of Sport, 161
Philosophy, defined, 156
Philosophy of kinesiology, 156–176
aesthetics, 162, 172–174
axiology, 162
career in, 174–176
defined, 156
degree in, 174–176
described, 156–160
epistemology, 162, 168–169
ethics, 162, 170–172
history of, 160–161
metaphysics, 161–162, 163–167
overview, 156
values, 169–170
Physical activity (PA), 19, 49, 126, 165, 172. *See also* Adapted physical activity (APA); Physical education (PE); Sociology of sport, exercise, and physical activity
ASD and, 397–400, 399*f*
defined, 126, 180, 232–233
experiences of, 31–35
healthy and disease populations need of, 113–114*b*
historical forms, 166
intrinsic reasons, 165–166
meaningful, 426–427
metaphysical consideration, 164–167
personal and cultural (*See* Personal and cultural physical activity)
sociological knowledge application to, 214–215
transtheoretical model of behavior change, 298–299, 298*t*
vs. exercise, 128–129
Physical Activity Guidelines for Americans, 203
2008 Physical Activity Guidelines for Americans, 232, 232*f*
Physical Activity Readiness Questionnaire (PAR-Q), 290, 291*f*
Physical activity relationship (PAR), 330–331
defined, 330
fields of, 330, 331*f*
potential of, 339–340
Physical culture, 42, 44
defined, 160
Physical education (PE). *See also* Physical activity (PA); Sport pedagogy
academic discipline of (1960–1980), 46–49
areas of specialization, 46–47
ASD and, 392–395, 394*f*
background, 8–9
components of program, 193
curriculum, 181
defined, 43–44, 180
historcal perspectives, 6, 42 (*See also* History, of kinesiology)
historical highlights of pioneers, 183–184*b*

history of, 182–188
instruction, 181
national standards, 181
philosophical orientations,
    187–188, 187*t*
place in curriculum, 165
scholarly field, 46
stereotypes, 48
subdisciplinary organizations,
    evolution of, 47–48, 47*t*
teaching, motor development
    and, 150
Physical education teacher education
    (PETE) program, 312
Physical fitness
defined, 131
health-related components of,
    131, 131*t*
skill-related components of, 131,
    131*t*, 132
Physical Fitness Research
    Laboratory, 123
Physical/occupational therapy,
    150–151
Physical Therapy, 61
Physical training, 42
Physical trauma, as stressor, 128
Physician clearance, 290, 292
Physiological adaptations, 120,
    129–130
Physiological approach, APA
    research, 256
Physiological mechanisms, 129
Physiological training adaptations, 130
Pistorius, Oscar, 172
Planning, for success, 419–420
Plantar flexion, MTC during,
    75, 77*f*
Play
defined, 156–157
as form of physical activity, 166
Play attitude, 44
Popular sport media, 267–268

Positive inclusion, strategies for
    awareness and appreciation,
    354–357, 355*f*
for fostering unity, 357–359
Posses, Nils, 235
Post-assessment, 300, 301*t*
Post-disaster trauma relief and life
    normalization, 358
Potential energy, 68
Power and performance sports, 275
Prepared, defined, 36
President's Council on Fitness, Sports
    & Nutrition in 2010, 124
President's Council on Physical Fitness,
    Sports, and Nutrition, 45
President's Council on Youth Fitness,
    123–124
The Principia, 59
Principle of overload, 133
Principle of progression, 134
Principle of reversibility, 134
Principles of exercise training, 132–134
The Principles of Physiology Applied to
    the Preservation of Health and
    to the Improvement of Physical
    and Mental Education, 121
Priority, defined, 375
Production in physical culture, 336
Professional, qualities of, 22*t*
Professional goals, 420–421, 426
Professionalism
defined, 21
survey of, 20–21
Professional network, 419–420
Professional training areas, 14
Profession of physical education
    (1900–1960), 44–46
Program assessment, in sport
    pedagogy, 193
Progress, assessment of, 422–423
Progression, principle of, 134
Promotion of gender equity, 358
Propulsive force, defined, 65

PSD. *See* Psychological skill development (PSD)

Psychological approach, APA research, 256–257

Psychological skill development (PSD), 102–104
 defined, 103
 delivery of programs, 104, 105*f*
 hierarchy of, 104, 105*f*
 myths about, 103–104

Psychology and Athletics, 93

Psychology of Coaching, 93

Psychophysiological orientation, in sport psychology, 98

Public Health, 418–427

Public Law 94-142, 311

Public sector, APA coordinator in, 250

Q

Qualitative research
 defined, 108
 in sport pedagogy, 195
 in sport psychology, 108

Quantitative research
 defined, 108
 in sport pedagogy, 194–195
 in sport psychology, 108

Quantum mechanics, 64

Questionnaire, health, 290, 291*f*

R

Race, 207, 223

Rarick, G. Lawrence, 145

Rathbone, Josephine, 123, 236, 237*f*

Reaction time, effect of, 93

Reasonable accommodation, 306

Recognition years, 125

Recovery exercise program, adapted fitness trainer in, 251

"Red Light, Green Light Dribble" game, 393, 401–402, 410–412, 411*f*, 412*f*

Reebok, 225

Reel, Justine J., 112–114*b*

Reevaluation, health and wellness, 300, 301*t*

Reeves, Keanu, 56

Reflective scrutiny, 158

Reflexive practice, 351

Reflexivity, 355

Regional Centers, 396

Regulars
 defined, 335–336
 life as, 335–337

Regulatory condition, 403

Reid, Greg, 234

Relative excellence, 386–387

Research
 motor behavior
  motor control, 147–148
  motor development, 148–149
  motor learning, 148
  during World War II, 144–145
 sport pedagogy, 200
 sport psychology, 95, 108, 109*t*

Research areas
 in APA, 254–257
  administrative and epidemiological approach, 254–255
  biomechanical approach, 255
  motor behavioral approach, 255–256
  pedagogical approach, 256
  physiological approach, 256
  psychological approach, 256–257
 in biomechanics, 87–88
 in exercise physiology, 136–138*t*, 139
 sport management, 276, 278–279*t*
 in sport pedagogy, 194–200, 195*t*

Research Quarterly, 122

Responsibility for learning, learner-centered approach, 25

Restoration, function
    extra IEP content for youth with
        disabilities, 309–326
        adapted physical activity, 315–320
        adapted physical education, 311
        adapted physical educator,
            312–315
        allied health professions,
            321–322, 322–324t
        career possibilities, 320–321
        therapeutic exercise and allied
            health, issues in, 324–326
    healthy balance, care for (case
        study), 304–309
    legislation, 306–309, 308t
    special education and related
        services, 307–309, 308t
Retirement community, adapted
        wellness program director at,
        251–252
Revenue generation, sport marketing
        and, 269–271
Reversibility, principle of, 134
Revision, health and wellness, 300, 301t
Revolt of the Black Athlete, 210
Robinson, Jackie, 171–172
Role model, 378
"Rolling-out-the-ball" methods,
        9–10, 9f
Roosevelt, Theodore, 184, 185f, 186b
Rotations, 72
Running, experiences from, 34

S
Sabermetrics, 278
Sacrifices
    defined, 375
    for excellence, 375–376
Safe space, 344–346
Sallis, Robert, 125
Sam, Michael, 172
Sarcomere length, 79–80, 81f
Sargent, Dudley, 183b

Schema theory, 145
Schmidt, Dick, 145
Scholarly field, of physical
        education, 46
Science and Medicine of Exercise and
        Sport, 124
"The Science of Sport"
        (sportsscientists.com), 36–37
Scientific principles, application of,
        9, 9f
    exercise programs, 12–13, 13f
Scientific Revolution, 59
Scripture, E. W., 93
Section 504 of the Rehabilitation
        Act of 19730, 306
Sedentary, defined, 286
Seguin, Edouard, 236
Self-assessment
    defined, 29
    learner awareness, 27
Self-development and sport
        protocol, 356
Self-image, 102f
Self-reflexive sensibility, 356
Self-regulatory skills, 93
Senior fall risk, 240
Service programs, APA, 242–245,
        243f, 244f
Sexual orientation, 364b
SFIA (ports & Fitness Industry
        Association), 219, 220
Shared excellence, 372, 389
Shaw, Gary, 210
Sherrill, Claudine, 234
Sherrington, Charles, 143
Shot put, throwing, 72, 73
Skill-related components of physical
        fitness, 131, 131t, 132
Skills, professional, 21–22, 22t
Slater-Hammel, Arthur, 94
SMART goals, 293, 294–296, 294t
Social cognitive theory, 100–101, 100f
Social cohesion, 106

Social currents, 215
Social demography, 218
Social facts, 214, 215
Social integration, 358
Social mobilizations, communication and, 359
Social-psychological orientation, in sport psychology, 98
Social rarity, 348–349
Social science, 235
Social world, 332
Society of Health and Physical Educators (SHAPE America), 180, 181, 188, 189
    evolution of, 43*t*
Sociocultural-based forms of movement, 11–12, 12*t*
Socioeconomic class, 223
Sociological imagination
    application to movement settings (case study), 223–227
        cultural conditions, 225–226
        emergent sport, 224–225
        historical context, 226–227
        structural conditions, 226
    defined, 206
    described, 211–212
    potential for, 212
    use of, 212–213
Sociological knowledge, application to sport and physical activity, 214–215
The Sociology of Sport, 210
Sociology of sport, exercise, and physical activity
    analytic knowledge technique, 218, 219, 221–223
    cultural theories, 217–218
    defined, 206
    degree in, 227
    experience knowledge techniques, 218, 219, 220–221
    history of, 209–211

    landscape knowledge techniques, 218, 219–220
    overview, 206–209
    questions related to, 211–213
    sociological imagination application to movement settings (case study), 223–227
    sociological knowledge application to, 214–215
    structural theories, 217
    theory and practice in, 216–223
Sociology of Sport Journal, 210
Sound philosophical arguments, 158
Special education, 235, 236
    and related services, 307–309, 308*t*
Specialists, in exercise psychology (educational backgrounds), 111–112*b*
Specialized movement forms, 12–13, 13*f*
    exercise programs, 12–13, 13*f*
    fundamental movement skills, 12, 13*f*
Special Olympics, 188
Spinal cord injury (SCI) recovery center, adapted fitness trainer in, 251
Sport, 159. *See also* Sociology of sport, exercise, and physical activity
    concept, 262
    sociological knowledge and, 214–215
    types of, 263
Sport, Culture, and Society: A Reader on the Sociology of Sport, 210
Sport, Ethics, and Philosophy, 161, 275
Sport and exercise biomechanics, 57, 84*t*, 85*t*
Sport consumer behavior, 271–272, 272*f*
Sport/exercise subdisciplines, 11
Sport facility management, 272–274, 273*f*
Sport for development, 344–345, 345*f*
Sport history, 21, 48–49

Sport industry. *See also* Sport
    management
  in United States, size and impact of,
    266–267
Sportization, 337
Sport law, 275–276
Sport management, 262–279
  academic journals, 265–266*t*
  career opportunities, 262*f*, 276, 277*t*
  defined, 262–263
  ethics, 274–275
  history, in United States, 263–266
  intercollegiate, interscholastic, and
    amateur athletics, 268–269
  overview, 262–263
  popular sport media, 267–268
  research areas, 276, 278–279*t*
  sport consumer behavior, 271–272
  sport facility management, 272–274
  sport law, 275–276
  sport marketing and revenue
    generation, 269–271
Sport Management Review, 274, 275
Sport marketing, and revenue
    generation, 269–271
Sport Marketing Quarterly, 271
Sport pedagogy. *See also* Physical
    education (PE)
  action research, 198–200, 198*f*
  analytic research, 200
  appropriate instruction, 190–193
  areas of research in, 194–200, 195*t*
  careers in, 194
  defined, 180
  degree in, 194
  descriptive research, 195–196
  experimental research, 196–198
  future directions, 201–203
  meaningful content, 189–190
  observational research, 196
  opportunity to learn, 189
  qualitative research in, 195
  quantitative research in, 194–195

  reasons to study, 188
  research and technology, 200
  student and program
    assessment, 193
Sport philosophy, 21
Sport physiology, 156. *See also*
    Philosophy of kinesiology
  defined, 120
Sport psychologist
  clinical, 97, 97*f*
  degree required for, 96–98
  educational, 97–98
Sport psychology, 21, 34. *See also*
    Exercise psychology
  application by field/occupation, 115*t*
  areas of practice, 95–96
  clinical, 97
  cognitive-behavioral orientation, 99
  consulting, 96
  defined, 92
  educational, 97–98
  history of, 92–95
  motivation, 99–102
  objectives, 92
  orientations in, 98–99
  psychological skill development,
    102–104
  psychophysiological orientation, 98
  qualitative research in, 108
  quantitative research in, 108
  research, 95
  research methods in, 108, 109*t*
  social-psychological orientation, 98
  sport psychologist, degree required
    for, 96–98
  teaching, 96
  team/group dynamics, 104–108
  vs. exercise psychology, 93*t*
Sport psychology consulting, 96
Sports and games, 9
Sports Biomechanics, 61
Sports & Fitness Industry Association
    (SFIA), 219, 220

Sports Illustrated, 267
Springfield College (Massachusetts), 123
Sputnik 1, 45
Spygate, 274
SSC. *See* Stretch-shortening cycle (SSC)
Standard of care, 114*b*
Statics, 65
Status quo, 214
Steinhaus, A. H., 123
Stranger, 331–332
Strategic planning, for success, 419–420
Stress
    defined, 128
    sources, 128
Stressors, 128
Stress resistance, 129–130
Stretch-shortening cycle (SSC)
    defined, 78
    MTC during, 78, 83
Stroke, 240, 293
Structural components, 212
Structural conditions, 226
Structural equation modeling
        (SEM), 278
Structural theories, sociology of
        sport, exercise, and physical
        activity, 217
Student assessment, in sport
        pedagogy, 193
Study skills, 23
Subdisciplinary organizations,
        evolution of, 47–48, 47*t*
Subdisciplines, 10–11, 11*t*, 21, 33–34,
        50. *See also specific entries*
Success, strategic planning for, 419–420
Suits, Bernard, 160, 167, 173
Summarizing, 26
Summative assessment, 193
Summer and Winter Olympic
        Games, 262
Super Bowl Sunday, 206
Supply, 128
Supply equals demand, 128

Survey(s), professionalism, 20–21
Swing patterns, 72–73
Systolic blood pressure, 290

T

Task cohesion, 106
TBI (traumatic brain injury), 304
Teacher-centered approach
    decisions about learning, 26
    described, 23–24
    vs. learner-centered, 23–24, 25*t*
Teacher movement, 190–191
Teacher's role, learner-centered
        approach, 25, 28
Teaching
    PE, motor development and, 150
    in sport psychology, 96
Teaching behaviors, 190
Teaching credential, 312
Team/group dynamics, 92, 104–108
    cohesion, 106–108, 107*f*
    formation of groups, 105–106
    team performance, factors
            influencing, 106–108, 107*f*
Teamwork, 20
Technology, sport pedagogy, 200
Test of Gross Motor Development-2
        (TGMD-2), 150, 401
Test of Performance Strategies
        (TOPS), 104
Theoretical period, biomechanics, 59
Therapeutic exercise, issues in, 324–326
Thorndike, Edward, 144
Throwlike patterns, 72
Time management, 23
Tissue mechanics, 65
TOPS (Test of Performance
        Strategies), 104
Torque
    defined, 65
    and exchange of energy, 66,
            68–70, 70*f*
    force and, 65–66, 66*f*, 67*f*

Tough Mudders, 225, 226
Tourist
    defined, 334
    life as, 333–335
"Toward a Sociology of Sport," 209–210
Training. *See also* Careers/career
        opportunities
    in APA, 245–254
        Aquatic Therapy and
            Rehabilitation Institute
            Certified (ATRIC), 253–254
        Certified Adapted Physical
            Educator (CAPE) certification,
            252–253
        Certified Inclusive Fitness Trainer
            (CIFT) certification, 253
        credentials/certifications,
            252–254
        working designations, 247–252
Training adaptations, 130
Transgender, 363*b*
Transition, 365*b*, 386
Transition services, 309
Transphobia, 365*b*
Transsexual, 365*b*
Transtheoretical model, of behavior
        change, 298–299, 298*t*
Traumatic brain injury (TBI), 304
Triceps surae group, 75
Trilling, Blanche, 183, 185, 185*f*, 186*b*
Tripartite Committee, 186*b*
Triplett, Norman, 92
True competition, 359
Turvey, Michael, 145

U

Ultrasound, 87
Uncertainty, 423–425
UNDP (United Nations Development
        Program), 345
UNICEF (United Nations Children's
        Fund), 345
United Nations (UN), 344

United Nations Children's Fund
        (UNICEF), 345
United Nations Development Program
        (UNDP), 345
United Nations Educational, Scientific
        and Cultural Organization
        (UNESCO), 344–345
United States
    history of exercise physiology in,
        121–125
    organized sport in, historical
        highlights, 186*b*
    size and impact of sport industry in,
        266–267
    sport management history in,
        263–266
Unity, in diversity, 357–359
University, APA researcher in, 251
University-based APA program,
        243–244, 243*f*
Unprofessional qualities, 21, 22*t*
    defined, 21
UN Sport for Development and Peace
        Working Group, 358
Upper extremity(ies), motions
        associated with flexion and
        extension patterns of, 70–72,
        71*t*, 72*f*
U.S. Census Bureau, 240, 266
U.S. Code of Federal Regulations
        (CFR), 321
U.S. Council for Exceptional
        Children, 236
U.S. Department of Health and
        Human Services, 203
U.S. Olympic Committee (USOC),
        95, 96
U.S. Surgeon General, 241

V

Values, 169–170
    extrinsic, 169
    intrinsic, 169

Velocity, MTC and, 82–83, 82*f*
Vesalius, Andreas, 58
Vineland Adaptive Behavior Scale, 396

W

Waist circumference, 293
Wait time, 192–193
Walking, 59
Walt Disney Pictures, 45
Warner Brothers, 56
Warren, John, 183b
Weight-bearing exercise, 297
Weiss, Paul, 160
Wellness. *See* Health and wellness
Whip patterns, 72–73
White House Task Force on Childhood
    Obesity Report to the
    President, 203
WHO. *See* World Health Organization
    (WHO)
Whole, defined, 30
Williams, Jean, 104
Williams, Jesse Feiring, 183
Wood, Thomas, 121, 183, 183*f*, 184b
Woodworth, R. A., 143
Work, defined, 68
Work–energy concepts, 68–69, 70*f*
Working designations, in APA,
    247–252

World Congress of Sport
    Psychology, 94
World Health Organization (WHO),
    239, 345
World War I, 44, 226
World War II, 45, 123, 184, 188,
    226, 236
    motor behavior research, 144–145

Y

Yates, Dorothy, 94
Yiannakis, Andrew, 210
York College of Pennsylvania's (YCP)
    Center for Professional
    Excellence, 20
Youth with disabilities, extra IEP
    content for, 309–326. *See also*
    Person with a disability
    adapted physical activity, 315–320
    adapted physical education, 311
    adapted physical educator, 312–315
    allied health professions, 321–322,
        322–324*t*
    career possibilities, 320–321
    therapeutic exercise and allied
        health, issues in, 324–326

Z

Zombie Runs, 225